DISASTER PSYCHIATRY

*Readiness, Evaluation,
and Treatment*

Second Edition

DISASTER PSYCHIATRY

*Readiness, Evaluation,
and Treatment*

Second Edition

Edited by
Frederick J. Stoddard Jr., M.D.
Craig L. Katz, M.D.
Grant H. Brenner, M.D.

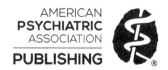

AMERICAN
PSYCHIATRIC
ASSOCIATION
PUBLISHING

Note: The authors have worked to ensure that all information in this book is accurate at the time of publication and consistent with general psychiatric and medical standards, and that information concerning medication dosages, schedules, and routes of administration is accurate at the time of publication and consistent with standards set by the U.S. Food and Drug Administration and the general medical community. As medical research and practice continue to advance, however, therapeutic standards may change. Moreover, specific situations may require a specific therapeutic response not included in this book. For these reasons and because human and mechanical errors sometimes occur, we recommend that readers follow the advice of physicians directly involved in their care or the care of a member of their family.

Books published by American Psychiatric Association Publishing represent the findings, conclusions, and views of the individual authors and do not necessarily represent the policies and opinions of American Psychiatric Association Publishing or the American Psychiatric Association.

If you wish to buy 50 or more copies of the same title, please go to www.appi.org/specialdiscounts for more information.

Copyright © 2025 American Psychiatric Association Publishing

ALL RIGHTS RESERVED

Second Edition

Manufactured in the United States of America on acid-free paper
28 27 26 25 24   5 4 3 2 1

American Psychiatric Association Publishing
800 Maine Avenue SW, Suite 900
Washington, DC 20024–2812
www.appi.org

Library of Congress Cataloging-in-Publication Data
Names: Stoddard, Frederick J., Jr. editor. | Katz, Craig L., editor. | Brenner, Grant H., editor. | American Psychiatric Association, issuing body.
Title: Disaster psychiatry : readiness, evaluation, and treatment / edited by Frederick J. Stoddard Jr., Craig L. Katz, Grant H. Brenner.
Other titles: Disaster psychiatry (Stoddard)
Description: Second edition. | Washington, DC : American Psychiatric Association Publishing, [2025] | Includes bibliographical references and index.
Identifiers: LCCN 2024026360 (print) | LCCN 2024026361 (ebook) | ISBN 9780873182508 (paperback ; alk. paper) | ISBN 9780873182522 (ebook)
Subjects: MESH: Stress Disorders, Post-Traumatic—therapy | Emergency Services, Psychiatric | Disasters | Crisis Intervention—methods | Disaster Victims—psychology | Survivors—psychology
Classification: LCC RC552.P67 (print) | LCC RC552.P67 (ebook) | NLM WM 172.5 | DDC 616.85/21—dc23/eng/20240809
LC record available at https://lccn.loc.gov/2024026360
LC ebook record available at https://lccn.loc.gov/2024026361

British Library Cataloguing in Publication Data
A CIP record is available from the British Library.

Dedicated to

Matilda, Jack, and Eve (Frederick J. Stoddard Jr.)

Linda, Maya, and Lev (Craig L. Katz)

Marina, Reyd, and Cameron (Grant H. Brenner)

*in gratitude for their support
and encouragement
from the beginning of this book*

Contents

PART I

PREVENTION AND READINESS

Grant H. Brenner, M.D.

PART II
EVALUATION
Craig L. Katz, M.D.

PART III

INTERVENTION

> Frederick J. Stoddard Jr., M.D.

Contributors

Jacob M. Appel, M.D., J.D., M.P.H.
Professor, Department of Psychiatry and Medical Education, Icahn School of Medicine at Mount Sinai, New York, New York

David R. Beckert, M.D.
Assistant Professor, Department of Psychiatry and Behavioral Sciences; Combined Psychiatry Neurology Residency Program Director, Medical University of South Carolina, Charleston, South Carolina

Grant H. Brenner, M.D.
Assistant Clinical Professor, Department of Psychiatry and Behavioral Science, Mount Sinai Beth Israel, New York, New York

Linda Chokroverty, M.D.
Assistant Clinical Professor, Department of Psychiatry and Behavioral Sciences and Pediatrics; Attending Psychiatrist, Albert Einstein College of Medicine, New York, New York

Kathleen A. Clegg, M.D.
Associate Professor, Department of Psychiatry, Case Western Reserve University School of Medicine, Cleveland, Ohio

Jonathan M. DePierro, Ph.D.
Associate Professor, Department of Psychiatry; Associate Director, Center for Stress, Resilience and Personal Growth, Icahn School of Medicine at Mount Sinai, New York, New York

Alisa R. Gutman, M.D., Ph.D.
Clinical Associate Professor, Department of Psychiatry, Perelman School of Medicine, University of Pennsylvania, Philadelphia, Pennsylvania

Genevieve Jing, M.D.
Psychiatry Resident, New York Medical College/NYC Health and Hospitals, New York, New York

Kristina Jones, M.D.
Attending Physician, Consultation-Liaison Psychiatry Service, Division of Psychiatry and Medicine, Montefiore Medical Center; Assistant Professor, Department of Psychiatry and Behavioral Sciences, Albert Einstein College of Medicine, Bronx, New York

Edward M. Kantor, M.D.
Associate Professor and Vice Chair for Education and Training and Residency Program Director, Department of Psychiatry and Behavioral Sciences, Medical University of South Carolina, Charleston, South Carolina

Craig L. Katz, M.D.
Clinical Professor of Psychiatry, Medical Education, System Design and Global Health, Icahn School of Medicine at Mount Sinai, New York, New York

Halley Kaye-Kauderer, M.D.
Psychiatry Resident, Department of Psychiatry, Icahn School of Medicine at Mount Sinai, New York, New York

Katherine A. Koh, M.D., M.Sc.
Psychiatrist, Massachusetts General Hospital and Boston Health Care for the Homeless Program; Assistant Professor of Psychiatry, Harvard Medical School; Co-chair, Disaster Readiness Committee, Massachusetts Psychiatric Society, Boston, Massachusetts

Sander Koyfman, M.D., M.B.A.
Chief Medical Officer, Languages of Care; Behavioral Health Medical Director, RiverSpring Health Plans; Clinical Psychiatrist, AthenaPsych, New York, New York

Helen Kyomen, M.D.
Clinical Assistant Professor, Department of Psychiatry, Boston University Chobanian and Avedisian School of Medicine; Adjunct Clinical Assistant Professor, Department of Psychiatry, Tufts University School of Medicine; Lecturer, Part-time, Department of Psychiatry, Harvard Medical School

Joseph P. Merlino, M.D., M.P.A.
Professor Emeritus, Department of Psychiatry, SUNY Health Sciences University College of Medicine, Brooklyn, New York

Anthony T. Ng, M.D., DFAPA
Medical Director, Community Services; Director, Neuromodulation Services, Northern Light Acadia Hospital, Bangor, Maine

Vinh-Son Nguyen, M.D.
Child and Adolescent Psychiatry Fellow, Boston Children's Hospital, Boston, Massachusetts

Srini Pillay, M.D.
Chief Medical Officer, Reulay, and Chief Executive Officer, NeuroBusiness Group, Cambridge, Massachusetts

Giuseppe Raviola, M.D., M.P.H.
Assistant Professor, Department of Psychiatry, Department of Global Health and Social Medicine, Harvard Medical School; Director, Chester M. Pierce Division of Global Psychiatry, Massachusetts General Hospital; Director, Mental Health, Partners in Health, Boston, Massachusetts

Robert Roca, M.D.
Professor and Vice Chair, Department of Psychiatry and Behavioral Sciences, The Johns Hopkins University School of Medicine, Baltimore, Maryland

Kenneth Sakauye, M.D.
Emeritus Professor of Psychiatry, University of Tennessee Health Science Center, Memphis, Tennessee

Kunmi Sobowale, M.D.
Assistant Professor, Department of Psychiatry and Biobehavioral Sciences, University of California, Los Angeles, Los Angeles, California

Frederick J. Stoddard Jr., M.D.
Professor, part-time, Department of Psychiatry, Harvard Medical School at the Massachusetts General Hospital, Boston, Massachusetts

Sho Takahashi, M.D., Ph.D.
Associate Professor, Department of Disaster and Community Psychiatry and Division of Clinical Medicine, Institute of Medicine; Manager, Department of Community and Disaster Assistance, Ibaraki Prefectural Medical Research Center of Psychiatry, University of Tsukuba, Tsukuba, Japan

Disclosures

The following contributors to this book have indicated a financial interest in or other affiliation with a commercial supporter, a manufacturer of a commercial product, a provider of a commercial service, a nongovernmental organization, and/or a government agency, as listed below:

Linda Chokroverty, M.D.: Employee, Montefiore Health Systems; consultant, New York City Department of Health and Mental Hygiene; funds for travel and conference attendance from Einstein/Montefiore Department of Psychiatry and Behavioral Sciences and New York State Office of Mental Health Workforce funding grant.

Jonathan M. DePierro, Ph.D.: Speaker fees, Ro Health Ventures (2022); royalties; Cambridge University Press; salary support from Springer related to editor-in-chief role for an academic psychiatry journal (2023).

Craig L. Katz, M.D.: Honoraria, Medical Society of the State of New York's Committee on Emergency Preparedness for disaster mental health trainings and webinars; National Trauma Consultant, Advanced Recovery Systems.

Kunmi Sobowale, M.D.: Advisory Board member, Little Otter; consultant, City University of New York.

The following contributors have indicated that they have no financial interests or other affiliations that represent or could appear to represent a competing interest with their contributions to this book: Jacob M. Appel, M.D., J.D., M.P.H.; David R. Beckert, M.D.; Grant H. Brenner, M.D.; Kathleen A. Clegg, M.D.; Alisa R. Gutman, M.D., Ph.D.; Genevieve Jing, M.D.; Kristina Jones, M.D.; Edward M. Kantor, M.D.; Halley Kaye-Kauderer, M.D.; Katherine A. Koh, M.D., M.Sc.; Sander Koyfman, M.D., M.B.A.; Helen Kyomen, M.D.; Joseph P. Merlino, M.D., M.P.A.; Anthony T. Ng, M.D., DFAPA; Vinh-Son Nguyen, M.D.; Srini Pillay, M.D.; Giuseppe Raviola, M.D., M.P.H.; Robert Roca, M.D.; Kenneth Sakauye, M.D.; Frederick J. Stoddard Jr., M.D.; Sho Takahashi, M.D., Ph.D.

Preface

Even more so than at the time of the first edition of this book in 2011, psychiatrists and other mental health professionals are increasingly active in disaster response. In the first edition, we highlighted the hundreds of psychiatrists who responded to the 9/11 attacks and such disasters as the Indian Ocean earthquake and tsunami in 2004, Hurricane Katrina in 2005, and the 2010 earthquake in Haiti. This new edition comes more than a decade later, prompted in large part by the coronavirus disease 2019 (COVID-19) pandemic that the entire world endured and that surely rendered every mental health professional a de facto, if not "official," disaster mental health professional. It was also prompted by the looming climate crisis with all of its many behavioral roots and mental health implications. And as we were writing, fires burned on Maui, floods overran Libya, and war broke out between Israel and Hamas. What more will happen to necessitate this book by the time it is read? Drawing from all that we have learned since the first edition and anticipating what lies ahead, we hope that this book remains more clinically oriented and practical than a textbook but explicit and practical in its discussion of the evidence base for recommendations for mental health evaluation and interventions.

There are varying definitions of *disaster*. The definition offered by the World Health Organization (1992) is brief and clear: a "severe disruption, ecological and psychosocial, which greatly exceeds the coping capacity of the affected community" (p. 2). Disasters may be caused by natural occurrences, or so-called acts of God (e.g., earthquakes, hurricanes, floods); by human-made accidental or technological events (e.g., airline crash, power plant explosion); or by willful human acts (e.g., mass shootings, terrorism (see Stoddard et al. 2011). The ultimate human-made disasters are through war (Massachusetts Medical Society 2024), especially use of nuclear weapons. An initial document by the Group for the Advancement of Psychiatry sought to identify psychiatric aspects of how to prevent nuclear war (Group for the Advancement of Psychiatry Committee on Social Issues 1964). Robert Jay Lifton classically documented the sequelae of the

Hiroshima and Nagasaki atom bombs. His most recent book warns of the far greater destructiveness of newer nuclear weapons and offers hope both after Hiroshima and the COVID-19 pandemic (Lifton 2023).

Although depictions of the psychological and emotional impacts of severe trauma on humans appear in ancient literature such as religious texts and Homer's *Iliad* and *Odyssey* (Shay 1994, 2002), approaches to clinical evaluation and treatment are relatively recent. *Soldier's heart*, a term dating from the Civil War era and a predecessor of what was later called *posttraumatic stress disorder*, was elegantly depicted in an episode of *Frontline* shown on American public television in 2005 (Aronson 2005). Although soldiers were initially the focus of clinical care, civilians eventually followed. After the 1942 Cocoanut Grove fire in Boston, which killed 492 people and left many people grieving the deaths of their young family members, papers on neuropsychiatric observations and complications and the symptomatology and management of acute grief by Erich Lindemann (1944), Stanley Cobb (Cobb and Lindemann 1943), and Alexandra Adler (1943) signaled the beginning of modern disaster psychiatry. Even earlier, classic work directly relevant to disaster psychiatry was done with both children and adults after the terror of the 1940 London Blitz (Freud and Burlingham 1943; Jones et al. 2006).

The field of disaster psychiatry has evolved to embrace a wide spectrum of clinical interests, including public health preparations and early psychological interventions; psychiatric consultation to surgical units; psychotherapeutic interventions to alleviate stress on children and families after school shootings, hurricanes, or civil conflict; and preparedness for climate change. Disaster psychiatry has an important role in emergency prevention, response, and recovery. Although disaster mental health is still a young field, research with adults and children is aiming to improve interventions. Research is slowly progressing in applying methods to accurately identify valid relationships—not merely associations—among preexisting risk factors, postdisaster mental health problems, and effective interventions (Norris et al. 2006; Pfefferbaum 1998; Pfefferbaum and North 2008).

Over the past three decades, the American Psychiatric Association (APA) has taken a leadership role in disaster preparedness and, at times, response. In particular, Robert L. Ursano, M.D., founder of the APA's Committee on Psychiatric Dimensions of Disaster, has taken on such a role, together with many other leaders in disaster response at the APA and internationally. Dr. Ursano; Ann E. Norwood, M.D.; Carol S. Fullerton, M.D.; and their colleagues at the Uniformed Services University of the Health Sciences played groundbreaking roles in educating mental health professionals about disasters, the need for disaster mental health training, and the need for their expertise. District branches of the APA in Massachusetts, New York, California, Louisiana, and several other states have actively contributed to training and responses to disasters near and far.

The APA has provided both basic and advanced training courses on disaster psychiatry. In times of disasters, the APA is a lead organization that works to coordinate and disseminate valuable and timely disaster psychiatry materials to professionals in the field and to facilitate the flow of information into and out of the organization. APA's website on disaster mental health (www.psychiatry.org/psychiatrists/practice/professional-interests/disaster-and-trauma) boasts a comprehensive range of references and resources.

In *Disaster Psychiatry: Readiness, Evaluation, and Treatment*, we synthesize information gathered from a variety of sources, including the peer-reviewed scientific literature; the clinical wisdom imparted by frontline psychiatrists, psychologists, and social workers; and the experiences of those who have organized disaster mental health services. The authors of the 21 chapters explain, using a biopsychosocial model, what a disaster is, how disasters relate to mental health, and how psychiatrists and other mental health professionals can effectively intervene to reduce suffering in such circumstances. Because informing mental health professionals about the evidence base for different best practices remains a central goal of this book, chapters are extensively referenced and present the level of scientifically validated research needed to support any recommendations. The book is divided into three parts for ease of use by mental health clinicians preparing for or responding to disasters: "Prevention and Readiness," "Evaluation," and "Intervention."

As noted, many psychiatrists and other mental health professionals have become acquainted with disaster psychiatry, and many may be experiencing some disaster fatigue now, especially in the shadow of the COVID-19 pandemic. Climate change, socioeconomic stresses, political dissension, and racism and ethnic strife add dimensions of uncertainty, not rare among disasters, that may cause vast suffering over many years. These stressors can have such insidious impact that the need for clinical disaster services, both acute and postacute, may not even be recognized. We hope that this updated clinical manual provides needed encouragement and support, based on accumulating evidence from treating disaster survivors, to those mental health professionals who may have experienced disaster fatigue as well as to those who have not.

Frederick J. Stoddard Jr., M.D.
Craig L. Katz, M.D.
Grant H. Brenner, M.D.

References

Adler A: Neuropsychiatric complications in victims of Boston's Cocoanut Grove disaster. JAMA 123:1098–1101, 1943

Aronson R: The Soldier's Heart [TV series episode]. Frontline, season 2005, March 1, 2005. Available at: www.pbs.org/wgbh/frontline/documentary/showsheart. Accessed July 26, 2023.

Cobb S, Lindemann E: Neuropsychiatric observations after the Cocoanut Grove fire. Ann Surg 117(6):814–824, 1943 17858228

Freud A, Burlingham DT: War and Children. New York, Medical War Books, 1943

Group for the Advancement of Psychiatry Committee on Social Issues: Psychiatric Aspects of the Prevention of Nuclear War (Report No 57). New York, Group for the Advancement of Psychiatry, 1964

Jones E, Woolven R, Durodie B, et al: Public panic and morale: Second World War civilian responses re-examined in light of the current anti-terrorist campaign. J Risk Res 9(1):57–73, 2006

Lifton RJ: Surviving Our Catastrophes: Resilience and Renewal from Hiroshima to the Covid-19 Pandemic. New York, New Press, 2023

Lindemann E: Symptomatology and management of acute grief. Am J Psychiatry 101:141–148, 1944 8192191

Massachusetts Medical Society: The Impact of War on Health, Human Rights, and the Environment. Virtual live webinar. Waltham, Massachusetts Medical Society, June 13, 2024

Norris FH, Galea S, Friedman MJ, et al: Methods for Disaster Mental Health Research. New York, Guilford, 2006

Pfefferbaum B: Caring for children affected by disaster. Child Adolesc Psychiatr Clin N Am 7(3):579–597, ix, 1998 9894056

Pfefferbaum B, North CS: Research with children exposed to disasters. Int J Methods Psychiatr Res 17(Suppl 2):S49–S56, 2008 19035441

Shay J: Achilles in Vietnam: Combat Trauma and the Undoing of Character. New York, Simon & Schuster, 1994

Shay J: Odysseus in America: Combat Trauma and the Trials of Homecoming. New York, Scribner, 2002

Stoddard FJ Jr, Gold J, Henderson SW, et al: Psychiatry and terrorism. J Nerv Ment Dis 199(8):537–543, 2011 21814075

World Health Organization: Psychosocial Consequences of Disaster: Prevention and Management. Geneva, Switzerland, World Health Organization, 1992. Available at: https://apps.who.int/iris/handle/10665/58986. Accessed July 26, 2023.

Acknowledgments

This second edition builds on the collaboration that led to the first edition: the Group for the Advancement of Psychiatry (GAP) and Disaster Psychiatry Outreach in New York. The volume was again initiated and written by the GAP Committee on Disasters, Trauma and Global Health, now chaired by Kathleen Clegg, M.D., and Grant Brenner, M.D. We are grateful to the past President of GAP, Calvin Sumner, M.D., and its Publications Board, chaired then by David Adler, M.D., for their reviews of the manuscript. We thank Joshua Morganstein, M.D., and James West, M.D., past and current chairs, respectively, of the APA Committee on the Psychiatric Dimensions of Disasters, for their review. We again express gratitude to the many colleagues acknowledged in the first edition, particularly Robert Ursano, M.D., founding Director of the Center for the Study of Traumatic Stress and Chairman of Psychiatry at Uniformed Services University from 1992 to 2017. The editors are grateful to American Psychiatric Publishing, especially to prior Editor-in-Chief Robert E. Hales, M.D., who helped choose the original title, and to Laura Roberts, M.D., M.A., current Editor-in-Chief, and her publications staff for careful guidance and support through the publication process.

PART I

PREVENTION AND READINESS

Grant H. Brenner, M.D.
Section Editor

1

Disaster Psychiatry Education

Frederick J. Stoddard Jr., M.D.
Craig L. Katz, M.D.
Grant H. Brenner, M.D.

> *Education is the most powerful weapon which you can use to change the world.*
> —Nelson Mandela

> *By failing to prepare, you are preparing to fail.*
> —Benjamin Franklin

Education in disaster psychiatry is the foundation for developing and improving psychiatric knowledge and skills in readiness for a disaster; evaluation and treatment before, during, and after disasters; and the *prevention* of some disasters before they wreak destruction (see Chapter 2, "Disaster Prevention and Climate Change"). It is also an imperative because the practice of disaster psychiatry entails many clinical and operational issues that are foreign to usual mental health practice, especially the effects of climate change. The need for these skills grows daily, and acquisition of these skills can be aided by excellent courses, guidelines, websites, and consultants. It is essential for psychiatrists and other health care personnel to communicate effectively (see Chapter 5, "Communication and Relationships"), to care for themselves under the stress of a disaster (see Chapter 6, "Rescuing Ourselves"), and to grasp the structure of disaster organizations (see Chapter 7, "Engaging in Disaster Response") as well as the complexity of disasters themselves (see Chapter 8, "Model for Adaptive Response to Complex Cyclical Disasters"). In the current chapter, we outline ways to learn about disaster psychiatry, with key topics described in the chapters that follow.

One of us (G.H.B.) writes,

> On the post-Covid note, I think a lot is happening there. It may be important on a collective level in some way to reflect on what has happened. I'm thinking of this as "the Lost Years" (dissociated) particularly for younger people perhaps given key developmental windows which were interrupted and/or altered. It may be important for people to work on [these] issues. This is coming up for us with new teens who came through late childhood online, and we are now adjusting back—and also is part of what I'm thinking about in writing to the general public [about] this back-to-school month [August–September 2023]. For adults, as well, and of course the massive loss of life.

How We Became Interested in Teaching About Disaster Psychiatry

When we began in this field, it barely existed. Each of us, the editors and most of our contributing authors as well, became interested from our personal experiences spanning early in our careers to recent events. One of us (F.J.S.) lost his father from an accident during his pediatric internship at Yale. Shortly thereafter, he developed an interest in grief and traumatic stress while working with burn teams providing psychiatric care and through research with children and adults with burns, some as a result of disasters, at Shriners Hospital for Children and Massachusetts General Hospital. Another one of us (G.H.B.) experienced maternal loss at age 9, after witnessing several years of cancer's toll, in addition to having an older sibling with a significant developmental disability. Two of us (C.L.K., G.H.B.) responded acutely in New York City through Mount Sinai School of Medicine to the devastation and human suffering of 9/11 and led acute psychiatric care through the Disaster Psychiatry Outreach program for many people affected by that event. In addition, one of us (C.L.K.) participates in longitudinal studies of resilience of the survivors of 9/11. All of us have been affected by recent losses of loved ones and workplace stress due to the coronavirus disease 2019 (COVID-19) pandemic, and we find that our resilience is enhanced by our supportive families, collegial relationships with one another, and physical exercise.

We first came together in the Group for the Advancement of Psychiatry (GAP) to pursue our interest in disaster psychiatry, to write about it in order to learn more and to educate colleagues and the health care professionals with whom we work. GAP's Report "Psychiatric Aspects of the Prevention of Nuclear War" (Group for the Advancement of Psychiatry 1964) was an early inspiring work that educated about the prevention of nuclear disaster. We find it very satisfying professionally to share our knowledge of disaster psychiatry with others, and to learn from them as well. Our wish to do so has been accelerated by the progression of climate change, its impacts on all living things and the Earth itself, our role in causing it, and the psychological barriers to taking decisive action not only to slow it but also to reverse its course.

Goals of Disaster Psychiatry Education

> *My first disaster experience occurred in response to Hurricane Hugo in 1989. One member of our medical team was from St. Croix, so a group of us joined in the response for medical care. I had no idea at the time as to how a psychiatrist could be effective in disaster response, but what I learned through that first exposure is that often there are no rules in the immediate aftermath of a disaster.*
> —Sandra Maass-Robinson, M.D. (Maas-Robinson 2023)

The goals of education in disaster psychiatry include providing knowledge and skills to prevent disasters from occurring; to improve readiness; and to aid in the evaluation and treatment of disasters before, during, and after they occur. The extent to which these goals may be achieved vary depending on the clinician's preceding depth of knowledge and the time frame for the curriculum.

Ideally, a regular disaster mental health curriculum would be part of all formal training and continuing medical education (CME) for mental health clinicians. For example, some psychiatry residencies and medical schools have a standard curriculum on disaster preparation and response covering both physical and mental health. Likewise, curricula are available for psychologists, social workers, nurses, physician assistants, and other professionals who may be called on. Table 1–1 lists trainings and other educational resources of which we are aware.

TABLE 1–1. Disaster mental health educational resources

American Medical Association Education in Disaster Medicine and Public Health Preparedness During Medical School and Residency Training H-2905.868 (last modified 2021)

American Nurses Association

- American Nurses Association: *Adapting Standards of Care Under Extreme Conditions: Guidance for Professionals During Disasters, Pandemics, and Other Extreme Emergencies.* New York, Center for Health Policy, Columbia University School of Nursing, 2008

- National Academy of Sciences, Engineering and Medicine, National Academy of Medicine, Committee on the Future of Nursing 2020–2030, et al: Nurses in disaster preparedness and public health response, in *The Future of Nursing 2020–2030: Charting a Path to Achieve Health Equity.* Washington, DC, National Academies Press, 2021

- National Healthcare Disaster Certification: this certification was retired in 2022, but clinicians who hold the NHDP-BC can maintain it through renewal; see www.nursingworld.org/our-certifications/national-healthcare-disaster

American Psychological Association Disaster Mental Health Training Courses

- American Psychological Association: Desire to Help in Trying Times: Responding to Disasters [video]. Washington, DC, American Psychological Association, 2019 (a clinician workshop exploring ethical principles in responding to disasters)

American Red Cross Disaster Mental Health Course to become an ARC Disaster Mental Health volunteer

- Disaster Mental Health Introduction (30-minute ARC course for prospective volunteers)

- Disaster Services: An Overview

- Disaster Mental Health Fundamentals

Center for the Study of Traumatic Stress Studies, www.cstsonline.org

Centers for Disease Control and Prevention: Crisis and Emergency Risk Communication (CERC) Training. Atlanta, GA, Centers for Disease Control and Prevention, 2018. Available at: https://emergency.cdc.gov/cerc/training/index.asp

Climate Psychiatry Alliance, www.climatepsychiatry.org

Coker TR, Gootman JA, Backers EP: *Addressing the Long-Term Effects of the COVID-19 Pandemic on Children and Families.* Washington, DC, National Academies Press, 2023 (available at: https://doi.org/10.17226/26809)

TABLE 1–1. Disaster mental health educational resources *(continued)*

Disaster and Trauma Resource Center Resources for Parents, Youth and Clinicians, American Academy of Child and Adolescent Psychiatry (available at: www.aacap.org/AACAP/Families_and_Youth/Resource_Centers/Disaster_Resource_Center/Home.aspx)

Federal Emergency Management Agency Emergency Management Institute, https://training.fema.gov

- Community Emergency Response Team via FEMA

International Society for Traumatic Stress Studies, https://istss.org/home

- ISTSS publications on earthquake-related trauma and hurricane-related trauma
- Other trauma-related online learning

Just In Time Disaster Training Library, Psychological First Aid [video] (available at: www.youtube.com/watch?v=JESzIr8yG9U)

Medical Reserve Corps: A national network of community-based volunteers; contact the MRC unit in each community

Morganstein JC, West JC: Disaster and Preventive Psychiatry: Protecting Health and Fostering Community Resilience. Washington, DC, American Psychiatric Association, May 19, 2023. Available at: https://education.psychiatry.org/Listing/Disaster-and-Preventive-Psychiatry-Protecting-Health-and-Fostering-Community-Resilience-6019. Accessed July 4, 2023.

National Association of Social Workers Disaster Response Network. www.naswnc.org

- Massachusetts Chapter: Disaster Resources for Social Workers and Clients, 2013 (available at: https://cdn.ymaws.com/www.naswma.org/resource/resmgr/imported/Temp_NASW-MA_disaster_resource_manual.pdf)

National Center for PTSD, www.ptsd.va.gov

National Child Traumatic Stress Network, www.nctsn.org

National Organization for Victim Advocacy Community Crisis Response Program, https://trynova.org/initiatives/community-crisis-response

National Voluntary Organizations Active in Disaster (a collection of organizations and volunteers), www.nvoad.org/resources-center

Skills for Psychological Recovery: Field Operations Guide—An evidence-informed modular approach to help children, adolescents, adults, and families in the weeks and months after a disaster and after the early period of psychological first aid or when more intensive interventions are needed

Ursano RJ, Fullerton CS, Weisaeth L, et al: *Textbook of Disaster Psychiatry*, 2nd Edition. Cambridge, UK, Cambridge University Press, 2017

Of special importance is Disaster and Preventive Psychiatry: Protecting Health and Fostering Community Resilience, a course first offered in 2023 by Joshua C. Morganstein, M.D., and James C. West, M.D., and available free from the American Psychiatric Association's online Learning Center (American Psychiatric Association 2023). This nine-module interactive course is the most comprehensive online training of this critical topic area, focusing heavily on public mental health principles to support individuals, families, and communities impacted by disasters, and it is highly informative to psychiatrists and allied health care professionals, disaster responders, and community leaders. The nine modules are Basic Concepts in Disaster and Preventive Psychiatry, Psychological and Behavioral Effects of Disasters, Risk and Vulnerability to Disasters, Public Health Approaches to Interventions and Disasters, Psychological First Aid, Risk and Crisis Communication, Leadership Consultation, Disaster Responders, and Disaster Preparedness. The course includes eight CME credits.

Many trainings are "just in time," offered to quickly prepare responders with less knowledge and experience eager to offer their services when a disaster is imminent or occurring. Several national and international organizations maintain a roster of trained, and sometimes certified, adult and child psychiatrists and other mental health and health care professionals. For example, the American Red Cross offers certification through its Disaster Mental Health Training and maintains a cadre of licensed mental health responders at the master's level of education or higher. Vibrant Emotional Health is another example, with programs including the 988 Suicide and Crisis Lifeline, the interdisciplinary Crisis and Emotional Care Team, and the Disaster Distress Helpline. Hospitals, clinics, and educational institutions may encourage or require their employees to complete periodic disaster training as part of the core curriculum.

Educational standards for disaster mental health education vary widely. Depending on the type of training and time available, disaster curricula cover a range and depth of subjects that combine subjects everyone has to be familiar with and elements that are either optional or best reserved for a future date (Table 1–2).

Disaster Education Beyond Mental Health

Although it is critical for mental health personnel, including clinicians and allied professionals, to be trained in at least basic disaster mental health principles in the service of prevention and preparedness, population-level education to prepare for disasters and education on how to respond to them are equally essential given the increasing roles of disaster and crisis

---

TABLE 1–2.   Elements of disaster mental health education

1.   Definitions of disaster and crisis
2.   Basic approach to milieu
3.   Psychological first aid
4.   Skills for psychological recovery
5.   Self-care
6.   Organizational considerations
7.   Mental and behavioral health considerations
8.   Special populations
9.   Collaboration

---

in our everyday lives. In fact, it is useful to incorporate basic disaster preparedness into the curriculum for health profession students as part of health and wellness education.

Public health initiatives already address basic elements of preparedness, such as campaigns in many cities and states and from not-for-profit organizations encouraging people to have "go kits" available in case of sudden need. Such kits are designed to cover basic needs for a brief period of time, including food, water, clothing, first aid, basic shelter and coverage (e.g., compact Mylar emergency blankets), cell phones, emergency beacons, and basic supplies. These kits can be assembled individually and are also available commercially.

Beyond including disaster preparedness in classes and schools, broad public health efforts are needed to educate and prepare the general public for what to do in the inevitable event of crisis, including developing awareness of the mental health implications of such events and the resources with which to address them. Advocacy with policymakers and the media may help achieve this before and, if necessary, after an event.

Conclusion

In this chapter we present a brief overview of educational needs and resources in disaster psychiatry and, more broadly, disaster mental health. Some of our life experiences that contribute to why we find it meaningful to educate others in disaster psychiatry are described. Readers are directed to the disaster psychiatry and mental health courses and trainings listed in Table 1–1 and, of course, to the chapters that follow for additional resources and information. Developing integrated approaches to education about mental health in disasters, including readiness, evaluation, and psychiatric as well as broader health interventions and treatments, is necessary from a public and global health perspective. At this point, our capacity to mount coherent and well-coordinated responses is hindered by a relative lack of consistency. The states of disaster training, preparedness, prevention, and response have advanced dramatically in the past few decades. We have the tools and knowledge to respond much more effectively. The key next steps include seeking consistency in organizing disaster responses; pursuing further training of disaster responders; and continuing to build, test, and evaluate response systems on the basis of shared understandings. Approaches require adaptation to local needs specific to the disaster, strong relationships and communication, and systems prepared to respond and support action on the ground when disaster strikes.

References

American Psychiatric Association: Disaster and Preventive Psychiatry: Protecting Health and Fostering Community Resilience. May 19, 2023. Available at: https://education.psychiatry.org/Public/Catalog/Details.aspx?id= GlVaoPKBEthDLXm8aE4E%2bA%3d%3d. Accessed October 1, 2023.

Group for the Advancement of Psychiatry Committee on Social Issues: Psychiatric Aspects of the Prevention of Nuclear War (Report No 57). New York, Group for the Advancement of Psychiatry, 1964

Maas-Robinson S: Disaster psychiatry needs you: how to get involved. Psychiatric News, March 27, 2023. Available at: https://psychnews.psychiatryonline.org/doi/full/10.1176/appi.pn.2023.04.3.40. Accessed October 1, 2023.

2

Disaster Prevention and Climate Change

Halley Kaye-Kauderer, M.D.
Craig L. Katz, M.D.

Disaster psychiatry has traditionally focused on preparing mental health professionals to respond to disasters. The following statement from the American Psychiatric Association captures this spirit:

> It is important to understand how psychiatric care can be integrated into disaster response systems in order to effectively provide medical assessment, treatment, and consultation. Proper education and training are critical for responding to disasters and are crucial to ensuring successful intervention. (American Psychiatric Association 2022)

The book chapters that follow seek to do just that—educate the aspiring disaster mental health professional on how to most effectively mobilize and intervene when disaster strikes. We have not found any writings on the role of mental health professionals in disaster mitigation, which is remarkable given that the target of all such mitigation is human behavior and choices. In this chapter, we optimistically explore how psychiatry might be able to help avert disasters.

An understanding of the causes of disasters has evolved significantly across history. In the earliest of times, disasters were thought to be the product of supernatural forces, acts of God over which humans had little or no sway. With the advent of science, disasters were instead seen as acts of nature, enabling humans to take precautions to reduce the impact of disasters such as through earthquake-proof buildings. In very recent times, however, disasters have come to be seen as acts of society and thereby resulting from human actions, intentional or otherwise (Voogd 2004). This is clear with so-called human-made disasters, including terrorist attacks such as 9/11 or technological ones such as nuclear disasters such as Chernobyl, but the concept can also be applied to how human choices and actions contribute to the impact of natural disasters.

The United Nations Office for Disaster Risk Reduction differentiates natural hazards from disasters, stating plainly that natural hazards such as floods, earthquakes, and volcanoes do not have to become disasters (United Nations Office for Disaster Risk Reduction 2022a). It elaborates with the example of volcanoes: if one erupts where no one lives, it is only a hazard. But if people choose to live near the volcano, then that eruption becomes a disaster. Importantly, in this context, we focus on the impact of a disaster specifically on human beings, not larger environmental consequences or effects on other sentient animals. It has even been written that "natural disasters do not exist" but rather are "caused by society and societal processes, forming and perpetuating vulnerabilities through activities, attitudes, behavior, decisions, paradigms, and values" (Kelman 2019). Therefore, all disasters are human-made. The U.N.-endorsed *Sendai Framework for Disaster Risk Reduction* elaborated even further on the inherently human makeup of disasters in declaring that its goal is to

> [p]revent new and reduce existing disaster risk through the implementation of integrated and inclusive economic, structural, legal, social, health, cultural, educational, environmental, technological, political and institutional measures that prevent and reduce hazard exposure and vulnerability to disaster, increase preparedness for response and recovery, and thus strengthen resilience. (United Nations Office for Disaster Risk Reduction 2022b, p. 12)

As such, disasters are caused by vulnerabilities arising from human action or inaction, and their impact correlates far more with those vulnerabilities than with the nature of the hazard itself. Therefore, whereas hazards such as earthquakes and tsunamis occur quickly and often suddenly, disasters are the result of a long storyline of societal choices (Kelman 2019). But a tragic end need not be inexorable.

In sum, disaster prevention does not involve outright prevention of hazards because, of course, earthquakes cannot be prevented from happening, nor, as yet, do we know how to eradicate the possibility of mass human violence. Instead, it involves mitigation of risks posed by hazards and preparation for an effective response when disasters inevitably occur (Voogd 2004). Examples of mitigation include reengineering the slopes of hillside villages in Hong Kong to reduce the likelihood of landslides during the rainy season (Choi and Cheung 2013) or use of a video game to train children in a seismically active region on how to respond during an earthquake (Musacchio et al. 2016).

Climate change, which was a major catalyst for publishing an updated version of this book and the responsibility for which is clearly laid at the feet of humankind, poses an urgent case in point for exploring how mental health professionals can prevent disasters. In this chapter, we start by reviewing existing literature that addresses the rate of climate change progression, the mental health consequences of the global climate crisis, and the vulnerabilities of certain populations in dealing with current and future climate change. We then home in on the role that human behavior plays in the emergence of disasters in order to establish a rationale for mental health professionals to intervene in the predisaster phase. Finally, we try to envision what this intervention might look like in the context of climate change. We hope to answer the all-important question of what role mental health professionals can play in the face of what is predicted to be one of the largest disasters that humanity has ever faced (Sheehan et al. 2017).

Background: Presenting the Problem of Climate Change

Climate change is a global crisis that threatens both human and planetary health. Although the causes and outcomes of climate change are complex, the crisis can be understood quite simply—our planet is getting warmer. As a result of these increasing temperatures, glaciers are shrinking; sea levels are rising and shifting structures; animals are moving to higher elevations; and we are experiencing more intense and more frequent heat waves, droughts, floods, and wildfires (Rosen 2021). In other words, weather patterns that seemed inviolable are changing and becoming more chaotic and extreme. Nearly 90% of scientists who study Earth's climate agree that humans have caused this change, and consensus exists among the most prominent scientific organizations such as the National Aeronautics and Space Administration (NASA) and the World Meteorological Organization (Cook et al. 2016). The cause of a warmer climate can be explained almost entirely by increasing greenhouse gases due to emissions from human activities (Zeebe et al. 2016). The impact of these gases will depend on the response and sensitivity of the Earth's climate system. Without significant reductions, experts predict that the annual average global temperature could increase by 9°F (5°C) or more by the end of this century (Reidmiller et al. 2017). Over the years to come, societies and ecosystems will suffer immense consequences, leading to profound effects on both environmental and human health. Changes will include depletion in biodiversity, mass displacement of communities, disruptions to food production and water availability, and destruction of infrastructure, to name a few.

Although climate change is a collective challenge, it has already begun to highlight and intensify existing inequalities on individual, community, and global levels. On a global level, poorer countries will be hit hardest because of their proximity to tropical and coastal regions, despite data showing that they emit only a fraction of the total greenhouse gases (Eckstein et al. 2019). In other words, they will experience more hazards, and these hazards may go on to spawn true disasters given that these countries have less developed infrastructure and access to resources at baseline. On community and individual levels, already marginalized and disadvantaged minorities are more susceptible to the impacts of climate change, even within wealthier countries (Norman and Henry 2015; Rudolph et al. 2015). These communities are often excluded in planning processes and are more affected by food insecurity, heat waves requiring reliance on electricity, changing agricultural conditions, weakened infrastructure, and inaccessible health care (Gamble et al. 2016). Given these inequalities, it is clear that we must center equity in the climate crisis conversation and develop cultural paradigms and global policies that ensure equitable distribution of the burdens and prevention of climate change.

Impact of Climate Change on Global Mental Health

Climate change has already begun and will continue to deeply impact global mental health. Although environmentalists, conservationists, and some political leaders have made climate change a priority for years, few mental health professionals have focused on its impact until more recently, when the number of articles investigating this relationship proliferated.

It is helpful to conceptualize disasters in the framework outlined by Berry et al. (2010), who characterized climate-related disasters as belonging to three categories: acute, sub-acute, and more existential or chronic disasters. Much of the existing literature focuses on the connection between direct exposure to acute disasters and ensuing mental health consequences (Ebi et al. 2021). These studies aim to highlight how acute and sudden events such as tornadoes, floods, or wildfires negatively impact mental health and largely agree that disasters lead to elevated levels of mood disorders such as anxiety and depression as well as acute stress reactions, posttraumatic stress disorders, sleep disruption, suicidal ideation or attempts, complicated grief, recovery fatigue, and substance abuse (Basu et al. 2018; Bryant et al. 2014; Fernandez et al. 2015; Galea et al. 2007; Nahar et al. 2014; Orengo-Aguayo et al. 2019). In fact, studies show that between 25% and 50% of people exposed to acute climate-related hazards will go on to experience negative mental health outcomes (Palinkas and Wong 2020). Further studies have identified risk factors for developing psychopathology, including the magnitude of the traumatic event, exposure to direct injury or death, lower socioeconomic status, younger age, history of psychiatric disease in self or family, and limited social support (Palinkas and Wong 2020).

Although this research is essential, questions still remain regarding the mental health impacts of sub-acute or chronic changes such as long-term droughts or heat waves, as well as the existential threat of more permanent changes to our physical and social environments, such as displacement of communities, migrant crises, and civilization conflict (Berry et al. 2010; Hayes et al. 2018; Palinkas et al. 2020). Studies reveal that chronic environmental change similarly disrupts mental well-being as the accumulation of small traumas and adversities (e.g., needing to work in more extreme conditions, deteriorating economic conditions, displacement from homes) leads to further helplessness, depression, anxiety, and psychological distress (Berry et al. 2010). Already, these changes have the greatest impact on vulnerable populations, including families and children. This makes intuitive sense because younger populations have lifelong exposure to changes in the environment. Research also suggests that the well-being of children may be more profoundly impacted given that children interact with the environment in unique ways, depend on stressed adults, possess only limited adaptive capacity, and have greater vulnerable biological sensitivity (Burke et al. 2018).

Perhaps most interesting is the question of how the existential threat of climate change may affect our individual and collective psyche. A report by the American Psychological Association and ecoAmerica proposed that the deterioration of the environment is already causing a sense of stress that influences the way individuals interact with their communities (Clayton et al. 2014). They have defined a new set of conditions called *psychoterratic syndromes*, which include *ecoanxiety* (anxiety associated with the threat of climate change), *ecoparalysis* (complex feelings of not being able to take effective action against climate change), *ecological grief* (grief felt in response to losses in the natural world), and *solastagia* (distress and isolation caused by the gradual removal of solace from one's home environment (Coffey et al. 2021). Among these ideas, ecoanxiety is the most studied, although a large systematic review found a discrepancy in the way it is defined (Coffey et al. 2021).

Overall, most studies support the American Psychological Association's definition of ecoanxiety as a "chronic fear of environmental doom" while also acknowledging its association with a range of adverse emotional reactions, including worry, fear, dread, and despair, as well as irritability, sadness, numbness, helplessness, hopelessness, guilt, frustration, uncertainty, and anger (Coffey et al. 2021). These psychoterratic syndromes may also connect to a broader fear of death and the difficulty of grappling with the impact of climate change on our own mortality. Terror management theory, which focuses on the evidence-based and characteristic ways this fear impacts human thought and behavior, may further drive individuals with anxiety to adopt worldviews that can both protect their self-esteem and lead to further maladaptive beliefs and defenses (Naidu et al. 2023). In other words, mortality salience can motivate individuals toward climate change mitigation or, counterproductively, can lead to further avoidance, denial, or minimization. Understanding the scope of these psychoterratic conditions is an important first step. But the question then becomes: Can ecoanxiety and its associated negative emotions be conceptualized on a spectrum of healthy psychological adaptations in response to threat? And furthermore, can we channel this into action?

Mental Health Services in the Aftermath of Disasters

Research has attempted to investigate and propose various mental health strategies for preparedness and response to disasters on local and global levels. Most studies focus on acute hazards and necessary steps for the development and implementation of accessible mental health services in the immediate aftermath of a disaster. Although there is no universal approach, groups such as the Sendai Framework for Disaster Risk Reduction, World Health Organization (WHO), and European Network for Traumatic Stress have established strategies and guidelines that focus on 1) monitoring and treating psychiatric diseases, especially for persons at high risk for decompensation; 2) strengthening individual and community resilience; and 3) training individuals in the community to deliver such services (Palinkas et al. 2020). Some evidence-based treatments to be discussed elsewhere in this book, such as trauma-focused cognitive-behavioral therapy, narrative exposure, and psychopharmacology, require formal psychiatric training, but many others do not.

WHO emphasizes the importance of task-shifting in areas where there is a shortage of mental health providers by calling on and training primary care–based nonspecialists or community workers such as teachers or spiritual leaders to aid in the delivery of such interventions. One large systematic review found that task-shared psychological interventions were associated with decreased depression severity and enhanced response and remission rates in low- and middle-income countries (Karyotaki et al. 2022).

Although there is no single established approach to psychological interventions that promotes resilience, most interventions focus on enhancing protective psychosocial factors such as cognitive reframing, building social support, developing coping skills, promoting purpose and optimism, and encouraging physical exercise (Kaye-Kauderer et al. 2021). Several programs exist to target these skills and factors, including Psychological First Aid (PFA), the Strengthening Families Program, Skills for Psychological Recovery, and Skills for Life Adjustment and Resilience (Palinkas et al. 2020). In fact, PFA, which is discussed in depth in Chapter 16 ("Psychological First Aid"), can be taught and carried out by anyone and may represent a great opportunity for task-sharing within places that have limited access to professional mental health care providers. However, although some studies have shown the utility and effectiveness of these programs, they are limited mainly to resource-rich settings and do not account for differences in both socioeconomic and cultural contexts. Recruitment of local community workers can help to ensure that these interventions prioritize cultural contexts while also ensuring sustainability and longevity of care that may persist long after the acute dangers and stresses subside.

When it comes to more subacute and chronic consequences of climate change, we must shift our attention toward strategies rooted in mitigation, adaptation, and harm prevention that move beyond just immediate responses to address longer-term secondary threats to economic stability, individual and community safety, and environmental sustainability. Implementing these programs in the postdisaster setting may be the first step, but following the trends seen in the rest of health care reform, we must shift our attention toward better strategies for primary and preventive mental health care. In the same way that stronger baseline infrastructure allows communities to better withstand disasters, stronger baseline mental health can similarly allow populations to be more resilient in the face of these disasters (Doyle et al. 2023). Importantly, we must develop and implement new approaches that intervene before the onset of crises, when we can be more deliberate, organized, and fair.

Preventive Mental Health Care

The United States and other countries are increasingly committed to preventing disease, or at least decreasing its severity, by focusing on vaccination; screening; patient counseling; and management of common chronic conditions such as high blood pressure, diabetes, and cardiovascular disease. Yet, even though 5 of the top 25 leading causes of disability and premature death worldwide are psychiatric conditions (Mokdad et al. 2018), little effort has been made to implement large-scale, sustainable preventive mental health care. Given the current difficulties in accessing mental health care, especially in places where access is limited, we must devote more attention to methods of prevention on local, national, and global levels. There is no easy way to do this. But what is clear is that we must allot more resources to the development, implementation, evaluation, and iteration of mental health programs designed to reduce risk factors and promote resilience. Many of these risk factors are complex, with evolving interactions among biological, psychological, social, and societal factors. For this reason, we must rely not only on physicians but also on public policymakers, clergy members, and teachers to work together to enact change.

In recent years, our understanding of resilience has expanded beyond just describing individual character traits to emphasizing its dynamic ability to be practiced and cultivated through evidence-based interventions. Although there is no single definition of resilience, it is generally understood as one's ability to bounce back after a disaster. Several experts have developed a "prescription" of resilience, further explained in Chapter 15 ("Vulnerability, Resilience, and Grief"), that includes the key factors of optimism, cognitive flexibility, altruism, finding a positive role model, facing fears, developing active coping skills, establishing a social network, attending to physical well-being, focusing on how one's mind is working emotionally and intellectually, and fostering strengths (Southwick and Charney 2018). Many resilience interventions help individuals cultivate protective psychosocial factors such as positive affect, spirituality, and supportive communities and develop better methods of cognitive reappraisal (Kaye-Kauderer et al. 2021). When it comes to climate change, these tools will be invaluable. For example, cognitive reappraisal, or the deliberate use of thoughts to reframe negative circumstances, can be used to reframe climate change as an opportunity to reexamine societal institutions and work environments, team up to combat a shared problem, and develop more robust and agile strategies for mitigating further damage.

Several environmental psychologists have begun to push the concept of resilience even further, asking whether people can do more than just bounce back from a disaster. Instead, they propose *transilience*, which emphasizes further ability to "persist, adapt flexibly, and positively transform in the face of climate change risks" (Nasi et al. 2022, p. 1). Their results highlight a positive association between transilience and enhanced climate-adaptive behaviors, greater support for environmental policies, increased intention to actually engage in collective action, and increased general well-being and resilience (Nasi et al. 2022). Much of this research draws on ideas of posttraumatic growth, defined as positive psychological growth through exposure to trauma and adversity. Specifically, when thinking about the environment, posttraumatic growth suggests that people may not just bounce back from an experienced disaster but may actually see opportunities for positive change. This may, in turn, encourage individuals to find a greater sense of meaning and may lead to reduced dissociative or denial reactions, ultimately facilitating climate change action. The relationships among resilience, transilience, and posttraumatic growth are equivocal, but together, they suggest that individuals and communities can find positive transformation in posttraumatic experiences over time.

Anxiety Into Action

The development of psychoterratic syndromes such as ecoanxiety and solastalgia (distress and isolation caused by the gradual removal of solace from one's home environment) comes from deep-rooted worry, concern, and helplessness associated with change in our surrounding environments. At times, the threat of climate change can feel almost insurmountable or fatalistic. But there is also an overwhelming sense that the consequences of climate change may not affect us, in this present and immediate moment, but rather may have impacts on a future self or a future generation. Our responsibility to something that is both difficult to detect on a day-to-day basis and future-facing may make us feel less responsible for mitigating any further change. Paradoxically, these same existential threats can also inspire humans to foster a sense of meaning and personal growth; to look toward the future with resilience-promoting perspectives such as optimism and altruism; and, perhaps most importantly, to collaborate to enact change against a slowly worsening climate crisis despite cultural or societal differences.

This is not to say that we should normalize reactions of fear, anxiety, or distress to climate disasters or become numb to a clear and present danger. It is crucial to differentiate normal responses of stress from more pathological and persistent mental health problems. Anxiety itself does not indicate an illness. However, if we can better identify individuals who have more resilience factors than risk factors, those who feel responsibility toward changing their individual and collective impacts, then we may be able to capitalize on healthy degrees of anxiety as an adaptive function toward future-oriented action. In fact, in a 2019 survey, people who reported ecoanxiety were more than twice as likely as those not reporting it to exhibit motivation toward changing their behavior to aid the climate change battle (Clayton 2020). Studies found that increased anxiety and distress related to the environment was a strong predictor of adaptive behavioral responses and ultimately led people to want to reduce their contribution to climate change. On the other hand, there was a sense that too much anxiety could lead to ecoparalysis. Lower anxiety levels may ultimately be related to existing coping strategies, self-efficacy, degree of direct or indirect experience, or processes of denial and disengagement. Further research is needed to investigate subgroups who are motivated toward adaptive behavior and climate activism.

We must also be careful to properly treat anxiety when it leads to dysfunction in key areas of life and, perhaps more importantly, to acknowledge that appropriate levels of anxiety may be dictated by socioeconomic and cultural contexts. Individuals who are more vulnerable to direct and immediate consequences from climate change, who may worry how they will cool their homes during extreme heat or provide food for their families in the midst of changing agricultural patterns, may not have the bandwidth or resources to engage in such coordinated efforts. Additionally, those living in economically disadvantaged conditions due to social inequality may not prioritize climate activism as much as those whose basic needs are met in daily life. In this sense, healthier forms of ecoanxiety are intimately tied to perceived threat and an individual's ability to cope and adapt.

One preventive psychiatry strategy calls on individuals and communities to take responsibility for protecting their environment through organized action. Studies have shown that individuals who engage in climate change mitigation efforts or ecotherapy report positive changes in mood, attention, cognition, and resilience. Furthermore, there is a direct correlation between happiness and environmental action (Clayton 2020). Another study emphasized the concept of *active hope*, which helps move hopeful but passive intentions into adaptive behaviors to actually mitigate climate change (Macy and Johnstone 2012). The authors further elaborated that active hope requires three crucial steps: acknowledging the scope of the problem, setting intentions, and engaging in actions. Thus, by engaging in climate change mitigation efforts, we attempt to help not only the environment but also our own psyches. Finally, these efforts might also enable us to combat more indirect outcomes of climate change such as civil unrest, economic instability, and population displacement by strengthening community identity and cohesion. If we can work to enhance the mental health of both individuals and communities at large now, we may even be able to change the course and magnitude of our global climate crisis. In fact, studies show that healthier individuals are

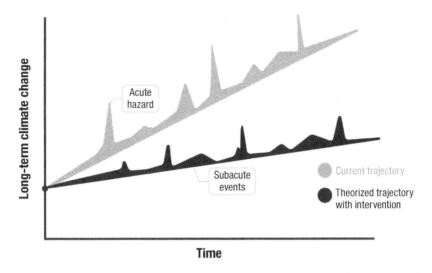

FIGURE 2–1. **Impact of preventive efforts on the trajectory of long-term climate change.**

better global citizens (Babey et al. 2020; Nelson et al. 2019), which means they may actually work harder to prevent further disasters. Perhaps, to heal the planet, we must first collectively heal ourselves.

Practical Implications for Mental Health Professionals

As mental health providers, we believe it is our responsibility to take the information presented here and use it for outreach and education and to enact change ourselves in order to "bend the curve" of long-term climate change (Figure 2–1). However, we cannot only prepare to respond to climate disasters; we also must reach back before they occur, using our professional pulpits to become role models, climate ambassadors, and preventive mental health care advocates (see related discussion in Chapter 5, "Communication and Relationships").

When it comes to outreach, the first step may be to step outside the hospital and office and into the community (Figure 2–2). This is in keeping with the dictum to see ourselves as humanitarians first, health professionals second, and mental health professionals last. Through town halls, local gatherings, and religious institutions, we can work to provide information and educate our communities about ongoing climate change and its inevitable impact not just on our mental health but on our lives. We can

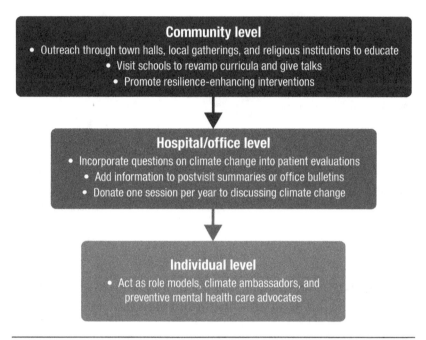

FIGURE 2–2. **Interventions for mental health providers on community, hospital/office, and individual levels.**

visit schools to advocate for including climate change and mental health prevention in curriculua, even giving talks ourselves. Importantly, given that so many people still deny the reality of climate change, we must address why this is the case and develop communication and intervention strategies to combat the processes of denial. Beyond just highlighting political divisions, mental health professionals can draw on research related to denial theory to highlight maladaptive patterns of avoidant coping and encourage adaptive patterns of acceptance and reappraisal (Clarke et al. 2019). We can also work to promote resilience-enhancing interventions (Kaufman and Feingold 2022) that simultaneously strengthen mental health and reduce the impact of climate change, at times drawing on social and conventional media outlets (Table 2–1). Helping to make our communities mentally healthier in general helps insulate our fellow citizens from the adverse mental health impacts of any disaster, climate-related or otherwise (Katz 2011).

Within the hospital and office, we can speak to our patients about their understanding of and interactions with climate change, perhaps incorporating these questions into new evaluations, follow-up review of

TABLE 2–1. **Examples of resilience-promoting behaviors in the face of climate change**

Resilience factors	Proposed interventions	Outcome
Cognitive flexibility and confronting fears	Schedule "worry time" related to the environment and psychoterratic syndromes into a regular routine	By scheduling worry time, we can transform intrusive ruminations that may be flooding us with negative thoughts into deliberate ruminations that we can consciously choose to face in a more controlled, thoughtful, and intentional way
Gratitude and positive affect	Three good things exercise: write down three good things about the environment that you are grateful for each day and why you are grateful for them	This exercise can allow for a greater appreciation for and savoring of the environment that might push us toward changing our behavior
Meaning, purpose, and social support	Volunteer and contribute to philanthropic organizations that align with your values in helping the environment	Committing to a mission can help strengthen our sense of purpose and agency while also fostering support from others with shared goals
Role models	Choose a climate change role model to emulate	By identifying role models with beliefs, attitudes, and behaviors that inspire us, we can follow in their pathways toward meaningful action

systems (e.g., presence of psychoterratic syndromes), social histories, and spiritual histories (e.g., connecting to something greater). We can even institute *environmental histories* (e.g., an individual's relationship with the environment) alongside traditional aspects of history-taking, such as social and psychiatric history. We may also choose to add additional resources or information packets to our postvisit summaries, on our office bulletin boards, or to our email signatures. We might even imagine a profession-wide national or international campaign on responding to climate change. For example, what if all mental health professionals donated one session per year to discussing climate change with their patients?

Conclusion: Taking a Step Back

Many individuals and organizations believe that climate change represents the most significant disaster facing society today. Its psychological impact is complex, with direct outcomes on mental health and well-being and indirect consequences that will change structures of societies and cultural traditions, shift economic plans and infrastructure, and further worsen existing socioeconomic inequalities. However, climate change is just one of many disasters that we currently face. Our globe continues to witness war and invasion, the evolving coronavirus disease 2019 (COVID-19) pandemic, immigration, and refugee crises, as well as more domestic disasters such as gun violence and school shootings. These ongoing disasters, like climate change, have far-reaching and existential threats that impact human behavior and interactions with our surrounding environments. Our hope is that mental health providers can draw on the raw material and research presented here and, with additional imagination and global discourse, further develop accessible, fair, and universal preventive mental health care around the world.

With the discussions in this chapter, we strive to highlight that mental health care providers do have a crucial role in both the immediate response and the aftermath of a disaster and in the disillusionment, adaptation, growth, and recovery processes. But equally important is our role in addressing the ongoing existential threats of climate change. Preventive mental health care may not just help to strengthen individual and global mental health but may also work to actually prevent or mitigate the disaster itself. In addition, we must specifically target our most at-risk populations, such as families and children, Indigenous peoples, and communities of color, who are already disadvantaged, and work to implement mental health programs that increase protective factors such as resilience, social support, positive coping mechanisms, and healthy living habits. Disasters, like climate change, represent a collective challenge and require a collective response.

References

American Psychiatric Association: Disaster Mental Health. Washington, DC, American Psychiatric Association, 2022. Available at: www.psychiatry.org/psychiatrists/practice/professional-interests/disaster-and-trauma. Accessed December 8, 2022.

Babey S, Wolstein J, Charles S: Better health, greater social cohesion linked to voter participation. Los Angeles, CA, UCLA Center for Health Policy Research, Health Policy Brief, September 2020. Available at: https://healthpolicy.ucla.edu/

publications/Documents/PDF/2020/VoterParticipation-PolicyBrief-sep2020.pdf. Accessed March 21, 2024.

Basu R, Gavin L, Pearson D, et al: Examining the association between apparent temperature and mental health-related emergency room visits in California. Am J Epidemiol 187(4):726–735, 2018 29020264

Berry HL, Bowen K, Kjellstrom T: Climate change and mental health: a causal pathways framework. Int J Public Health 55(2):123–132, 2010 20033251

Bryant RA, Waters E, Gibbs L, et al: Psychological outcomes following the Victorian Black Saturday bushfires. Aust N Z J Psychiatry 48(7):634–643, 2014 24852323

Burke SEL, Sanson AV, Van Hoorn J: The psychological effects of climate change on children. Curr Psychiatry Rep 20(5):35, 2018 29637319

Choi KY, Cheung RW: Landslide disaster prevention and mitigation through works in Hong Kong. Journal of Rock Mechanics and Geotechnical Engineering 5(5):354–365, 2013

Clarke EJ, Ling M, Kothe EJ, et al: Mitigation system threat partially mediates the effects of right-wing ideologies on climate change beliefs. J Appl Soc Psychol 49(6):349–360, 2019

Clayton S: Climate anxiety: psychological responses to climate change. J Anxiety Disord 74:102263, 2020 32623280

Clayton S, Manning C, Hodge C: Beyond Storms and Droughts: The Psychological Impacts of Climate Change. Washington, DC, American Psychological Association and ecoAmerica, 2014

Coffey Y, Bhullar N, Durkin J, et al: Understanding eco-anxiety: a systematic scoping review of current literature and identified knowledge gaps. J Clim Chang Health 3:100047, 2021

Cook J, Oreskes N, Doran PT, et al: Consensus on consensus: a synthesis of consensus estimates on human-caused global warming. Environ Res Lett 11(4):048002, 2016

Doyle SJ, Feingold JH, Van Gilder TJ: Modeling the future of prevention in primary mental health care: a narrative literature review. AJPM Focus 2(3):100092, 2023 37790673

Ebi KL, Vanos J, Baldwin JW, et al: Extreme weather and climate change: population health and health system implications. Annu Rev Public Health 42:293–315, 2021 33406378

Eckstein D, Künzel V, Schäfer L, et al: Global Climate Risk Index 2020. Bonn, Germany, Germanwatch, 2019

Fernandez A, Black J, Jones M, et al: Flooding and mental health: a systematic mapping review. PLoS One 10(4):e0119929, 2015 25860572

Galea S, Brewin CR, Gruber M, et al: Exposure to hurricane-related stressors and mental illness after Hurricane Katrina. Arch Gen Psychiatry 64(12):1427–1434, 2007 18056551

Gamble J, Balbus J, Berger M, et al: Populations of concern, in The Impacts of Climate Change on Human Health in the United States: A Scientific Assessment. Washington, DC, U.S. Global Change Research Program, 2016, pp 247–286

Hayes K, Blashki G, Wiseman J, et al: Climate change and mental health: risks, impacts and priority actions. Int J Ment Health Syst 12(1):28, 2018 29881451

Karyotaki E, Araya R, Kessler RC, et al: Association of task-shared psychological interventions with depression outcomes in low- and middle-income countries: a systematic review and individual patient data meta-analysis. JAMA Psychiatry 79(5):430–443, 2022 35319740

Katz C: Disaster psychiatry: good intentions seeking science and sustainability. Adolesc Psychiatry 1(3):187–196, 2011

Kaufman SB, Feingold J: Choose Growth: A Workbook for Transcending Trauma, Fear, and Self-Doubt. New York, TarcherPerigree, 2022

Kaye-Kauderer H, Feingold JH, Feder A, et al: Resilience in the age of COVID-19. BJPsych Adv 27(3):166–178, 2021

Kelman I: Axioms and actions for preventing disasters. Prog Disaster Sci 2:100008, 2019

Macy J, Johnstone C: Active Hope: How to Face the Mess We're in Without Going Crazy. Novato, CA, New World Library, 2012

Mokdad AH, Ballestros K, Echko M, et al: The state of US health, 1990–2016: burden of diseases, injuries, and risk factors among US states. JAMA 319(14):1444–1472, 2018 29634829

Musacchio G, Falsaperla S, Bernhardsdóttir A, et al: Education: can a bottom-up strategy help for earthquake disaster prevention? Bull Earthq Eng 14(7):2069–2086, 2016

Nahar N, Blomstedt Y, Wu B, et al: Increasing the provision of mental health care for vulnerable, disaster-affected people in Bangladesh. BMC Public Health 14(1):708, 2014 25011931

Naidu PA, Glendon AI, Trevor J: Climate change risk and terror management theory. J Risk Res 26(1):19–36, 2023

Nasi VL, Jans L, Steg L: Can we do more than "bounce back"? Transilience in the face of climate change risks. J Environ Psychol 86:101947, 2022

Nelson C, Sloan J, Chandra A: Examining Civic Engagement Links to Health. Santa Monica, CA, RAND Corporation, 2019

Norman AW, Henry HL: Eiscanoids, in Hormones, 3rd Edition. San Diego, CA, Academic Press, 2015, pp 171–188

Orengo-Aguayo R, Stewart RW, de Arellano MA, et al: Disaster exposure and mental health among Puerto Rican youths after Hurricane Maria. JAMA Netw Open 2(4):e192619–e192619, 2019 31026024

Palinkas LA, Wong M: Global climate change and mental health. Curr Opin Psychol 32:12–16, 2020 31349129

Palinkas LA, O'Donnell ML, Lau W, et al: Strategies for delivering mental health services in response to global climate change: a narrative review. Int J Environ Res Public Health 17(22):8562, 2020 33218141

Reidmiller DR, Avery CW, Easterling DR, et al (eds): Impacts, Risks, and Adaptation in the United States: Fourth National Climate Assessment, Vol II. Washington, DC, National Oceanic and Atmospheric Administration, 2017

Rosen J: The Science of Climate Change Explained: Facts, Evidence and Proof. The New York Times, April 19, 2021. Available at: www.nytimes.com/article/climate-change-global-warming-faq.html. Accessed March 21, 2024.

Rudolph L, Gould S, Berko J: Climate Change, Health, and Equity: Opportunities for Action. Oakland, CA, Public Health Institute, March 2015. Available at: https://climatehealthconnect.org/wp-content/uploads/2017/03/Climate-

Change-Health-and-Equity-Opportunities-for-Action.pdf. Accessed March 21, 2024.

Sheehan MC, Fox MA, Kaye C, et al: Integrating health into local climate response: lessons from the U.S. CDC climate ready states and cities initiative. Environ Health Perspect 125(9):094501, 2017 28934724

Southwick SM, Charney DS: Resilience: The Science of Mastering Life's Greatest Challenges. New York, Cambridge University Press, 2018

United Nations Office for Disaster Risk Reduction: What is UNDRR? Geneva, Switzerland, United Nations Office for Disaster Risk Reduction, 2022a. Available at: www.stopdisastersgame.org. Accessed December 8, 2022.

United Nations Office for Disaster Risk Reduction: Sendai Framework for Disaster Risk Reduction 2015–2030. Geneva, Switzerland, United Nations Office for Disaster Risk Reduction, 2022b, p. 12. Available at: www.undrr.org/implementing-sendai-framework/what-sendai-framework. Accessed December 8, 2022.

Voogd H: Disaster prevention in urban environments. European Journal of Spatial Development 2(4):1–20, 2004

Zeebe RE, Ridgwell A, Zachos JC: Anthropogenic carbon release rate unprecedented during the past 66 million years. Nat Geosci 9(4):325–329, 2016

3

Needs Assessment

Craig L. Katz, M.D.
Sho Takahashi, M.D., Ph.D.

If disaster constitutes a community-level trauma, then, in many respects, the disaster psychiatrist's patient is the community. Psychiatric care ultimately occurs at the level of individual disaster survivors, but disaster-related ministrations begin with the recognition that a community has been stricken. If the community is the patient, then it makes sense that any disaster mental health intervention begins with an evaluation of the community. In this chapter, we describe the type of information to be gathered in a needs assessment, review what existing disaster psychiatry response guidelines say about how to gather the information, discuss the practical considerations involved in conducting a needs assessment, and provide an example from Japan's efforts following the March 2011 (3/11) triple disaster involving an earthquake and resultant tsunami and nuclear reactor meltdown in that country's northeastern Tohoku region.

Figure 3–1 outlines the flow of the disaster psychiatry needs assessment and can serve as a guide for the detailed material to be discussed in this chapter. In reviewing this flowchart, the disaster psychiatrist can see that systems-level needs assessment and planning are integral to all phases of the response. The midline arrows create a visual sense of what the needs assessment truly is—the backbone of all phases of disaster response. Whether involved in information gathering and logistical planning, a needs assessment mission, or a clinical deployment, the disaster psychiatrist will be working either toward or from a needs assessment.

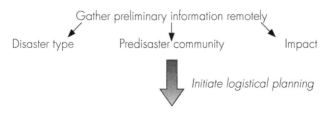

Gather preliminary information remotely

Disaster type   Predisaster community   Impact

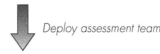

Initiate logistical planning

Establish estimate of human and financial resources available for a response

Establish or confirm local liaison(s)

Establish scope of needs assessment

Identify methods of needs assessment—qualitative and/or quantitative?

Ensure safety and logistics of assessment team

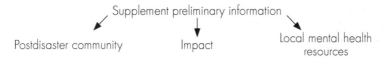

Deploy assessment team

Liaison with local contacts—health, education, community,
government, other response agencies

Supplement preliminary information

Postdisaster community   Impact   Local mental health
                                                resources

Establish need for a clinical response

Establish plan for clinical response ⟶ Share information

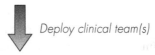

Deploy clinical team(s)

Assess impact and reassess plan

Reassess need for ongoing acute response or future postacute response

**FIGURE 3–1.   Flowchart for conducting a disaster psychiatry
                 needs assessment.**

Information Relevant to a Disaster Psychiatric Response

Three essential categories of information about a given disaster are relevant to launching a disaster psychiatry response: 1) basic facts of the general disaster type, including relevant science as well as extant knowledge about its psychiatric aspects; 2) information about the impact on the community; and 3) background information about the predisaster community.

Disaster Type

It is not clear whether types of disasters—considered broadly as human-made versus natural or in more specific terms such as earthquakes versus aviation disasters—can be linked to particular types or extent of psychopathology. Common wisdom suggests that human-made events cause more psychiatric problems than do natural disasters, although careful review of the literature and clinical experience call this reasoning into question (Garakani et al. 2004). The disaster mental health professional, therefore, should not approach a given disaster with any assumptions about whether it is likely to be more or less distressing than other disasters because myriad details about the event and the stricken community bear on its mental health impact.

On the other hand, various types of disasters may engender very different reactions and concerns among survivors. For example, earthquakes involve a literal shake-up of one's entire world and raise such concerns as the unpredictability of nature, persistence through aftershocks, and even anger about human beings' role in assuring structural safety. Being armed with this information can help psychiatrists anticipate what will be on people's minds. Contrast this with a radiological disaster, which involves issues of an invisible, unfamiliar, and potentially stigmatizing threat. In the 3/11 triple disaster in Fukushima, Japan, an earthquake and tsunami led to the meltdown of nuclear reactors at the Fukushima Daiichi power plant, and among the factors associated with postdisaster depression were concerns about the genetic effects of radiation (Oe et al. 2016).

In addition to the psychological themes common to a given disaster type, psychiatrists should have general information about the disaster for two reasons. First, they need to understand the areas of potential concern for their own safety and involvement. For example, during the 2001 anthrax scare in New York City, psychiatrists were invited to assist staff at the headquarters of the television networks that were affected. Information on the spread of anthrax was obtained to reassure volunteer psychiatrists that it was safe to meet with potentially exposed staff because human-to-human spread does not occur. Second, knowledge about disasters permits psychiatrists to be more effective mental health professionals. This is akin to the situation of consultation-liaison psychiatrists who, to be truly helpful, must understand the medical problems of the patients for whom they provide consultation. Excellent "Hazard Information Sheets" are available at www.ready.gov/be-informed.

Disaster Impact

The particulars of an event fill in the broad outline of disaster type. Relevant information is best obtained via situation reports generated by disaster response agencies. Disaster mental health professionals who work within the disaster response system and in collaboration with emergency management agencies and other responders will have access to these reports, which provide regular updates on all facets of an event, sometimes several times per day during the acute phase. In the example of an intentional anthrax exposure via aerosolization, a situation report should provide information regarding where the exposure was found to have occurred or at least which areas public health authorities believe to be free of the agent or are working to sterilize. Logistical information can also be obtained in this manner, shaping how disaster mental health professionals can travel to the affected area and where they may work, remain in communication, and, if relevant, safely live.

Beyond providing safety and logistical information, detailed data about a disaster can also shape when it makes clinical sense to deploy. When the environment has not stabilized sufficiently to reduce some of the immediate stresses placed on survivors, the role of the psychiatrist is limited. When the stresses are too high, emphasis should be placed on resources that can reduce the intensity of the stresses rather than on assisting people with coping. As discussed in Chapter 16, "Psychological First Aid," meeting survivors' basic needs for safety and comfort is an essential early intervention that has physical and psychological benefits. During this phase, disaster mental health professionals should expect to function more as humanitarians or physicians than as traditional mental health clinicians, which may or may not be considered a good use of resources.

Finally, determination of the magnitude of the mental health impact of a disaster lies at the core of the information needed by the disaster psychiatrist. This may involve a community-level assessment of symptoms or behavioral changes during the acute phase and of disorders during the postacute phase. This information helps to guide the size of an eventual clinical program.

Predisaster Community

The third pillar of information that shapes a disaster mental health response consists of background facts about the stricken community. Gathering information about the community's political, social, economic, and cultural history is comparable to obtaining a complete psychosocial history from an individual patient. The impact of an event on a community cannot be fully gauged without knowing about the strength and vitality that preceded it. As discussed in Chapter 12, "Adult Psychiatric Evaluation," it is well established that preexisting psychosocial problems predispose a disaster survivor to a psychopathological reaction (Katz 2011). If the problems are great before an event, it is to be expected that the risk will be worse afterward. It is also worth noting that the freedom to conduct a needs assessment and to conduct it freely cannot be assumed when working in stricken communities within authoritarian states.

Knowledge about the predisaster community not only helps predict needs but also provides context for how the disaster psychiatrist will function. Working in an environment where there was a robust public health and mental health system before a disaster is entirely different from working in a situation where this was lacking. The difference influences the possibility of collaborations in the field and the ultimate goals of a disaster psychiatry mission: Will disaster mental health professionals be able to partner with local mental health professionals, other health professionals, or others such as spiritual care providers or teachers? Will their goal be to help restore or supplement a previously functioning system of psychiatric care, or are they faced with the more daunting challenge of effectively having to create such a system? What is the community's experience with and attitude toward mental health?

The World Health Organization (WHO) has created an instrument for establishing the nature and details of a local mental health system, the Assessment Instrument for Mental Health Systems (WHO-AIMS; World Health Organization 2005). This instrument includes 156 items to be assessed across six different domains: legislative and policy framework, mental health services, mental health in primary care, human resources, public education and links with other sectors, and monitoring and research. The results provide a comprehensive picture of a local mental health system. The WHO-AIMS offers guidance with identifying sources of data for establishing these items, and WHO will even provide an Excel database into which these data can be entered and guidance for writing a summary report of the data.

Importantly, the purpose of the WHO-AIMS is to collect information with which to improve the mental health systems of countries or regions.

It was not designed for use in disaster settings, where the aim would be to either restore or build a mental health system, and its breadth and depth might suggest why. Nonetheless, it is valuable for several reasons. First, it presents a framework for the kind of information the disaster psychiatrist would ideally have available when planning and implementing a disaster response. Second, the WHO-AIMS is available in a brief form (Table 3–1) that is more practical for completion in the pressurized disaster environment. Finally, WHO publishes findings from the countries it has surveyed with the WHO-AIMS, providing an invaluable platform from which the disaster mental health professional can work (World Health Organization 2023). Currently, 78 reports are available.

Disaster Psychiatry Guidelines

A number of authoritative guidelines have been published that provide varying levels of detail about how to provide psychiatric, or what tends to be called *psychosocial*, care in the disaster setting. These are wide-ranging documents meant to address all facets of care. We briefly review them here from the perspective of conducting a needs assessment.

Inter-Agency Standing Committee Guidelines

The Inter-Agency Standing Committee (IASC) was established in 1992 by the United Nations (UN) to coordinate the efforts and expertise of various UN and nongovernmental agencies involved in humanitarian assistance. In 2007, the IASC's Task Force on Mental Health and Psychosocial Support in Emergency Settings developed guidelines to help response agencies "plan, establish and coordinate a set of minimum multisectoral responses to protect and improve people's mental health and psychosocial well-being in the midst of an emergency" (Inter-Agency Standing Committee 2007, p. 3). These guidelines delineated 11 major areas of intervention and described minimal and comprehensive levels of response for each. One of these domains consists of assessment, monitoring, and evaluation.

Amplifying what we have already discussed as essential information relevant to planning a disaster mental health response, the IASC guidelines specified six different types of information to be collected as part of a needs assessment (Table 3–2). Some important points were made in the guidelines concerning conducting an assessment. First, the assessment determines not only how a response should look but also whether it is needed at all. A desire to help can sometimes erroneously translate into an assumption that psychiatric help is needed and perhaps even that help of a certain kind is needed.

TABLE 3–1. Items from the brief version of WHO-AIMS 2.2

Item code	Item title
B1–1.1.1	Last version of mental health policy
B2–1.1.3	Psychotropic medicines included on the essential medicines list
B3–1.2.1	Last version of the mental health plan
B4–1.3.1	Last version of mental health legislation
B5–1.4.2	Inspecting human rights in mental hospitals
B6–1.5.1	Mental health expenditures by the government health department
B7–1.5.2	Expenditures on mental hospitals
B8–1.5.4	Free access to essential psychotropic medicines
B9–2.1.1	Existence and functions of a national or regional "mental health authority"
B10–2.1.2	Organization of mental health services in terms of catchment areas/service areas
B11–2.2.1	Availability of mental health outpatient facilities
B12–2.2.2	Users treated through mental health outpatient facilities
B13–2.2.6	Children and adolescents treated through mental health outpatient facilities
B14–2.3.2	Users treated in day treatment facilities
B15–2.4.1	Availability of community-based psychiatric inpatient units
B16–2.4.2	Beds in community-based psychiatric inpatient units
B17–2.4.6	Time spent in community-based psychiatric inpatient units per discharge
B18–2.5.2	Beds/places in community residential facilities
B19–2.6.2	Availability of mental hospital beds
B20–2.6.3	Change in beds in mental hospitals
B21–2.6.6	Involuntary admissions to mental hospitals
B22–2.6.7	Long-stay patients in mental hospitals
B23–2.6.10	Physical restraint and seclusion in mental hospitals
B24–2.7.3	Long-stay patients in forensic units
B25–2.8.2	Number of beds/places in other residential facilities
B26–2.9.1	Availability of psychosocial interventions in mental hospitals
B27–2.9.3	Availability of psychosocial interventions in mental health outpatient facilities

TABLE 3–1. Items from the brief version of WHO-AIMS 2.2 (continued)

Item code	Item title
B28–2.10.1	Availability of medicines in mental hospitals
B29–2.10.3	Availability of medicines in mental health outpatient facilities
B30–2.11.1	Psychiatry beds located in or near the largest city
B31–3.1.2	Refresher training programs for primary health care doctors
B32–3.1.5	Interaction of primary health care doctors with mental health services
B33–3.1.7	Availability of medicines to primary health care patients in physician-based primary health care
B34–3.2.3	Refresher training programs for primary health care nurses
B35–3.2.4	Refresher training programs for nondoctor/nonnurse primary health care workers
B36–3.2.6	Mental health referrals between non-physician-based primary health care to a higher level of care
B37–3.3.3	Interaction of mental health facilities with complementary/ alternative/traditional practitioners
B38–4.1.1	Human resources in mental health facilities per capita
B39–4.1.4	Staff working in or for mental health outpatient facilities
B40–4.1.5	Staff working in community-based psychiatric inpatient units
B41–4.1.6	Staff working in mental hospitals
B42–4.2.2	Refresher training for mental health staff on the rational use of psychotropic drugs
B43–4.2.3	Refresher training for mental health staff in psychosocial (nonbiological) interventions
B44–4.4.1	User/consumer associations and mental health policies, plans, or legislation
B45–4.4.2	Family associations involvement in mental health policies, plans or legislation
B46–4.4.8	Other nongovernmental organizations involved in community and individual assistance activities
B47–5.1.4	Professional groups targeted by specific education and awareness campaigns on mental health
B48–5.3.1	Provision of employment for people with serious mental disorders
B49–5.3.2	Primary and secondary schools with mental health professionals
B50–5.3.8	Mental health care of prisoners
B51–5.3.9	Social welfare benefits

TABLE 3–1. Items from the brief version of WHO-AIMS 2.2 *(continued)*

Item code	Item title
B52–6.1.5	Data transmission from mental health facilities
B53–6.1.6	Report on mental health services by government health department
B54–6.2.2	Proportion of health research that is on mental health

Note. WHO-AIMS = World Health Organization Assessment Instrument for Mental Health Systems.
Source. Reprinted from "Brief Version of Items for WHO-AIMS 2.2," in *World Health Organization Assessment Instrument for Mental Health Systems,* Version 2.2 (WHO-AIMS 2.2). Geneva, Switzerland, World Health Organization, 2005, pp. 58–59.

TABLE 3–2. Categories of information for assessment in Inter-Agency Standing Committee guidelines on mental health and psychosocial support in emergency settings

Relevant demographic and contextual information

Experience of the emergency

Mental health and psychosocial problems

Existing sources of psychosocial well-being and mental health

Organizational capacities and activities

Programming needs and opportunities

Source. Inter-Agency Standing Committee 2007.

Second, IASC guidelines underscore that any assessment needs to be done in a collaborative fashion with local health and mental health professionals, governments, communities, relief agencies, and other stakeholders. Mental health responders coming from outside a stricken community should neither act nor appear to act as though they are expert diagnosticians who can paternalistically ascertain the local mental health needs. The affected population should be involved in defining what is distress and what is well-being.

A third and related suggestion in the IASC guidelines is that needs assessments should be shared. Ideally, these needs assessments would be shared with a disaster psychiatry coordinating body that oversees mental health efforts in a disaster setting. This means that given the humanitarian implications of the situation, agencies should not try to maintain their assessments as proprietary. It also means that any given disaster psychiatry response team should research whether a mental health needs assessment has already been done and disseminated before launching into an assessment.

Finally, the IASC recommends that a "rapid" assessment be completed within 1–2 weeks of a disaster, focusing on the experience of survivors. A more comprehensive evaluation of all six domains of information listed in Table 3–2 would follow later. This stepwise approach appears reasonable but may be overly optimistic. It may be problematic in at least two regards. First, limited disaster psychiatry resources may render it difficult to launch a response within 1–2 weeks. During this time, a more reasonable approach might be to research historical background about the affected community, much of which can be done prior to travel to the community. Second, mental health needs are likely to be especially fluid in the early days and weeks after a disaster, such that an evaluation done in the first 1–2 weeks may become rapidly outdated. Monitoring such shifts and targeting mental health resources appropriately may not be possible with limited resources, and a more pragmatic approach might be to conduct an initial assessment after several weeks to a month or more, when the initial stresses of impact have subsided and postdisaster life has assumed a relative rhythm, and to then consider reassessing that assessment several weeks or months beyond that.

World Health Organization Guidelines

The WHO's "Rapid Assessment of Mental Health Needs of Refugees, Displaced and Other Populations Affected by Conflict and Post-Conflict Situations" (RAMH) includes specific assessment guidelines for use in conflict or complex humanitarian emergencies (World Health Organization 2001). Although focused on conflict situations, this tool may be tailored for assessing needs in any catastrophic situation. Similar to the IASC guidelines, the RAMH emphasizes collecting information across seven areas: information about the conflict; description of the affected populations; mental health needs; cultural, religious, socioeconomic, and political aspects of the affected communities; cultural responses to trauma; mental health resources; and recommendations. The RAMH includes a six-page tool that specifies the information to be collected within each of these seven domains. Unlike the IASC guidelines' focus on the initial 1–2 weeks, the RAMH suggests that an assessment be done once basic survival needs are addressed.

The RAMH's recommendations are more operationalized than those of the IASC guidelines. For example, the RAMH specifies the composition of the RAMH team. It suggests that the team be multidisciplinary, consisting of at least one mental health professional and both local and international members. Experts in crisis situations and refugee mental health are deemed essential. Of note, the RAMH allows for and even expects the inclusion of non–mental health professionals who can be trained as evaluators. This expectation arises from the reality that many situations lack sufficient mental health professionals but also suggests that even when more resources are available, psychiatrists may not need to be the evaluators of the affected community.

The RAMH also underscores that one or more agencies must invite the assessment. Although WHO may recommend the assessment, a government, another UN agency, a nongovernmental organization, or a funding source also may request it. This point highlights that disaster mental health professionals ought not to just show up and embark on assessing a situation for logistical, political, financial, and even clinical reasons. The information will have a much greater impact if it is collected collaboratively.

The RAMH also lays out three broad sources of information for the needs assessment. The RAMH team should contact central and regional authorities, which include ministries of health, education, and social welfare; representatives of agencies, associations, services, and universities, which span UN agencies in the affected country, nongovernmental organizations, churches, and even youth associations; and intersectoral sectors, which include health care providers, existing mental health care providers, teachers and professors, and law enforcement representatives. In the chaos of postconflict or other disasters, having access to a list of potential contacts from each of these three categories can render a needs assessment much more organized and efficient.

Disaster Psychiatry Outreach

Table 3–3 provides an even more concise framework for conducting a postdisaster needs assessment based on the experience of one of us (C.L.K.) while leading an organization previously known as Disaster Psychiatry Outreach and now known as the Crisis Emotional Care Team (www.vibrant.org/whatwe-do/advocacy-policy-education/crisis-emotional-care). Although not as exhaustive as the WHO-AIMS or the IASC or RAMH guidelines, this framework is proposed as a pragmatic alternative when only a basic disaster mental health needs assessment is possible because it is brief and commonsense enough to be used without any preparation.

Practical Considerations

In the remainder of this chapter, we focus on practical concerns in undertaking a needs assessment. The ranges of possible circumstances, disas-

TABLE 3–3. Assessment items for use with a stricken community

Assessment item	Predisaster	Acute disaster	Postacute disaster
Living conditions			
Travel			
Communication			
Government			
Educational system			
Emergency system			
Public health system			
Mental health system			
Religion			
Economy			

ters, and even resources render it difficult to lay out a one-size-fits-all approach to assessment. However, a number of issues apply across most possibilities.

For several related reasons, it is especially important for assessment teams without a prior relationship with a community to work with local liaisons at the very outset. First, this partnership will enable the team to get the fullest possible picture of the community's culture and history. Second, it will better ensure integration of whatever future mental health resources are deployed into the community, which may be wary of outside help—mental health or otherwise. Third, working with local partners will help to keep the focus on local priorities. Finally, it will pave the way for what should be the eventual goal of any large-scale disaster mental health intervention: fully handing over the programming to the local community.

Another fundamental consideration in shaping a needs assessment is its scope, which can be looked at in terms of time and space. Regarding time, will the assessment have as its focus the acute period or the longer-term postacute period? To some degree, the answer to this question lies in the ambitions or resources of the response agency. It is certainly easier to focus on the acute period, both in terms of information needed and eventual resources. On the other hand, some circumstances require a longer-term commitment, particularly international responses, where building of partnerships with local counterparts is essential but labor-intensive (Silove and Bryant 2006).

On the matter of space, disaster psychiatry planning requires consideration of the possible breadth of the efforts and the potential size of the mental health footprint. The "patient" requires identification. Will the needs of an entire country or region be the concern, or will the focus be much narrower, even limited to assisting one institution? For example, Calderon-Abbo (2008) described the efforts to reopen and even expand the inpatient mental health services offered by several New Orleans hospitals following Hurricane Katrina. Conceivably, a disaster psychiatry mission could meaningfully choose to focus on revitalizing and staffing the inpatient psychiatric services of just one hospital. Or consider the case of the heavily damaged Soso area of Fukushima after 3/11. The inpatient-focused psychiatric system in the area was inadequate for community psychiatric care prior to the disaster and then suffered heavy damage from 3/11. This became an opportunity to build back from the destruction in the direction of a system oriented toward community and outpatient use (Fukunaga and Kumakawa 2015).

The techniques of assessment can vary as well. Will the assessment or scouting team be conducting a scientifically rigorous study of mental health needs or relying more on an observational approach to assessment? Epidemiological studies of postdisaster mental health needs abound in the literature, but these studies take enormous planning and oversight because of the practical, ethical, and scientific challenges of working in a postdisaster environment (North et al. 2002). The immediacy of needing to forecast disaster-related needs and services may not afford the luxury of time required to address these challenges. Publication-quality scientific rigor may not be possible or necessary when clinical and service needs beckon.

Therefore, to assess need, a disaster psychiatry assessment team typically relies on liaison with local professionals and community leaders as well as on its own clinical impressions. For example, Humayun (2008) described a team consisting of a psychiatrist and three trainees who worked for 3 weeks at a 650-bed hospital following the 2005 Pakistan earthquake; the team used clinical work as the medium for assessing need while ministering to what were deemed to be high-risk patients. There are many similar examples of several-person assessment teams that rely on what is essentially qualitative data gathering done amid clinical work (e.g., Choudhury et al. 2006; Math et al. 2006). Even if needs assessments are unlikely to be epidemiological in quality, they do not need to rely solely on clinical impressions. Screening and assessment tools can be used to improve diagnostic accuracy while also permitting reliance on non–mental health professionals to administer them in an effort to capture a larger sample (Connor et al. 2006).

One final consideration in conducting a disaster psychiatry needs assessment involves the resources available for responding. For example, researchers calculated that providing full mental health services to populations affected by Hurricanes Katrina and Rita for up to 30 months after the disasters would have cost $1,133 per capita, a total of $12.5 billion for the affected populations (Schoenbaum et al. 2009). Finances are an important consideration because the IASC guidelines are explicit in discouraging, on ethical grounds, the collection of information that will not be used toward future services (Inter-Agency Standing Committee 2007). Ultimately, information gathering should be proportionate to the capacity for future services as much as can realistically be foreseen in order to avoid using information for purposes other than promised (i.e., academic publication) and overtaxing affected communities with surveys.

The Example of Japan's Disaster Psychiatry Assistance Teams

Japan's disaster psychiatry assistance teams (DPATs) exemplify an organized approach to disaster mental health needs assessment. We have found no other reports of such teams that have been organized to respond to mental health needs in acute phases of disasters in such a specialized and sophisticated manner. Before DPATs, the disaster psychosocial support system had an unclear chain of command, but since the DPATs were established, the system has changed to an efficient, rational, and systematic disaster psychosocial support system.

Following 3/11, several organizations and institutions, such as universities with psychiatry departments, academic associations, and nongovernmental organizations, implemented disaster medical services involving the creation of mental health care (*kokoro no care* in Japanese) teams, which carried out support work in the disaster-affected areas. However, a lack of coordination among the teams, as well as their varied composition, led to confusion when providing assistance. Drawing on these experiences, the disaster medical assistance team (DMAT) system was modified to consider psychiatric needs, and officially approved DPATs, which are dispatched to provide mental health support services to people in disaster areas, were established in 2013 (Takahashi et al. 2020). The Ministry of Health, Labor, and Welfare set up a DPAT head office in Tokyo and established DPATs in each prefecture and in designated cities in Japan. The number of teams across Japan has been gradually increasing, and as of April 2023, the DPAT reconnaissance teams have been maintained by 106 medical institutions, and the number of prefectural DPAT team members maintained by each municipality has been maintained at 3,654 as of the end of 2021, according to the Ministry of Health, Labor and Welfare Scientific Research Report (Fussa et al. 2023). Meanwhile, the support activities of DPATs have expanded since 3/11 as various disasters, such as volcanic eruptions, landslides, floods, earthquakes, and the coronavirus disease 2019 (COVID-19) pandemic, occurred.

A DPAT consists of about five people (composed of one psychiatrist, two nurses, and two logistics personnel for administrative work, for example). Each team is dispatched to a site to conduct support activities for approximately 1 week. An initial DPAT reconnaissance team arrives in the disaster area within 48 hours (somewhat later than the DMAT), sets up a DPAT coordination headquarters, coordinates with the DMAT, coordinates the dispatched teams, and provides initial services at evacuation shelters for approximately a week. Given the especially exhausting nature of this early work, they are then relieved by a second DPAT, which, in coordination with government agencies, fire departments, police departments, and defense forces, conducts support activities for up to several months or until there is no further need. Their efforts last longer than those of DMATs. After that, the regional DPATs that follow continue the support activities in 1-week rotations, although initial consultations to DPATs appear to peak within 1 week of activation (Takahashi et al. 2020) (Figure 3–2). The main activities of a DPAT are 1) responding directly or indirectly to the psychological problems experienced by residents at evacuation shelters in a disaster area, 2) coordination of the transport of patients from psychiatric hospitals whose functionality has been affected by the disaster, and 3) support for disaster relief workers.

Japan's disaster mental health information collection system used to be a disaster mental health information support system, which was very useful for gathering detailed psychiatric information. However, it was hampered by being DPAT-only, which made it difficult to share information with other disaster response teams. DPAT members are now able to collect data on disaster operations for inclusion in Japan–Surveillance for Post Extreme Emergencies and Disasters (J-SPEED), which is similar to the WHO's Emergency Medical Team Minimum Data Set and includes mental health. Mental health data can be entered by registered disaster response team members, including DPAT members, via smartphone apps and computers, and data are shared in real time with full privacy protection via the Emergency Medical Information System (EMIS). The EMIS is an information network among medical institutions, including base hospitals for disaster management, medical-related organizations, fire departments, health centers, and municipalities, as well as among the national and prefectural governments. Its purpose is to collect and provide information related to disaster medical care, including the activities

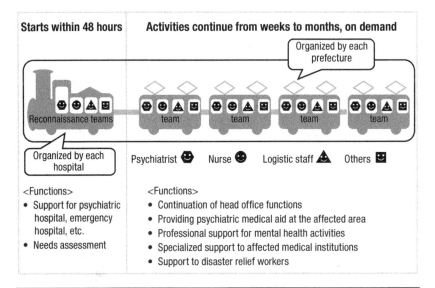

FIGURE 3–2. Roles of the reconnaissance disaster psychiatric assistance team (DPAT) and subsequent DPATs.

of medical institutions in and out of disaster-stricken areas, at the time of a disaster. As a result, it is now possible to identify and share mental health needs in real time, providing for a rational and informed mental health response to disasters (Kubo et al. 2019; Yumiya et al. 2022).

Conclusion

Systems-level assessment lays the groundwork for an effective clinical response by disaster mental health professionals, enabling them to render maximal assistance without contributing to the chaos of the situation. In the inevitable rush to help a disaster-stricken community, psychiatrists can apply the principles of their usual clinical practice by first assessing the "patient" (i.e., the community) before launching into interventions. A collaborative and methodical approach to systems-level assessment will yield the most useful information, especially when such an approach is guided by awareness of the potential resources and scope of the eventual clinical response. We can look to Japan's DPATs as a model for such an approach.

References

Calderon-Abbo J: The long road home: rebuilding public inpatient psychiatric services in post-Katrina New Orleans. Psychiatr Serv 59(3):304–309, 2008 18308912

Choudhury WA, Quraishi FA, Haque Z: Mental health and psychosocial aspects of disaster preparedness in Bangladesh. Int Rev Psychiatry 18(6):529–535, 2006 17162693

Connor KM, Foa EB, Davidson JRT: Practical assessment and evaluation of mental health problems following a mass disaster. J Clin Psychiatry 67(Suppl 2):26–33, 2006 16602812

Fukunaga H, Kumakawa H: Mental health crisis in northeast Fukushima after the 2011 earthquake, tsunami, and nuclear disaster. Tohoku J Exp Med 237(1):41–43, 2015 26329988

Fussa Y, Tachikawa H, Tateishi S, Gomyo S: Research to strengthen the functions of the Disaster Psychiatric Assistance Team (DPAT) and to consider responses to sever disasters (such as the Nankai Trough earthquake). Tokyo, Ministry of Health, Labor and Welfare Scientific Research, 2023. Available at: https://mhlw-grants.niph.go.jp/project/170605. Accessed July 2, 2024.

Garakani A, Hirschowitz J, Katz CL: General disaster psychiatry. Psychiatr Clin North Am 27(3):391–406, 2004 15325484

Humayun A: South Asian earthquake: psychiatric experience in a tertiary hospital. East Mediterr Health J 14(5):1205–1216, 2008 19161095

Inter-Agency Standing Committee: IASC Guidelines on Mental Health and Psychosocial Support in Emergency Settings. Geneva, Switzerland, Inter-Agency Standing Committee, 2007. Available at: https://interagencystandingcommittee.org/iasc-task-force-mental-health-and-psychosocial-support-emergency-settings/iasc-guidelines-mental-health-and-psychosocial-support-emergency-settings-2007. Accessed January 20, 2023.

Katz CL: Disaster psychiatry: good intentions seeking science and sustainability. Adolesc Psychiatry 1:187–196, 2011

Kubo T, Yanasan A, Herbosa T, et al: Health data collection before, during and after emergencies and disasters—the result of the Kobe Expert Meeting. Int J Environ Res Public Health 16(5):893, 2019 30871037

Math SB, Girimaji SC, Benegal V, et al: Tsunami: psychosocial aspects of Andaman and Nicobar islands. Assessments and intervention in the early phase. Int Rev Psychiatry 18(3):233–239, 2006 16753660

North CS, Pfefferbaum B, Tucker P: Ethical and methodological issues in academic mental health research in populations affected by disasters: the Oklahoma City experience relevant to September 11, 2001. CNS Spectr 7(8):580–584, 2002 15094694

Oe M, Maeda M, Nagai M, et al: Predictors of severe psychological distress trajectory after nuclear disaster: evidence from the Fukushima Health Management Survey. BMJ Open 6(10):e013400, 2016 27798033

Schoenbaum M, Butler B, Kataoka S, et al: Promoting mental health recovery after hurricanes Katrina and Rita: what can be done at what cost. Arch Gen Psychiatry 66(8):906–914, 2009 19652130

Silove D, Bryant R: Rapid assessments of mental health needs after disasters. JAMA 296(5):576–578, 2006 16882965

Takahashi S, Takagi Y, Fukuo Y, et al: Acute mental health needs duration during major disasters: a phenomenological experience of disaster psychiatric assistance teams (DPATs) in Japan. Int J Environ Res Public Health 17(5):1530, 2020 32120917

World Health Organization: Rapid Assessment of Mental Health Needs of Refugees, Displaced and Other Populations Affected by Conflict and Post-Conflict Situations. Geneva, Switzerland, World Health Organization, 2001

World Health Organization: WHO-AIMS Version 2.2—Assessment Instrument for Mental Health Systems. Geneva, World Health Organization, 2005

World Health Organization: WHO-AIMS Country Reports. Geneva, Switzerland, World Health Organization, 2023. Available at: https://extranet.who.int/mindbank/collection/type/whoaims_country_reports/all?page=all. Accessed January 20, 2023.

Yumiya Y, Chimed-Ochir O, Taji A, et al: Prevalence of mental health problems among patients treated by emergency medical teams: findings from J-SPEED data regarding the West Japan Heavy Rain 2018. Int J Environ Res Public Health 19(18):11454, 2022 36141727

4

Technology

Anthony T. Ng, M.D., DFAPA
Sander Koyfman, M.D., M.B.A.

Emotional health is now widely considered to be an integral part of disaster preparedness and response. However, access to general and specialized psychiatric care remains a challenge even outside of disasters because of workforce shortages and other factors. Among trained psychiatrists and mental health professionals, only some receive training in disaster work (see Chapter 1, "Disaster Psychiatry Education"), contributing to a deficit of disaster-trained professionals available to respond to disasters and the needs that may overwhelm communities both short and long term.

At the same time, technology has continued to evolve significantly. Almost nowhere has that evolution been as impactful as in health care. In this chapter, we attempt to cover some of the common use cases, opportunities, and challenges of technology use in disaster response. Nearly every facet of delivery of care, from direct clinical care to supportive functions, now has technological components. When effective, technology in health care in general and disaster mental health relief work in particular can play an important role by providing immediate access to rapidly changing information, resources, and support for individuals and responders impacted by disaster. Providing just-in-time content can play a crucial role in allowing individuals to better adjust to fluid environments. Table 4–1 lists some websites that may be useful in providing updated information.

TABLE 4–1. List of helpful websites

	Organization	Websites and Apps
Disaster Mental Health	American Psychiatric Association	www.psychiatry.org/psychiatrists/practice/professional-interests/disaster-and-trauma
Disaster Preparedness, Response, and Recovery	Substance Abuse and Mental Health Services Administration	www.samhsa.gov/disaster-preparedness
Center for the Study of Traumatic Stress	Uniformed Services University	www.cstsonline.org
What Is Child Trauma?	National Child Traumatic Stress Network	www.nctsn.org/what-is-child-trauma
Resources for Survivors and the Public Following Disaster and Mass Violence	National Center for PTSD	www.ptsd.va.gov/understand/types/resources_disaster_violence.asp
Disaster and Trauma Resource Center	American Academy of Child and Adolescent Psychiatry	www.aacap.org/aacap/Families_and_Youth/Resource_Centers/Disaster_Resource_Center/Home.aspx
Natural Disasters	Centers for Disease Control and Prevention	www.cdc.gov/natural-disasters
PFA Mobile	Veterans Affairs Mobile Store	https://mobile.va.gov/app/pfa-mobile
Multilingual resources	Languages of Care	www.languagesofcare.org

Note. PFA=Psychological First Aid.

Technology Throughout the Disaster Cycle

Perspectives on the role of technology can be viewed from the four disaster phases as illustrated in the Model for Adaptive Response to Complex Cyclical Disasters (Brenner and Clegg 2022): anticipation, impact, adaptation, and growth and recovery (see Chapter 8, "Model of Adaptive Response to Complex Cyclical Disasters"). In the *anticipation* phase, or the pre-event phase, educational materials on crisis response, including stress reactions, distress behavior, and coping skills, can be gathered and integrated into educational websites (see Table 4–1). During this phase, it is helpful to familiarize patients, clinicians, and the community with digital technology to be used in the event of disasters to establish credible communication channels in case of disaster. Stakeholders need to be aware of and familiar with these technological resources because adoption of new resources under stress of an acute disaster would be exponentially more difficult. Predisaster planning tools should be incorporated as part of general psychiatric care whenever possible. Hard copies of disaster mitigation plans integrated into treatment planning should be given to individuals in case of network disruptions.

The *impact* phase of the cycle is often the most intense phase. People and groups may have little ability to assess overall impact beyond the immediate line of sight. Isolation and lack of knowledge of the fate of loved ones significantly amplify the mental health risk of negative impacts for individuals. It is important to appreciate the varying level of disaster exposure to determine appropriate digital interventions and optimize them. During this period, significant challenges to the use of digital psychiatric care are likely, with general deprioritization of emotional health care in the face of immediate needs. In situations where infrastructure is disrupted and the community is displaced because of loss of homes or work, it will be helpful to promote various messaging modalities to tell others that individuals may be safe or where resources may be located. Resources must take into account cultural and language needs. Quick tips on self-care, either as education files or apps, that have been previously developed in the anticipation phase may be distributed. It is important to realize that during the impact phase, individual abilities to prioritize or manage complex tasks may be compromised, and level of retention may be limited. As such, any digital tools need to be easy to find and simple to use. Whenever possible, consistent content should be available with just a few clicks and through multiple channels.

Brief support and counseling sessions via telepsychiatry can be implemented. Although the focus may be on the immediate survivors and first responders, digital tools can be helpful for secondarily impacted individuals such as friends and families and the community as a whole. Televideo town hall meetings can be held to promote community coping and healing as well as to ensure consistent access to lifesaving information. Successful implementation of digital clinics requires effective facilitation strategies that take into account features of the technology itself, the needs of its end users, and the clinical content of deployment (Connolly et al. 2021).

The *adaptation* phase immediately following the impact phase is characterized by an increased sense of safety and stability and the opportunity to begin acute recovery. In this phase, individuals and communities realize the limits of disaster assistance. People may feel abandoned, especially given delays in aid or unfulfilled promises of aid. Digital interventions can offer needed continuity during this period. The ability to safely interact with digitally assisted community spaces such as social media platforms and other virtual support groups can offer important opportunities for reentering social spaces. Ongoing psychoeducation about disaster stress, postdisaster psychiatric illnesses or exacerbation of preexisting illness, and patient coping and interventions could be shared and coordinated through various channels. Possible opportunities for digital tools to support individual and community recovery include screening tools and telepsychiatry. It is likely that at this point, there will be some transition to more regular psychiatric service delivery, and familiarity with what was and what could be available going forward could promote continuity of care and a sense of safety.

The last phase to be described in this cycle, *growth and recovery*, is marked by a restoration of previous or new routines, accompanied by the feeling of things being "back to normal" for some groups. This stage may offer an opportunity for digital platforms to further reinforce resilience with continued psychoeducation and promotion of wellness skills and behavior.

Table 4–2 summarizes the role of telepsychiatry in the various phases of the Complex Cyclical Disasters model.

Role of Conventional Technology

Landline telephones remain an effective tool for communication. Many health entities call patients to check in on them and remind them of appointments. This can be done by live staff or via automated calls; however, for checking in, a staff caller likely will be better received (McClean et al. 2016). In addition, many communities rely on telephones for crisis communications. Telephones, especially cell phones, can become overwhelmed in the acute aftermath of a disaster, but they remain a valuable tool for people to connect, learn of the whereabouts of their loved ones,

---

TABLE 4–2. Roles of telepsychiatry in the phases of the Complex Cyclical Disasters model

---

Anticipation

Training in postdisaster psychiatry issues

Developing competence in the use of culturally aware telepsychiatry

Learning to manage safety issues

Developing supportive infrastructure

Creating licensing and regulatory guidelines

Creating emergency protocols for the use of telepsychiatry, with clear delineation of roles and responsibilities

Impact

Consultation with medical providers

Consultation with other mental health professionals

Consultation with disaster human services providers or organizations

Just-in-time-training continuously tailored to the response environment

Monitoring of wellness in disaster responders

Direct triage, evaluation, and intervention

Adaptation

Ongoing consultation with medical providers, including primary care physicians and emergency physicians

Ongoing training and education of stakeholders

Ongoing triage, evaluation, and intervention

Growth and recovery

Ongoing consultations with providers, health care entities, and community stakeholders

Direct evaluation and intervention

Analyzing evaluation and treatment data from previous phases for opportunities

---

and obtain general information. Such information, especially learning about the safety of friends and loved ones, can be protective of mental health. The telephone can also be a means of asynchronous medical and psychiatric care.

In the United States, rollout of the national three-digit mental health crisis hotline #988 and corresponding Disaster Distress Helpline number 1-800-985-5990 has allowed both call and text access, in multiple languages, to communities impacted by disasters (Table 4–3). A public information campaign has led to a significant increase in use even before full integration into provider disaster planning.

TABLE 4–3.   List of crisis helplines

Name of hotline	Description	Number
988 Suicide and Crisis Lifeline	Three-digit dialing code that routes callers to the 988 Suicide and Crisis Lifeline	988
Disaster Stress Hotline	Provides immediate crisis counseling for people who are experiencing emotional distress related to any natural or human-caused disaster	1-800-985-5990
Physician Support Line	Psychiatric help for U.S. physicians and medical students to discuss immediate life stressors	1-800-409-0141

Public radio has been traditionally used worldwide as a communication tool in disasters and public health emergencies, especially around disaster preparedness, risk awareness, and risk reduction (International Federation of Red Cross and Red Cresent Societies 2013). Radio has been used after disasters to provide information about disaster relief efforts and public health behavior to stay healthy. Radio has also been used to inform the community where to find medical services, such as which hospitals are open and whether temporary medical units such as field hospitals were available (Hugelius et al. 2016a). Radio can promote resilience by increasing a sense of normalcy and promoting social connectedness and effective coping (Hugelius et al. 2016b) as well as being a tool for disseminating general personal resilience and self-care information.

Telemedicine in Disaster Mental Health

One of the more established technological tools that received much attention and even special accommodation in the midst of the coronavirus disease 2019 (COVID-19) pandemic is telepsychiatry. Telepsychiatry has also played a role in addressing disaster needs; it can help alleviate patient surge and access challenges by being a workforce multiplier even in war zones (Lee et al. 2023). Both supervision and direct services can be done remotely, which can help reduce stress on providers locally. Telepsychiatry makes it possible for clinicians to access psychiatric expertise in specialty areas such as trauma, disaster psychiatry, substance abuse, specific topics in psychopharmacology, or cross-cultural psychiatry or to address specific needs of populations such as the LGBTQ+ community, children, or older adults (Ng 2010). Telepsychiatry can also promote online support groups and forums that can provide a sense of community and connection for individuals who may be feeling particularly isolated in the aftermath of a disaster.

Telepsychiatry has been used in conflicts and various disaster situations both nationally and globally, most predominantly during the COVID-19 pandemic (Carretier et al. 2023; Chaudhry et al. 2022; Garshnek and Burkle 1999; Kannarkat et al. 2020) and in conflict zones, as has been done extensively in Ukraine (Lee et al. 2023). Telepsychiatry had been considered in the planning of pandemic responses and became a widespread reality with the COVID-19 pandemic. Many organizations quickly adapted telepsychiatry to maintain care for existing patients, extend care to new patients, and protect their workforce at the same time (Di Carlo et al. 2021).

As telepsychiatry played a significant role in meeting the psychiatric needs of communities during the pandemic, several issues were brought to light, such as challenges related to economic and infrastructure disparities (e.g., access to necessary hardware, sufficient broadband) and simple privacy. Accommodations needed to meet specific needs of older adults and physical barriers due to medical and developmental disabilities are just a few examples noted at scale due to pandemic-induced rapid growth and reduced access to acceptable alternatives. Digital literacy may be variable with end users and providers, and acceptance of the use of telepsychiatry may vary widely between patients and clinicians (Barton et al. 2007).

Both users of telemedicine and providers who decline to use telemedicine have reported dislike of the loss of personal contact with patients. Some clinicians have reported difficulty in picking up nuances and emotions (May et al. 2001). Payment issues also restrict the type and location of reimbursable telemedicine services (Kim 2004). Lack of support has shown to be the major source of implementation failure in digital integration, including telemedicine (Greenhalgh et al. 2017). Last, many providers have reported difficulties coping with the level of social isolation inadvertently triggered when the trip to the office and associated social interactions along the way significantly drop off.

Despite these challenges, telepsychiatry will likely continue to play a significant role in disaster psychiatry, offering an extremely rapid and relatively safe way to deploy clinical expertise to a disaster zone. As such, telemedicine should be a routine part of disaster training and resource allocation (Garshnek and Burkle 1999). The Lancet Commission on Global Mental Health recommended that digital interventions such as telemedicine should be adopted alongside traditional in-person treatments (Patel et al. 2018). Combined, or so-called hybrid, use may help resolve stigma related to mental health treatment and practical challenges with engagement between the clinician and patient that have been noted in exclusive use of technology platforms, where access challenges may affect adoption.

Mobile Communications

The role of smartphones in daily life has increased significantly in sync with technological advancements, and smartphones now have a ubiquitous presence. The UN's International Telecommunication Union has provided its first estimate of regional and global ownership, revealing that 73% of the world's population older than age 10 years owned a cell phone in 2022 (International Telecommunication Union 2022). Mobile communication places a variety of tools in a user's hands, with tremendous implications for psychiatry. From basic voice to text messaging, to apps and general internet access, all may be readily available in a portable platform. When the critical access issues of connectivity are addressed (potentially requiring advocacy on the part of mental health care workers), many additional uses are ready to deliver mental health solutions.

Mobile technology can be used to gather data and monitor the mental health needs of a community following a disaster, helping governments and aid organizations respond equitably to the needs of those affected. Importantly, technology can be used to facilitate building of supportive group environments to reduce both individual and social distress (Richters et al. 2008).

Mobile implementations do not need to depend on complex interfaces to be effective. Text messaging has become a significant tool in health care. Messaging is accessible and easy to use and is already widely adopted by users. Text messaging can be used for reminders, short pieces of information, self-monitoring, and patient engagement (McClean et al. 2016). Text messages have been used to promote the use of CBT skills by military service members experiencing subthreshold posttraumatic stress disorder (PTSD) symptoms (Roy et al. 2015) or to help youth reach out for help while in distress (e.g., The Trevor Project, www.thetrevorproject.org; New Jersey Quit Line, www.njquitline.org/momsquitconnection; NYC Well, 1-888-NYC-WELL). Additional uses specific to disasters are likely to come to the fore, such as access to the Disaster Distress Hotline (www.samhsa.gov/find-help/disaster-distress-helpline).

Social Media

Social media, despite some well-publicized risks (Alonzo et al. 2020), can play an important role in offering channels of communication and support after disasters. When social media is used as an active communication tool, rather than to passively observe others, it can promote connectedness while minimizing risks of overexposure to harmful and retraumatizing content. Establishing credible channels of communication through social media well ahead of a disaster should be included in disaster preparedness and response road maps. Most internet users in many countries, both developing and developed, use some sort of social networking. These platforms can potentiate the reach and engagement of communities after a disaster. For example, Facebook's Safety Check feature can play a vital role in disaster response by allowing individuals to let friends and families know they are safe during disasters (Gleit et al. 2014).

Although in-person support is ideal, social media can provide support to individuals after a disaster, with an even more pronounced benefit for younger users. On the other hand, because of the abundance of information on social media platforms, it is important to appreciate the varying perspectives of information being presented, some more accurate than others. People posting this information may have a number of conflicting motivations, including blatantly fraudulent ones. Better understanding of such dynamics can potentiate helpful content and ensure that messages reach as wide an audience as possible when needed.

Mobile Apps

The development of smartphone applications has grown exponentially in recent times. In 2019, researchers identified 1,435 mobile apps related to mental health, of which 449 addressed anxiety issues, 450 addressed depression, 282 addressed schizophrenia, 124 addressed self-harm, and 140 addressed substance use disorders (Larsen et al. 2019). Mobile apps can provide information and resources on disaster-related mental health issues, such as PTSD and grief, as well as tips for self-care and coping, distress behavior monitoring, and promotion of resilience factors (Kuhn et al. 2017). One study found that veterans who used an app called PTSD Coach experienced a decrease in PTSD symptoms from the first to the last assessment, with approximately one-third of users experiencing clinically significant improvements (Hallenbeck et al. 2022). Mobile apps can be used to share information about local resources such as emergency shelters, medical facilities, and mental health services. This can help individuals quickly find the support they need. The use of digital navigators such as mobile apps has been helpful in promoting and navigating care (Wisniewski and Torous 2020).

Digital Therapeutics

Digital therapeutics consist of software that provides evidence-based interventions to prevent, manage, or treat a medical disorder. A relatively new entrant in the health care space, digital therapeutics hold the promise of being prescribed, or self-administered in a way akin to over-the-counter medications. As such, clinicians should consider the impact of these interventions. Similar to the way we now collect information about exercise, over-the-counter medications, therapies, and other interventions, we should be disciplined about inquiring whether a patient is benefiting from a self-directed digital therapeutic. The gains from such use may dissipate if the app is not available because of internet outages or an inability to charge devices. Without a clear *digital treatment history*, a patient may experience needless distress when alternatives are not readily available. For example, if a child living with autism spectrum disorder is permitted to use a digital tool to help with distress of a physical examination, lack of a smartphone can lead to an avoidable incident of distress. For other patients, appropriate meditation software can help management of their anxiety.

Artificial Intelligence

The role of artificial intelligence (AI) has received an increased level of attention in all areas of life, including mental health. By using a model called machine learning, which is based on a large variety of computer algorithms, data analysis can assist with psychiatric diagnosis, symptom tracking with individualized treatment, disease course projection, and adjustments and education. AI can be available through the internet, smartphone applications, or digital gaming (Pham et al. 2022). Examples of AI application include Woebot, an application that automates the process of cognitive-behavioral therapy (Fiske et al. 2019). Although AI requires ongoing maturation as it continues to address various concerns such as privacy, racial biases, and cultural nuances, as well as fidelity of data quality that drives the algorithms, it has the potential to provide rapid support in disasters because of its low cost and high accessibility.

On the other hand, as we enter an uncharted AI-enabled future, we can only speculate about a need for human-enabled fact-checking to assist AI in creating the most meaningful reference library when it comes to scientific knowledge. In addition, going forward, health care providers entering medicine will need additional training to help navigate an ever-expanding universe of knowledge. We imagine new graduates will be required to demonstrate ability to critically assess publicly available content—including AI-generated content—just as rigorously as they assess scientific articles.

Electronic Health Records

Electronic health records (EHRs), have become a significant component in the provision and management of health care today, ranging from the private practitioner to large health care systems. Advanced EHR systems can help to improve application of evidence-based care though effective use of the accumulated data. EHRs have the potential to collate clinical data that can be helpful for illness surveillance as well as supporting computerized decision support to guide care (Van Eaton et al. 2014). EHRs provide an important access tool through patient portals where patients can interact with their treatment team about their illnesses and treatment, which can be crucial post disaster. EHRs present both challenges and opportunities in the general claims-based data flows, including improving interoperability, creation of durable data flags when patients change doctors and insurance, and integration of relief organization–directed services.

Discussion of basic infrastructure needed to deliver many of the technologies included here is beyond the scope of this chapter, but it is critically important to promote reliable use of these tools in the field. Other issues to consider are the varying levels of tech literacy, concerns about security and privacy, and the fine balance between use of technology and the need for personal contact. Technology's success in the postdisaster environment likely rests on its ability to support that connection, not replace it. Additional references for innovative use of technology in disasters are provided in Table 4–4.

Conclusion

Technology can have a positive impact in disaster mental health by providing a variety of tools and resources that can help individuals cope with the emotional and psychological effects of a disaster. Planning and thoughtful mitigation as well as care integration measures can help decrease any technology-driven disruptions. It is important for future program development and outcome studies to examine the direct clinical implications of technology in disaster psychiatry as well as the increasing influence of technology on the individual and societal resiliencies in communities. Consideration of language and culture in technology offerings remains an important consideration for effective community utilization of offered resources.

TABLE 4–4. **Studies of uses for technology in disaster response**

Subject of study	Description	Reference
Crisis informatics	Use of technology during crises and disasters and its impact on the social, societal, and sociotechnical dynamics of those events	Palen and Anderson (2016)
Crisis informatics and social media	Use of social media during disasters, including potential benefits and challenges	Reuter et al. (2018)
Management of misinformation	Examination of the spread of misinformation on Twitter following the 2013 Boston Marathon bombing and the challenges of managing rumors and false information during a crisis	Starbird et al. (2014)
Data analytics and disaster management	Potential uses of big data analytics in disaster management, including using data from social media and other sources to inform disaster response and recovery efforts	Zhang et al. (2019)
Mobile crowd sensing	Potential of mobile crowd sensing as a tool for disaster management, including the use of smartphones and other mobile devices to collect and share information during a crisis	Al-Rodhaan and Al-Dhelaan (2021)
Drones in disaster response	Potential uses for search and rescue operations, damage assessment, and delivery of supplies and medical aid	Datta and Pal (2021)
Social media for disaster management	Use of social media in Jordan, including the challenges and opportunities associated with its use and the implications for disaster response and recovery efforts	Khasawneh et al. (2021)
Artificial intelligence (AI)	Comprehensive review of the application of AI in disaster management, including the use of machine learning and other techniques to analyze data, predict disasters, and inform response efforts	Wang et al. (2021)

References

Alonzo R, Hussain J, Stranges S, Anderson KK: Interplay between social media use, sleep quality, and mental health in youth: a systematic review. Sleep Med Rev 56:10414, 2020 33385767

Al-Rodhaan MA, Al-Dhelaan AM: Applications of mobile crowd sensing in disaster management. J Netw Comput Appl 178:103004, 2021

Barton PL, Brega AG, Devore PA, et al: Specialist physicians' knowledge and beliefs about telemedicine: a comparison of users and nonusers of the technology. Telemed e-Health 13(5):487–499, 2007 17999611

Brenner G, Clegg K: Model for Adaptive Response to Complex Cyclical Disasters. New York, Vibrant Emotional Health, 2022. Available at: https://chroniccyclicaldisasters.info. Accessed July 8, 2024.

Carretier E, Bastide M, Lachal J, et al: Evaluation of the rapid implementation of telehealth during the COVID-19 pandemic: a qualitative study among adolescents and their parents. Eur Child Adolesc Psychiatry 32(6):963–973, 2023 36370315

Chaudhry S, Weiss A, Dillon G, et al: Psychosis, telehealth, and COVID-19: successes and lessons learned from the first wave of the pandemic. Disaster Med Public Health Prep 16(5):1785–1788, 2022 33588969

Connolly SL, Kuhn E, Possemato K, et al: Digital clinics and mobile technology implementation for mental health care. Curr Psychiatry Rep 23(7):38, 2021 33961135

Datta S, Pal S: Disaster response: utilizing drone technology for post-disaster relief operations. Geocarto Int 36(2):155–168, 2021

Di Carlo F, Sociali A, Picutti E, et al: Telepsychiatry and other cutting-edge technologies in COVID-19 pandemic: bridging the distance in mental health assistance. Int J Clin Pract 75(1):e13716, 2021 32946641

Fiske A, Henningsen P, Buyx A: Your robot therapist will see you now: ethical implications of embodied artificial intelligence in psychiatry, psychology, and psychotherapy. J Med Internet Res 21(5):e13216, 2019 31094356

Garshnek V, Burkle FM Jr: Applications of telemedicine and telecommunications to disaster medicine: historical and future perspectives. J Am Med Inform Assoc 6(1):26–37, 1999 9925226

Gleit N, Zeng S, Cottle P: Introducing safety check. Facebook Newsroom, October 15, 2014. Available at: https://about.fb.com/news/2014/10/introducing-safety-check. Accessed March 25, 2024.

Greenhalgh T, Wherton J, Papoutsi C, et al: Beyond adoption: a new framework for theorizing and evaluating nonadoption, abandonment, and challenges to the scale-up, spread, and sustainability of health and care technologies. J Med Internet Res 19(11):e367, 2017 29092808

Hallenbeck HW, Jaworski BK, et al: PTSD Coach Version 3.1: a closer look at the reach, use, and potential impact of this updated mobile health app in the general public. JMIR Ment Health 9(3):e34744, 2022 35348458

Hugelius K, Gifford M, Örtenwall P, et al: Disaster radio for communication of vital messages and health-related information: analysis from the Haiyan Typhoon, the Philippines. Disaster Med Public Health Prep 10(4):591–597, 2016a 26940871

Hugelius K, Gifford M, Ortenwall P, et al: "To silence the deafening silence": survivor's needs and experiences of the impact of disaster radio for their recovery after a natural disaster. Int Emerg Nurs 28:8–13, 2016b 26724170

International Federation of Red Cross and Red Cresent Societies: World Disaster Report 2013: focus on technology and the future of humanitarian action. Geneva, Switzerland, Internal Federation of Red Cross and Red Cresent Societies, 2013

International Telecommunication Union: Internet more affordable and widespread, but world's poorest still shut off from online opportunities. Geneva, Switzerland, International Telecommunication Union, November 30, 2022. Available at: www.itu.int/en/mediacentre/Pages/PR-2022-11-30-Facts-Figures-2022.aspx#:~:text=Mobile%20phone%20ownership%20continues%20to,a%20mobile%20phone%20in%202022. Accessed March 25, 2024.

Kannarkat JT, Smith NN, McLeod-Bryant SA: Mobilization of telepsychiatry in response to COVID-19: moving toward 21st century access to care. Adm Policy Ment Health 47(4):489–491, 2020 32333227

Khasawneh M, Al-Bdour A, Al-Ajlouni F: Use of social media for disaster management in Jordan: an exploratory study. Telematics and Informatics 64:101593, 2021

Kim YS: Telemedicine in the USA with focus on clinical applications and issues. Yonsei Med J 45(5):761–775, 2004 15515185

Kuhn E, Kanuri N, Hoffman JE, et al: A randomized controlled trial of a smartphone app for posttraumatic stress disorder symptoms. J Consult Clin Psychol 85(3):267–273, 2017 28221061

Larsen ME, Huckvale K, Nicholas J, et al: Using science to sell apps: evaluation of mental health app store quality claims. NPJ Digit Med 2:18, 2019 31304366

Lee J, Petrea-Imenokhoeva M, Naim H, et al: Rapid deployment of telehealth in a conflict zone: supporting the humanitarian needs in Ukraine. NEJM Catalyst 4(3), 2023

May C, Gask L, Atkinson T, et al: Resisting and promoting new technologies in clinical practice: the case of telepsychiatry. Soc Sci Med 52(12):1889–1901, 2001 11352414

McClean SM, Booth A, Gee M, et al: Appointment reminder systems are effective but not optimal: results of a systematic review and evidence synthesis employing realist principles. Patient Prefer Adherence 10:479–499, 2016 27110102

Ng AT: Use of telepsychiatry: implications in disaster, in Hidden Impact: What You Need to Know for the Next Disaster: A Practical Mental Health Guide for Clinicians. Edited by Stoddard FJ, Katz CL, Merlino JP. Sudbury, MA, Jones & Bartlett, 2010, pp 187–194

Palen L, Anderson KM: Crisis informatics: an emerging perspective on the social, societal, and socio-technical dynamics of crises. Int J Hum Comput Stud 107:1–4, 2016

Patel V, Saxena S, Lund C, et al: The Lancet Commission on global mental health and sustainable development. Lancet 392(10157):1553–1598, 2018 30314863

Pham KT, Nabizadeh A, Selek S: Artificial intelligence and chatbots in psychiatry. Psychiatr Q 93(1):249–253, 2022 35212940

Reuter C, Hughes AL, Kaufhold MA: Social media in crisis management: an evaluation and analysis of crisis informatics research. Internation Journal of Human-Computer Interaction 34(4):86–99, 2018

Richters A, Dekker C, Scholte WF: Community based sociotherapy in Byumba, Rwanda. Intervention (Amstelveen) 6(2):100–116, 2008

Roy MJ, Highland KB, Costanzo MA: GETSmart: guided education and training via smart phones to promote resilience. Stud Health Technol Inform 219:123–128, 2015 26799892

Starbird K, Maddock J, Orand M, et al: Rumors, false flags, and digital vigilantes: misinformation on Twitter after the 2013 Boston Marathon Bombing. iConference 2014 Proceedings, 2014. Available at: https://faculty.washington.edu/kstarbi/Starbird_iConference2014-final.pdf. Accessed March 26, 2024.

Van Eaton EG, Zatzick DF, Gallagher TH, et al: A nationwide survey of trauma center information technology leverage capacity for mental health comorbidity screening. J Am Coll Surg 219(3):505.e1–510.e1, 2014 25151344

Wang Q, Yang Y, Liu H, et al: A review of the application of artificial intelligence in disaster management. Saf Sci 141:105250, 2021

Wisniewski H, Torous J: Digital navigators to implement smartphone and digital tools in care. Acta Psychiatr Scand 141(4):350–355, 2020 31930477

Zhang X, Huang J, Huang Z, et al: Use of big data analytics in disaster management. Nat Hazards 99(1):1–19, 2019

5

Communication and Relationships

Grant H. Brenner, M.D.
Katherine A. Koh, M.D., M.Sc.

Vignette: The Pros and Cons of Constant Digital Connectivity

Dr. V, a primary care doctor, is a displaced person living in a refugee camp. He is the only one of his family to escape from a war-torn country after the abrupt withdrawal of foreign-occupying forces. He has been living in the camp for several weeks while his status being is decided, and he is trying to help out the local medical team in any way he can. However, he has grown increasingly despairing as the situation at home gets worse and worse. He is in direct contact with his wife and can speak with his children but has no way to help them escape. In the meantime, people in the camp as well as back home continue to use cell phone–based apps to share videos and stories, including images of murder and violence happening in real time. There is no clear way to advise people on what to do—limiting exposure makes sense from a stress-mitigation perspective, but asking them to risk missing critical information regarding loved ones is problematic. Regardless, short of taking away access to technology or internet service, it is unlikely refugees would limit their use of their phones. In addition, it is very boring in the camp, and even with activities planned, phone use is a main source of entertainment and distraction, a part of everyday normal life.

Importance of Communication During Disasters

Communication is a dynamic, complex concept central to effective disaster response, where the devil is in the details, even if we wish we could easily understand one another and work together. Used well, communications knit communities together in times of safety and crisis. Good communications are the foundation of solid relationships, shaped by social, emotional, and organizational intelligence. It is critically important for leaders (see Chapter 7, "Engaging in Disaster Response"), collaborating partners, and stakeholders to strive for effective communication practices.

Where does communication come into play during disasters? The classic and oft-cited five essential elements of psychosocial care (Hobfoll et al. 2007) are essential in mass casualty events for establishing and maintaining 1) a sense of safety, 2) calming, 3) a sense of both self-efficacy and community efficacy, 4) connectedness, and 5) hope. Responsive information exchange is the foundation on which the essential elements depend, creating a communication ecosystem (see section "Ecological Communications"). Such an ecosystem can optimize all stages of the disaster management cycle by facilitating information sharing, decision-making, and effective action. For more details on the disaster management cycle, see Chapter 8 for an overview of the recently developed Model of Adaptive Response to Complex Cyclical Disasters.

Given that disasters and crises are escalating because of climate change and geopolitical events, the role of conventional and technology-driven communication (see Chapter 4, "Technology") has become ever more important. Misunderstandings drive conflict and interfere with coordinated responses, risking systemwide failure where everyone is talking but it seems like no one is communicating effectively. Despite progress, not enough people are speaking the same language when it comes to disaster response and preparation. Mistakes beget more mistakes, and morale plummets, further degrading function. Even when communication channels are open, dissemination of misinformation, and even disinformation (deliberately false information, such as for political manipulation), is still possible.

Communication Models

Contemporary communication models highlight the complex, evolving, and interdependent nature of disaster and crisis. In this section, we outline several models, review theoretical underpinnings, and discuss future directions.

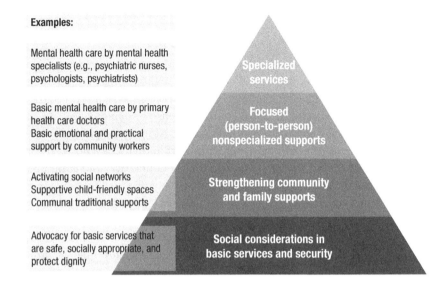

Examples:

Mental health care by mental health specialists (e.g., psychiatric nurses, psychologists, psychiatrists)

Basic mental health care by primary health care doctors
Basic emotional and practical support by community workers

Activating social networks
Supportive child-friendly spaces
Communal traditional supports

Advocacy for basic services that are safe, socially appropriate, and protect dignity

Specialized services

Focused (person-to-person) nonspecialized supports

Strengthening community and family supports

Social considerations in basic services and security

FIGURE 5–1. Intervention pyramid for mental health and psychosocial support in emergency situations.

The U.S. Federal Emergency Management Agency (FEMA) emphasizes the need to shift from a *government-centric* approach to a *whole community* approach (Federal Emergency Management Agency 2013; Spialek and Houston 2018). To be successful, local stakeholders' participation in crisis management must be fully integrated into the broader context while identifying, preserving, and honoring local experience and expertise. This begins and ends with effective multilateral communications. The Inter-Agency Standing Committee (2021) guidelines use the intervention pyramid for mental health and psychosocial support in emergency situations to describe how different levels of intervention sit on one another (Figure 5–1). Communication is, at all levels, essential, and speed and agility are enhanced by seamless, low-error *comms* (a term often used as shorthand).

Ecological Communications Models in Disaster Work

Communication is a living system with an ecology all its own. We cannot completely predict and control how such systems evolve, and sometimes, efforts to force things along can lead to problems. When navigating the complex ecology of crisis, it is essential to embrace uncertainty, leveraging what poet John Keats called *negative capability*—when a person "is capable of being in uncertainties, mysteries, doubts, without any irritable reaching after fact and reason" (as quoted by Rollins 1958)—with both predictable linear and suddenly discontinuous nonlinear structural elements (see Chapter 8). Liu and Zhao (2022) highlight that communication is critical for disaster communication ecology, serving to regulate uncertainty and helping stakeholders make sense of experiences and access three types of support: emotional, informational, and physical.

Media system dependency theory (in which individuals choose information sources according to circumstance and familiarity) and communication infrastructure theory (in which people are embedded in community information structures) suggest that there are nested levels of communication ecology: micro and meso levels. The micro level consists of granular, multidirectional communications among various groups, including friends, family, local governance and first responders, and other community members. These communications are especially important in groups with limited access to institutional resources, such as racial or ethnic minority communities. The meso level consists of two elements: news media and community-based organizations. Media outlets are critical for information sharing, with local media especially relevant for the communities in which they reside. Community-based organizations also serve as a hub for information sharing and notably serve to partner with external groups during disasters and in driving preparedness.

Developed interpersonal networks, or relationships, offer many advantages for streamlining crisis management. Rich networks are associated with more active emotional support seeking, a larger media network is associated with more informational and emotional support seeking, and richer organizational support is associated with physical support seeking. When evaluating crisis situations and planning for disasters, analysis of the communication ecology is foundational.

Operational Closure: You Can't Make the Dream Work Without Teamwork

The authors of Chapter 7 go into more detail on staff organization, but a few words here are helpful in contextualizing communications. According to Celikler and Kern (2022), several factors shape how disaster response organizations are structured, including 1) leadership style, 2) level of experience and related leader qualities, 3) incident type, 4) individual team member capabilities, 5) duration of the response, and 6) the physical location of team activities. In this context, "communication is understood as a

TABLE 5–1. Communication objectives and factors in disaster management teams

Objectives of meetings in disaster management teams
- Communicate measures adopted to date
- Assign orders and available resources (personnel, material)
- Check the success of measures and the processing status of orders
- Generate an overview of operation-related developments

Individual-centered social factors
- Understanding of roles, role delimitation, and role expectations
- Use of language (e.g., stylistic devices, idioms, dialectal coloration)
- Use of technical language and terminology

Team-centered social factors
- Professional and social familiarity or personal closeness and informality
- Transparency of decisions
- Precision with which information is passed on

Organizational influencing factors
- Number of participants in team meetings
- Orientation toward standards (e.g., with regard to communication channels, forms, command structures and legal mandates)
- Structuring of team meetings

Technological influencing factors
- Acceptance of communication systems
- Number and utilization of communication channels
- Distraction caused by communication systems

Source. Adapted from Celikler and Kern 2022.

dimension of social interaction or action in the context of which events in the organizational environment are given meaning…" (Celikler and Kern 2022, p. 3), requiring repetition and experimentation to continuously improve and adapt. Celikler and Kern (2022) define three *fields of action*—human, organizational, and technological—at which communications take place. It is important to consider these fields in the analysis, design, and implementation of communications processes, as highlighted in Table 5–1.

Coproduction of Knowledge Model

The coproduction of knowledge model (Lejano et al. 2021) focuses on areas where improved communications are required, drawing on ethnographic and political theories. Imperiale and Vanclay (2021) noted that "[p]aternalistic attitudes on the part of some authorities, particularly administrative ones, rather than learning in the field, can end up 'perpetuating business-as-usual and exacerbating the social pre-conditions of disasters'" (cited in Lejano et al. 2021, p. 1). Crisis learning is inherently responsive, based in feedback loops and mutuality rather than being a simple matter of expertise transmitted from above. Coproduction of disaster knowledge follows suit: stakeholders are more likely to be part of a network rather than a hierarchy. Outside experts, such as disaster mental health responders who are not locally based, are dependent on communities to fill them in on what affected individuals need, how they work, who they are, and what they already know. There is no one-size-fits-all solution, so disaster work has become fundamentally relational. Simultaneously, communities wishing to leverage the experience and resources of expert groups need to be able to receive knowledge from external groups, some of whom are not familiar with local customs or culture. Knowledge coproduction takes place across the cycle of disasters, from preparation to response and recovery and to reflection on lessons learned.

In the coproduction model, risk knowledge is

1. Democratized—not the sole property of the expert but rather shared and open source
2. Translated into the language of the affected community, both literally, as in the case of a refugee camp where posters and signs must be available in several applicable languages or the case of local responses where many languages are spoken, and figuratively or idiomatically rendered into an everyday conversational form rather than a distancing technical form
3. Decentered and leveled, authentically embracing the recognition that *everyone* has expertise

The coproduction of risk knowledge is a three-legged stool based on 1) Indigenous or local knowledge, 2) social learning, and 3) narrative. Indigenous and local knowledge, including that of traditional healers and communal wisdom, is partly recognized in formal response systems, defined as "a cumulative body of knowledge, practice, and belief, evolving by adaptive processes and handed down through generations by cultural transmission" (Berkes 2018, p. 7). Without deeply embracing and integrating this knowledge, experts quickly find themselves befuddled as to why their efforts fail seemingly without cause or why community leaders may appear receptive only to politely fail to follow up as the outside experts thought they had all agreed. Culture is not merely knowledge but also unique ways of seeing and interpreting fundamental aspects of physical and social reality. If we do not connect on cultural levels, we are not inhabiting quite the same realities, which leads to misunderstandings and avoidable mistakes.

Social learning is complex, with information being transmitted generationally via myriad channels that outsiders may not grasp. "Learning from direct observation of devastation from disaster effects and sensing risks from signs and signals do not necessarily result in cognitive and behavioral changes without leadership, social and moral institutions, and the needed follow up processes" (Lejano et al. 2021, p. 5). A lot of learning is "muscle memory" for communities and systems, passed on implicitly but not codified or formally retained. Unless knowledge is made explicit and captured in durable ways, learning from experience and skill transfer are less effective than they otherwise could be. Communities often have deep generational knowledge pertaining to signs of impending disaster and ways of responding and bouncing back that potentially are based in spiritual and mythic knowledge as well as technical knowledge and communal activity (Lejano et al. 2021).

It is critical to memorialize knowledge and action steps during and after disasters through real-time capture and review and synthesis following deployments to capture lessons learned in mutually understandable and sustainable ways. This can be accomplished through various media, from codified, written manuals to rules and regulations, to word of mouth and community mythos, to signs with symbols pointing toward shelters from storms or avenues of escape from rising tides, to QR codes and URLs posted with links to robust digital resources, and in many other ways. Multiple layers of feedback (*loop learning*) are required in order to retain information in local, governmental, and nongovernmental groups. Narrative models ground coproduction of knowledge. Having a shared set of stories—not just anecdotes of shared adversity, loss, and triumph but also stories of who we are and how we work together—is the tapestry that holds knowledge and weaves in resilience during provident times and through adversity.

On a basic level, technical knowledge must be translated into culturally congruent and accessible forms; otherwise, it is meaningless. This *social capital* creates resilience through trust, shared experiences, and, ultimately, meaningful relationships. They conclude, "Narrative forms of communication, especially when used in everyday language, encourages plurivocity, which simply means many narrators participating in telling a collective story in their own voice" (Lejano et al. 2021, p. 7).

Risk Communication

Risk communication is an evidence-based approach to designing communications in high-stress situations. Risk communication is intended to lead to the best outcomes in disaster response and preparedness by shaping messaging at different crisis phases to increase prosocial, adaptive behaviors and decisions; reduce ineffective communication; and quell needless anxiety and uncertainty while maintaining trust and connection.

Part of risk communication involves looking back on prior events to see what worked and what did not work. To that end, Dehghani et al. (2023) conducted a qualitative study of Iranian public health officials to draw out key elements identified by various stakeholder groups working together over a long span of time. Analysis revealed 479 codes—basic themes—that were cleaned of redundancy and distilled into a final set of five categories and 19 subcategories. The five categories were as follows:

1. Situation analysis, including evaluation of information conditions, risk monitoring and warning, functional and process situation, and audience analysis
2. Establishment and management of risk communication, including risk information, communications, planning and policymaking, process management and execution, and content of information
3. Education and training for experts, senior and middle managers, the community, and media owners
4. Monitoring and evaluation, including control over processes when possible, and documentation
5. Logistics, including human resources, funds, infrastructure, and coordination and organization

For each subcategory, the full analysis by Dehghani et al. (2023) details specific action steps required. For example, community education and training (category 3) includes teaching people how to correct rumors, and documentation (category 4) includes monitoring communications and updating databases developed to memorialize and codify important information relevant to the response.

Incident Command System (www.ready.gov/incident-management) is another example of how operational design and communication go hand in hand. In the United States, emergency management uses the same basic layout across events to facilitate communication and teamwork by establishing a common structure, or *org chart* spelling out the structure for incident management and command (Figure 5–2). This provides a solution to the all-too-familiar problem in which stakeholder groups cannot inter-

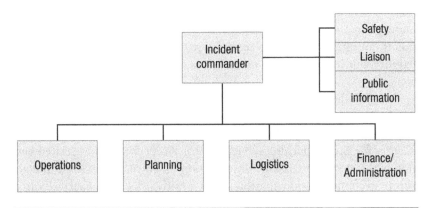

FIGURE 5–2. Incident management tree.

Source.   Ready.gov: Incident Management. Washington, DC, U.S. Department of Homeland Security, September 7, 2023. Available at: www.ready.gov/incident-management. Accessed March 26, 2024.

face by establishing a common framework for working together. In this way, standard operating procedures dictate the reporting structure for multiple stakeholder groups involved in a response, allowing individuals who have never worked together to align more easily by sharing an organizational schema and common language to designate key functions.

The incident commander (IC) is the "chief executive officer" of the whole response, and other leaders (who themselves may be designated ICs for their local groups) report to that person for their organizations. At the next layer, coordination is according to function. For example, a health supplies unit might coordinate with a group providing clothing and personal supplies to assemble a single care package for families, and logistics and operations would oversee distribution. In this way, external groups seeking to offer supplies and services are able to efficiently integrate into the response by interfacing appropriately within the incident management framework rather than disrupting function.

Risk Communication Framework

The term *risk communication* is used in disaster response planning to describe effective communication before, during, and after a crisis (Center for Mental Health Services 2002). It encompasses exchange of information with individuals (e.g., patients), groups (e.g., schools), businesses (those impacted or threatened), public agencies (e.g., first responders such as police and fire departments), and the news media (via the internet, radio, or TV). Psychiatrists and mental health teams may be consulted or hold leadership positions from which they may facilitate effective communication about risk (Norwood et al. 2005). Effective risk communication is not directly related to the concept of risk management in terms of liability, but it can mitigate other forms of risk as well as improve outcomes.

In 2002, the Center for Mental Health Services at the Substance Abuse and Mental Health Services Administration (SAMHSA) issued "Communicating in a Crisis: Risk Communication Guidelines for Public Officials" (Center for Mental Health Services 2002). According to an updated version of this document, risk communication "involves the effective and accurate exchange of information about health risks and hazards—often during an emergency—that advances risk awareness and understanding and promotes health-protective behaviors among individuals, communities, and institutions" (DiClemente and Jackson 2016, p. 1; Substance Abuse and Mental Health Services Administration 2019). The same document notes that

> Sound and thoughtful risk communication can assist public officials in preventing ineffective, fear-driven, and potentially damaging public responses to serious crises, such as unusual disease outbreaks and bioterrorism. Moreover, appropriate risk communication procedures foster the trust and confidence that are vital in a crisis situation. (Substance Abuse and Mental Health Services Administration 2019, p. 5)

The same principles public officials use to communicate during crisis are essential tools in disaster mental health response. A key role psychiatrists often play is to provide ad hoc risk communication information and training to leadership during deployments" (Substance Abuse and Mental Health Services Administration 2019, p. 20). Risk communication recommendations from the guidelines are summarized in Table 5–2.

Risk communication is based in psychology and neuroscience, grounded by four psychological models explaining how understanding and interpretation are distorted under high-stress conditions: 1) the risk perception model, 2) the mental noise model, 3) the negative dominance model, and 4) the trust determination model (Covello 2009). Descriptions of each model are provided in Table 5–3.

A carefully constructed risk message can be demonstrated by contrasting two different ways to communicate to the public a brief and effective message about the risk for posttraumatic stress disorder (PTSD) following a disaster. One way to discuss risk is to recite all of the diagnostic criteria, but the message to increase awareness of PTSD would get lost. A better approach is to advise disaster victims to consider the possibility that they may have developed PTSD and to seek mental health support if they feel that

TABLE 5–2. Risk communication recommendations

1. Ease public concern
2. Give guidance on how to respond
3. Stay on message
4. Deliver accurate and timely information
5. Develop goals and messages that are simple, straightforward, and realistic
6. Deliver information with brevity, clarity, and effectiveness

Source. Adapted from Center for Mental Health Services 2002.

TABLE 5–3. Risk communication models

Model	Description
Risk perception	People tend to detect threat as an inherent bias. The tendency increases when stress is high; higher cortical functions diminish and basic systems kick in.
Mental noise	Stress decreases information processing, limiting our ability to make sense of complex messages. Messages need to be simplified, assuming we can handle only three pieces of information at a time (vs. the usual 7 ± 2) and assuming that education level is effectively four grades lower than one's actual educational level. Messages should have three points, in 27 words, spoken in about 9 seconds.
Negative dominance	Negative information stands out more and is more salient. On average, people emphasize loss more than gain, scanning for threats. More positive messages are needed to balance out the negative, even more so in crisis. Use a 3:1 template in which least three positive pieces of information are given for each negative one.
Trust determination	Trust is considered to be the most important factor in risk communication, the foundation of all communication and collaboration. Trust takes time to build up but is easy to lose. Betrayal makes trust even harder to regain, making traumatic experiences more damaging. Factors contributing to trust include 1) caring, empathy, compassion, and listening; 2) expertise, competence, knowledge, and credibility; 3) openness, honesty, and transparency; and 4) accountability, perseverance, dedication, commitment, objectivity, fairness, responsiveness, and consistency.

their initial fight-or-flight reaction will not go away; at the same time, it should be noted that pathology is very uncommon, and most people recover without developing PTSD. Repeating the word "trauma" excessively can also be problematic. Such words as distress, adversity, strain, or challenge may be less likely to invoke negative dominance. Positive terms such as *opportunity* and *growth* also need to be used carefully and at the right times to avoid doing more harm than good. Invoking opportunity, growth, and related concepts may be premature, increasing distress for survivors who are dealing with acute loss. This can undermine trust, evoking anger toward responders, and induce feelings of guilt and/or inadequacy.

During disasters, public communication about mental health is essential. Helpful information should be provided by reliable sources, including psychiatrists and other health professionals. The lack of accurate, reliable public communication adds insult to injury, risking exacerbation of damage from the disaster itself. In addition, the media might transmit traumatic experiences (see, e.g., Schlenger et al. 2002) and increase the risk of mental health problems.

The Media

Psychiatrists and other health professionals communicate information about disaster risks to their patients, to their communities, and through the media. As community leaders, psychiatrists and other health professionals are often asked for advice and may provide information in advance that helps to prepare their communities for disasters of various types (Beard and Kantor 2004; Bennett et al. 1999). They also may be consulted by journalists for health information to clarify risks (e.g., regarding PTSD) to their audiences or for advice for parents or schools on what to tell children and how to protect them (American Academy of Child and Adolescent Psychiatry 2023; Fassler 2003; Rauch 2009; Morganstein 2023; Stoddard and Menninger 2004; Teichroeb 2006) or for caretakers responsible for protection and care of fragile elderly individuals. In many cases, depending on the context, it is best to minimize sharing information 1) without media training or official authorization and 2) if the media contact is unknown or may have unclear intentions. This is especially true in today's cancel culture environment, where words can be easily taken out of context to the detriment of the speaker and the audience.

Communication About Risk in Preparation for Disasters

Communication about risk during crisis is complicated by multiple factors, as discussed earlier. When communicating with affected individuals and communities, it is essential to follow best practices, as summarized in

---

TABLE 5–4. Guidelines for communicating with patients and other disaster survivors

---

1. Listen to, respect, and respond to the fears, anxieties, and uncertainties of patients; they want to know that the doctor cares before they care what the doctor knows.

2. Recognize that people are risk averse and, when upset, often fixate on negatives. Be extremely careful in offering up the five "N" words—no, not, never, nothing, none—and words with negative connotations that can add to rather than lessen fear.

3. Offer authentic statements of caring, empathy, and compassion while also taking time to listen. Back up your statements with actions.

4. Be honest, ethical, frank, and open, recognizing that there are limits on what needs to be disclosed.

5. Avoid mixed or inconsistent verbal and nonverbal messages.

Table 5–4. Formal training in risk communication is recommended (see Chapter 1, "Disaster Psychiatry Education"). Preparing to communicate with media and leaders is of critical importance. Mental health professionals should 1) provide information about the human factors associated with the event, their time course, and ways to obtain help (Myers and Zunin 2000); 2) educate about the stages of grief (disbelief and shock, symptoms of grieving, and acceptance of loss); and 3) describe bereavement after unnatural death, which is marked by somatic, posttraumatic, depressive, and substance craving symptoms, as well as discuss the fact that bereavement may be prolonged. Preparatory communications should also teach about the stresses of first responders and of persons engaged in body recovery and indicate how leaders and media representatives may best monitor and manage their own stress, educate others, and seek help when needed. Most important, public education is not beneficial if it creates a self-fulfilling prophecy of distress and dysfunction. It is important to refine messages that emphasize the fact that most survivors are resilient.

Protective Factors

If a population's resilience can be reinforced by public education, both providing hope and enhancing resiliency, the primary prevention of adverse psychological consequences could conceivably render disasters less damaging (Charney 2004; Shalev 2004; Stoddard 2009; Watson et al. 2006). When fear is proportional and time-limited and individuals have good emotional regulation and self-care, acute and chronic distress are mitigated.

Communication About Risk During Disasters

Part of communication about risk in the wake of disasters occurs among psychiatrists themselves to help them function effectively (see Chapter 6, "Rescuing Ourselves"). Risk communications by definition address areas of vulnerability as well as strength among special populations within the community, with tailored messaging developed, tested, and implemented to suit varying stakeholder groups.

Communication About Risk After Disasters

Although it is tempting to assume that psychological risk after disasters is proximal to the event, in this age of distance travel and electronic communications, the "proximal" areas to consider in providing public communication about the event may extend for long distances, even across the world. Vincent T. Covell, commissioner of the Department of Health and Mental Hygiene in New York City from 1998 to 2002, wrote that "one important lesson learned from [9/11] is that terrorism creates health impacts that reach far beyond the immediate boundaries of a disastrous event, because people will, whenever possible, seek to leave the immediate area and return to their homes" (Covello 2001). These individuals may seek help in communities far from the event, and other people are affected by televised images or by what they see on the internet.

In a postdisaster interview, a mental health professional should attempt to decrease public fears and confusion by providing clear and accurate information. Education about the actual risks, such as PTSD and depression (Bills et al. 2008), and instruction on how to decrease risk enhance feelings of control and familiarity with disasters. Instruction in active coping techniques, including Psychological First Aid (Brymer et al. 2006) and Skills for Psychological Recovery (Berkowitz et al. 2010), is helpful. Such instruction should include restoring familiar routines, providing for basic needs, bolstering problem-solving skills, promoting positive activities, managing difficult reactions, promoting adaptive cognitive skills, and establishing strong social connections. Collaboration between mental health professionals and primary health care providers is an important model for prevention and provision of services to large numbers of people. Learning to identify vulnerable locations and populations can assist in public communications that may be effective in countering the potential impact of disasters or terrorist events.

Mental Health Professionals as Ambassadors

When people think of mental health professionals, they may often imagine private office and hospital settings and related traditional treatment models. However, in acute and ongoing disaster preparedness and response, professionals work in other roles that may involve no direct clinical care, including consultative work, administration, entrepreneurship, and humanitarian and social justice activism work.

In all these roles, it is of paramount importance for mental health professionals to comport themselves in a professional, amiable, and helpful manner in the service of providing assistance, increasing recognition of mutual interdependence with other responders, and mitigating stigma directed against mental health. Creating a self-sustaining collaborative process requires the thoughtful nurturing of an atmosphere of safety and mutual respect and, furthermore, the balancing of frequently competing needs of diverse individuals and groups to accomplish broader overlapping goals (Brenner 2009; Disaster Psychiatry Outreach 2008).

In various senses, the disaster mental health professional serves as an emissary and representative of the field, entering into literal and metaphorical foreign territory where mental health perspectives are not necessarily native. The intent is to be an ambassador of goodwill whenever possible, while also pursuing myriad other goals. All professionals must take up ambassadorship uniquely and individually, making use of their unique skills and traits as a person across roles. There is no one recipe for doing this, only heuristic guidelines and complementary frameworks for understanding that are not within the usual purview of psychiatric training.

A specific factor that is important to note is the (often accurate) perception that psychiatrists tend to overpathologize, identifying disease and disorder where none is present. Monitoring countertransference to the disaster context is important to make sure we are compensating for our biases, notably cultural and political ones, while also honoring our personal motivations for engagement in the work.

Conclusion: Catalyzing Collaboration

One of the most important functions that a disaster psychiatrist can serve is to facilitate the development of short- and long-term collaborative processes for the groups with whom the professional is working. In the acute phases of disaster, collaboration is comparatively easy to achieve because the senses of immediacy and urgency demand a pragmatic focus. This situation parallels an acute care setting (e.g., operating room, emergency department, intensive care unit) in which people temporarily set aside differences to work on clear tasks. As time wanes and the situation passes into the postacute phases, the sense of acuity dissipates, interorganizational agendas begin to predominate, and individual burnout increases. This leads to the erosion of existing collaborative processes and prevents their ongoing development. Several strategies can be employed in an effort to sustain collaboration under such circumstances, as noted in Chapter 7.

A potential problem arises when outside disaster psychiatrists enter an affected community, offering assistance out of genuine goodwill but potentially alienating and marginalizing local professionals. The following case vignette demonstrates some problems that can result from lack of collaboration.

Vignette: A Cautionary Tale for Outside Responders

Following Hurricane Katrina, a large group of outside responders descended on New Orleans to offer assistance. Among this group were disaster mental health professionals, including psychiatrists from distant health care systems and from national professional organizations. This help was appreciated and useful, but some local psychiatrists reported that although they themselves had the requisite skills and willingness to offer assistance, they were not contacted by the outside organizations and were left out of planning and response. Several years later, these local psychiatrists continued to report significant feelings of resentment, potentially undermining future collaboration.

Ideally, local resources are contacted by various external groups in the planning and preparation stages so that relationships can be established in advance. Even better, regional and national networks of volunteer disaster responders lay a foundation for easy communication and coordination with the affected community in times of heightened needs to create a communication ecology. If such systems are not in place, difficulties can arise beyond the time of the disaster, undermining the collaborative spirit and, ultimately, stunting preparedness and systemic intelligence.

Disaster preparedness and response are grounded in effective communication. We cannot naively share information and trust that the message will get through. As an ecological process, the more stakeholder groups present, the greater the risk of miscommunication—but the greater the rewards from solid communication. Miscommunication is costly, undermining trust and shared wins, preventing the development of effective long-term collaboration and leading to potentially fatal mistakes. Having a nuanced and bespoke approach to communication, while also establishing an overarching framework that diverse groups can join, is at the heart of effective shared planning and action.

References

American Academy of Child and Adolescent Psychiatry: Terrorism and war: how to talk to children (No 87). Washington, DC, American Academy of Child and Adolescent Psychiatry, updated September 2023. Available at: www.aacap.org/AACAP/Families_and_Youth/Facts_for_Families/FFF-Guide/Talking-To-Children-About-Terrorism-And-War-087.aspx. Accessed August 8, 2024.

Beard R, Kantor E: Managing the Message in Times of Crisis: Risk Communication and Mental Wellness in Disaster Health Care. Charlottesville, VA, University of Virginia Medical Reserve Corps, Public Relations Office, University of Virginia Health System, 2004

Bennett P, Coles D, McDonald A: Risk communication as a decision process, in Risk Communication and Public Health. Edited by Bennett P, Calman K. Oxford, UK, Oxford University Press, 1999, pp 207–221

Berkes F: Sacred Ecology, 4th Edition. New York, Routledge, 2018

Berkowitz S, Bryant R, Brymer M, et al: Skills for Psychological Recovery: Field Operations Guide. Washington, DC, National Center for PTSD; Los Angeles, CA, National Child Traumatic Stress Network, 2010. Available at: www.ptsd.va.gov/professional/treat/type/skills_psych_recovery_manual.asp#:~:text=Skills%20for%20Psychological%20Recovery%20(SPR,post%2Ddisaster%20stress%20and%20adversity. Accessed July 6, 2024.

Bills CB, Levy NAS, Sharma V, et al: Mental health of workers and volunteers responding to events of 9/11: review of the literature. Mt Sinai J Med 75(2):115–127, 2008 18500712

Brenner G: Fundamentals of collaboration, in Creating Spiritual and Psychological Resilience: Integrating Care in Disaster Relief Work. Edited by Brenner G, Bush D, Moses J. New York, Routledge, 2009, pp 3–17

Brymer M, Jacobs A, Layne C, et al: Psychological First Aid: Field Operations Guide, 2nd Edition. July, 2006. Los Angeles, CA, National Child Traumatic Stress Network; Washington, DC, National Center for PTSD. Available at: www.nctsn.org/resources/psychological-first-aid-pfa-field-operations-guide-2nd-edition. Accessed July 6, 2024.

Center for Mental Health Services: Communicating in a Crisis: Risk Communication Guidelines for Public Officials. Rockville, MD, Substance Abuse and Mental Health Services Administration, 2002. Available at: https://store.samhsa.gov/sites/default/files/pep19-01-01-005.pdf. Accessed October 14, 2010.

Charney DS: Psychobiological mechanisms of resilience and vulnerability: implications for successful adaptation to extreme stress. Am J Psychiatry 161(2):195–216, 2004 14754765

Celikler JM, Kern EM: Factors influencing communication structures and processes in disaster management teams: fields of action and design options. Int J Disaster Risk Reduct 78:103153, 2022

Covello VT: Lessons learned from the front lines of risk and crisis communication: 21 guidelines for effective communication by leaders addressing high anxiety, high stress, or threatening situations. Presented as part of keynote address, U.S. Conference of Mayors Emergency, Safety, and Security Summit, Washington, DC, October 2001

Covello VT: Principles of risk communication, in Creating Spiritual and Psychological Resilience: Integrating Care in Disaster Relief Work. Edited by Brenner GH, Bush DH, Moses J. New York, Routledge, 2009, pp 39–74

Dehghani A, Ghomian Z, Rakhshanderou S, et al: Components of health system preparedness in disaster risk communication in Iran: a qualitative study. Int J Disaster Risk Reduct 84:103462, 2023

DiClemente RJ, Jackson JM: Risk communication, in International Encyclopedia of Public Health, 2nd Edition. Atlanta, GA, Emory University, 2016, pp 378–382

Disaster Psychiatry Outreach: The Essentials of Disaster Psychiatry: A Training Course for Mental Health Professionals (course syllabus). New York, Disaster Psychiatry Outreach, 2008

Fassler D: Talking to Children About War and Terrorism: Tips for Parents and Teachers. American Psychiatric Association News Release. Washington, DC, American Psychiatric Association, March 5, 2003. Available at: www.uua.org/families/war-talking. Accessed August 8, 2024.

Federal Emergency Management Agency: National strategy recommendations: Future disaster preparedness. Washington, DC, U.S. Department of Homeland Security, 2013

Hobfoll SE, Watson P, Bell CC, et al: Five essential elements of immediate and mid-term mass trauma intervention: empirical evidence. Psychiatry 70(4):283–315, discussion 316–369, 2007 18181708

Imperiale AJ, Vanclay F: Conceptualizing community resilience and the social dimensions of risk to overcome barriers to disaster risk reduction and sustainable development. Sustainable Development 29(5):891–905, 2021

Inter-Agency Standing Committee: Guidance: Mental Health and Psychosocial Support in Emergency Settings: Monitoring and Evaluation With Means of Verification, Version 2.0. Geneva, Switzerland, Inter-Agency Standing Committee, September 2021. Available at: https://app.mhpss.net/?get=393/iasc-common-monitoring-and-evaluation-framework-for-mental-health-and-psychosocial-support-in-emergency-settings-with-means-of-verification-version-2.0.pdf. Accessed April 23, 2023.

Lejano RP, Haque CE, Berkes F: Co-production of risk knowledge and improvement of risk communication: a three-legged stool. Int J Disaster Risk Reduct 64:102508, 2021

Liu W, Zhao X: How communication ecology impacts disaster support seeking in multiethnic communities: the roles of disaster communication network size, heterogeneity, and localness. Mass Communication and Society 26(5):773–800, 2022

Morganstein J: Caring for our families in difficult times: protecting mental health and wellbeing during terrorism, war, and other disasters. Washington, DC, American Psychiatric Association, October 24, 2023. Available www.psychiatry.org/news-room/apa-blogs/caring-for-our-families-in-difficult-times. Accessed August 8, 2024.

Myers D, Zunin L: Phases of disaster, in Training Manual for Mental Health and Human Service Workers in Major Disasters, 2nd Edition (DHHS Publ No ADM 90-538). Edited by DeWolfe D. Washington, DC, U.S. Government Printing Office, 2000

Norwood AH, Sermons-Ward L, Blumenfield M: Crisis communication: the role of psychiatric leaders in communicating with the media and government officials at the time of disaster, terrorism and other crises. Presented at the Speaker-Elect Forum, American Psychiatric Association, Washington, DC, November 10, 2005

Rauch PK: Talking With Children About Upsetting News Events. Boston, MA, MassGeneral Hospital for Children, 2009. Available at: www.massgeneral.org/children/talking-with-kids-about-upsetting-news. Accessed July 26, 2024.

Rollins HE: The Letters of John Keats. Cambridge, UK, Cambridge University Press, 1958, pp 193–194

Schlenger WE, Caddell JM, Ebert L, et al: Psychological reactions to terrorist attacks: findings from the National Study of Americans' Reactions to September 11. JAMA 288(5):581–588, 2002 12150669

Shalev A: Appraisal of terrorism: the media and the spectators. Presented at the Committee on Terrorism and Disasters, Group for Advancement of Psychiatry, Westchester, NY, March 16, 2004

Spialek ML, Houston JB: The development and initial validation of the citizen disaster communication assessment. Communication Research 45(6):934–955, 2018

Stoddard FJ: Book review: intervention and resilience after mass trauma. Psychiatr Serv 60(7):997–998, 2009

Stoddard FJ, Menninger EW: Guidance for parents and other caretakers after disasters or terrorist attacks, in Disaster Psychiatry Handbook. Edited by Hall RCW, Ng AT, Norwood AE. Washington, DC, American Psychiatric Association, 2004, pp 44–56

Substance Abuse and Mental Health Services Administration: Communicating in a Crisis: Risk Communication Guidelines for Public Officials. SAMHSA Publication No PEP19-01-01-005. Rockville, MD, Substance Abuse and Mental Health Services Administration, 2019. Available at: https://store.samhsa.gov/product/communicating-crisis-risk-communication-guidelines-public-officials/pep19-01-01-005. Accessed July 6, 2024.

Teichroeb R: Covering Children and Trauma: A Guide for Journalism Professionals. New York, DART Center for Journalism and Trauma, 2006. Available at: https://dartcenter.org/content/covering-children-trauma. Accessed July 6, 2024.

Watson PJ, Ritchie EC, Demer J, et al: Improving resilience trajectories following mass violence and disasters, in Interventions Following Mass Violence and Disasters: Strategies for Mental Health Practice. Edited by Ritchie EC, Watson PJ, Friedman MJ. New York, Guilford, 2006, pp 37–53

6

Rescuing Ourselves

Self-Care for Disaster Responders and Health Care Workers

Kathleen A. Clegg, M.D.
Joseph P. Merlino, M.D., M.P.A.

Vignette: *A COVID Cookbook*

The negative impact on nursing staff during the coronavirus disease 2019 (COVID-19) pandemic has been well documented. Nursing staff were left to serve as caregivers to critically ill patients, often as surrogate family members, as well given the isolation restrictions imposed for much of the early outbreak. Nurses were overwhelmed and exhausted. When they got home, they did not want to talk to their loved ones about what they had done and seen, so the phone group sessions they had with mental health clinicians such as me (J.P.M.) were all the more important to them for solace. Over time, it struck me that the most common theme was food: "What I'm making for dinner." "What are you making?" "I have this great recipe." "Have you ever tried this or that?" Given the tremendous ethnic variety in our staff makeup, a wide range of meals were discussed. Wanting to help the nurses feel empowered, I suggested to the nursing director that we facilitate production and publication of *A COVID Cookbook,* and they contributed a bounty of mouth-watering recipes that they could share with one another as well as the wider community. As a result of this collaborative effort, we all felt a sense of great accomplishment in the midst of an awful situation. It helped us get up the next day and continue our important work.

In addition to making recommendations for self-care for disaster responders, we aim to broaden the scope of these recommendations to apply also to health care providers, particularly in the aftermath of the COVID-19 pandemic. Health care workers providing care during the COVID-19 pandemic experienced trauma and demonstrated high prevalence estimates of moderate depression (21.7%), anxiety (22.1%), and PTSD (21.5%) (Li et al. 2021). The impact of the COVID-19 pandemic has been profound and far-reaching, and the well-being of health care providers is no exception. The extent of severe disease and death in the population, the scarcity of necessary equipment, the lack of adequate staffing necessitating long working hours, and the difficult decisions that had to be made contributed to moral injury. *Moral injury* can occur when health care providers must make decisions that go against their long-held beliefs and commitment to healing (American Psychiatric Association 2020). In fact, as of the time of this writing, COVID-19 continues to claim 187 deaths per week in the United States (Centers for Disease Control and Prevention 2024), but the impact varies greatly on the basis of the region of the country. In some places, people are moving on from the pandemic, but for others, COVID-19 remains an ongoing threat.

In this chapter, we discuss the positive and negative impacts that disaster response can have at the individual level. We draw some similarities between the issues faced by disaster responders and those faced by health care workers, particularly since the beginning of the COVID-19 global pandemic. Both disaster response and providing health care during the COVID-19 pandemic require the ability to manage severe job-related stresses and balance one's own needs and the needs of others within a rapidly changing organizational culture (Cherepanov 2022). Health care providers took care of patients with COVID-19 who were dying in numbers not seen by most health care providers in their lifetimes, while grappling with the ongoing risk of becoming infected themselves or exposing vulnerable family members to a potentially lethal disease. The excessive exposure to death, the perceived threat of death for oneself or loved ones, and repeated exposure to information about risks and vulnerability made health care work potentially traumatic.

There has been debate about whether the pandemic was characteristic of a disaster, which is defined as a moral threat to a large group of people that disrupts resources, services, and social networks. In fact, a third of health care workers appraised the COVID-19 pandemic as traumatic (Olson et al. 2022). Unlike disasters that are the result of a single event, such as a natural disaster, in which there are identifiable phases of recovery, the COVID-19 pandemic spanned several years, with periodic waves of greatly increased transmission of the disease, resulting in spiking numbers of hospitalization and deaths. Complex cyclical disasters (see Chapter 8, "Model for Adaptive Response to Complex Cyclical Disasters") push communities and their members through recurring phases of anticipation, impact, and adaptation before a recovery phase can begin (Vibrant Emotional Health et al. 2022).

Disaster responders and health care workers cannot take care of others if they cannot take care of themselves. The often-referenced analogy of putting on one's own oxygen mask first in an emergency on an airplane in order to be able to assist a child with their oxygen mask is fitting. Responders and health care workers cannot be of service to others if they are endangered or depleted.

In addition to the numerous reports of the massive toll that disasters including COVID-19 have caused, there is increased interest in the potential for posttraumatic growth for survivors and responders. This topic is discussed in the last section of the chapter.

Self-Awareness: Knowing One's Limits

Persons responding to disasters may be of a psychological makeup referred to in the literature as a *rescue personality*: one who is "inner-directed, action oriented, obsessed with performance, traditional, socially conservative, easily bored, and highly dedicated" (Mitchell and Bray 1990, p. 20); has difficulty saying no; is a risk taker; and can be addicted to trauma. Disaster responders often show a high capacity for empathy, which puts them at higher risk for compassion fatigue or secondary traumatic stress disorder (Figley 1995). The vulnerability of health care providers to burnout and compassion fatigue has increased as a result of the COVID-19 pandemic, affecting health care providers' well-being and quality of life. As a result, the quality of care provided has been reduced, and the shortage of health care providers already present in the United States and around the world has intensified (Lluch et al. 2022). For example, DePierro et al. (2021), reporting on the ongoing work of the Mount Sinai Center for Stress, Resilience, and Personal Growth, found that health care workers described the pandemic as their "most stressful life event," with more than half reporting symptoms of depression and posttraumatic stress, 65% reporting anxiety, and 13.2% screening positive for alcohol misuse.

Table 6–1 lists some recommendations for self-care of individuals providing services during a disaster. Important in self-care is being aware of one's own emotions and the effects of others' emotions on oneself. Much has been written about this topic, in particular the concept of *emotional intelligence* as "the ability to manage ourselves and our relationships effectively" (Goleman 2000, p. 6). The four major skills that make up emo-

---

TABLE 6–1. Planning and training to support the well-being of disaster responders and health care workers

---

Once the decision has been made to respond to a disaster, the Centers for Disease Control and Prevention (2018) offers specific recommendations to persons preparing to respond to a disaster, including the following:

1. Try to learn as much as possible about what your role will be.

2. If you will be traveling or working long hours, explain this to loved ones who may want to contact you. Come up with ways you may be able to communicate with them. Keep their expectations realistic, and take the pressure off yourself.

3. Talk to your supervisor and establish a plan for who will fill any urgent ongoing work duties unrelated to the disaster while you are engaged in the response.

4. Make plans for your household, childcare, and pet care needs if you will be away from home.

Psychiatrists and other mental health clinicians who want to become directly involved as responders in a future disaster should receive adequate training from a recognized source, such as the American Red Cross, the American Medical Association, or a local university or medical center (American Red Cross 2010).

---

tional intelligence are self-awareness, self-management, social awareness, and relationship management. Possessing the self-awareness to recognize that physically responding to a disaster may not be the appropriate response for some individuals is extremely important.

An important part of preparation is the development of a self-care plan. This secondary prevention plan has several components, including those listed in Table 6–2. Although these recommendations apply to individuals responding to a disaster, many of the same principles apply to health care workers responding in the midst of an ongoing disaster such as the COVID-19 pandemic.

Caring for Staff

Responders are advised to take the time to prepare a care plan for their clinical work setting, be it an office, a clinic, or a hospital (Merlino 2010b). Policies and procedures to respond to a crisis are best developed on both individual and organizational levels *before* a disaster strikes. When leadership pays more attention to staff morale and development, there is a corresponding growth in the knowledge of the cost *to caregivers* of caring, with myriad associated demands for enhanced resources on

TABLE 6–2. Self-care plan

Component	Description
Physical care	Maintaining the health of one's body through adequate diet, exercise, sleep, and rest is critical.
Psychological care	One should attempt to achieve an overall balance of work, outside interests, recreation, meditation/spirituality, and personal time.
Social/interpersonal care	Connection with others is restorative and involves educating social contacts about one's needs. Working with a team is an effective strategy to ensure positive social contacts.
Balance	In determining how much and what kind of disaster work to do, one needs to set and maintain appropriate and realistic boundaries.
Getting help when needed	Help can take the form of peer support, supervision, or consultation; personal therapy can be of benefit during or after one's disaster work experience.

Source. Yassen 1995.

many levels (Stamm 1999). The type of support negatively associated with posttraumatic stress disorder (PTSD) is emotional support received from supervisors and colleagues, including acting as a confidant, listening, and offering sympathy to the victim in a traumatic episode (D'Ettorre et al. 2020). Risk factors for PTSD among disaster responders are provided in Tables 6–3 and 6–4.

Psychosocial interventions are helpful in reducing the negative impact of a pandemic on health workers' well-being. Comprehensive programs that integrate visible and accessible mental health support with in-service training, enhanced team and institutional support, infection control measures, protective equipment, and increased provision of personnel and resources may be especially impactful. Interventions delivered with greater frequency and intensity and of longer duration were more effective at reliably improving clinically significant distress as compared with single-session interventions. Treatments based on current best practices using evidence-based interventions were found to be most effective (Ottisova et al. 2022); therefore, cognitive-behavior therapy (CBT) for PTSD and CBT approaches to anxiety and depression are the recommended treatment approaches. Early intervention is recommended for those with the highest mental health burden on embedded screenings.

TABLE 6–3.   Organizational pretrauma risk factors for PTSD

- Heavy workload
- Poor training on traumatic events in hospital settings
- Lack of cohesiveness among workers, which suggests possible areas for staff management
- General lack of training in disaster and crisis management

TABLE 6–4.   Organizational posttrauma risk factors for PTSD

- Lack of social support from managerial staff and colleagues
- Unavailability of debriefing after traumatic episodes
- Negative coping
- Burnout symptoms and depression

Being Prepared

Responders who are educated about and trained on disaster response perform better in the field, experience lower levels of stress, are likely to be more resilient, and are likely to grow psychologically in response to the stress of disaster experience (Merlino 2010a).

Stress and Reactions to It

Even with the best preparation, disaster responders will experience emotional challenges (International Critical Incident Stress Foundation 2021; Substance Abuse and Mental Health Services Administration 2022). Common reactions to major trauma can involve physical, cognitive, emotional, and behavioral responses (Table 6–5). Common physical symptoms include digestive issues, headaches, fatigue, being easily startled, and rapid heart rate. Cognitive effects can include being more or less alert than usual, having difficulty concentrating, and having difficulty making decisions or solving problems. Emotional symptoms can include feeling heroic or invulnerable, denial, anxiety, guilt, sadness, and anger. Behavioral reactions can include being unable to rest or relax, crying, isolating, increased or decreased appetite, and substance use.

As research into the field of trauma response grows, it is increasingly apparent that the effects of a traumatic event go well beyond the victims who immediately and directly experience the event. It is important for re-

TABLE 6–5. Normal reactions to trauma

Type of reaction	Reactions
Physical	Headache, loss of appetite, sleep impairment, nausea
Emotional	Irritability, anxiety, anger, guilt, fear
Behavioral	Withdrawal, emotional outbursts, unwillingness to leave scene until work is done, denying need for rest

sponders to develop emotional intelligence to better prepare for dealing with trauma. As stated in the section "Self-Awareness: Knowing One's Limits," two of the key skills of emotional intelligence are self-awareness and self-management (Bradberry and Greaves 2009). Self-monitoring is a key ingredient for self-care, tracking both expected and more intense responses with associated help-seeking planning.

Secondary traumatic stress, compassion fatigue, and vicarious victimization are potential adverse consequences of disaster relief work. Developing and practicing a self-care plan provides some protection against these overlapping outcomes but does not always prevent them. *Secondary traumatic stress* and secondary traumatic stress disorder are conceptualized as akin to primary traumatic stress (acute stress reaction) and primary traumatic stress disorder (Figley 1995). However, secondary trauma reactions are experienced by another person, such as a significant other or someone providing care to a directly traumatized individual, whereas primary reactions are directly experienced by the traumatized person. Secondary traumatic stress is also referred to as secondary victimization, vicarious traumatization, or emotional contagion (Miller et al. 1988).

Burnout is a syndrome of physical, emotional or attitudinal exhaustion characterized by impaired work performance, fatigue, insomnia, depression, and increased susceptibility to physical illness. This syndrome is generally considered to be a stress reaction to unrelenting performance and emotional demands stemming from one's occupation (Campbell 2009). *Compassion fatigue* can emerge suddenly or without warning. Compassion fatigue and burnout manifest in a variety of ways, subsuming symptoms across multiple domains. Cognitive symptoms include difficulty concentrating, reduced self-esteem, apathy, and trauma preoccupation; emotional symptoms can include feeling powerless, sadness, numbness, being reactive, and feeling depleted. Behavioral symptoms can include irritability, sleep and appetite difficulties, fatigue, and hypervigilance. Spiritual sequelae can include questioning meaning and purpose, decreased self-satisfaction, loss of faith, or skepticism regarding prior religious beliefs. Impact on personal relationships can include withdrawal, increased conflict or mistrust, reduced interest in sex and closeness, being overprotective of offspring, and blaming others. Somatic symptoms, such as tachycardia, shortness of breath, dizziness, musculoskeletal pain, and increased perspiration can occur. Finally, performance at work can be negatively impacted because of decreased morale, task avoidance, low motivation, detachment, difficulty keeping work commitments, and withdrawal from coworkers (Figley 2002).

Success in convincing disaster responders that they can and should avail themselves of mental health care can be aided by "depsychologizing" their symptoms by relating to the individuals in a medicalized manner, normalizing their signs and symptoms as much as possible, and focusing on function rather than feelings (Katz 2010). Guidance from the Centers for Disease Control and Prevention (CDC) further describes the conditions disaster responders may encounter and how to prevent and mitigate these conditions, as described in Table 6–6.

The skills described in Table 6–6 can prove extremely useful for preventing or at least mitigating the effects of burnout, compassion fatigue, and vicarious trauma that are very real risks for disaster responders and health care workers. Systemic review and meta-analysis across 21 countries demonstrated high prevalence estimates of moderate depression (21.7%), anxiety (22.1%), and PTSD (21.5%) among health care workers during the COVID-19 pandemic (Li et al. 2021). Another review of the global prevalence of mental health problems among health care workers during the COVID-19 pandemic found pooled prevalence for PTSD, anxiety, depression, and distress of 49%, 40%, 37%, and 37%, respectively (Saragih et al. 2021).

Another threat to the well-being of responders and health care workers further defined during the COVID-19 pandemic is the impact of moral injury, defined as distress (due to guilt, shame, disgust, withdrawal, and self-condemnation) following situations involving moral transgressions. These could be due to one's own actions; another's actions; or perceptions of betrayal from leaders, colleagues, or others (Hall et al. 2022). Potentially morally injurious or distressful events in health care workers and responders during the COVID-19 pandemic included six themes (Table 6–7).

Returning Home

Sooner or later, responders to a disaster will return home. The CDC estimates that approximately one-third of aid workers will report depression shortly after arriving home; in addition, more than half have reported predominantly negative emotions once home (Substance Abuse and Mental

---

TABLE 6–6. CDC guidance to prevent and mitigate burnout and secondary traumatic stress

---

Stress during a crisis

Responders experience stress during a crisis. When stress builds up, it can cause the following:

- *Burnout*—feelings of extreme exhaustion and being overwhelmed

- *Secondary traumatic stress*—stress reactions and symptoms resulting from exposure to another individual's traumatic experiences rather than from direct exposure to a traumatic event

It is important to recognize the signs of both of these conditions in yourself and other responders to be sure those who need a break or need help can address these needs.

Coping techniques such as taking breaks, eating healthy foods, exercising, and using the buddy system can help prevent and reduce burnout and secondary traumatic stress.

Signs of burnout

- Sadness, depression, or apathy
- Easily frustrated
- Blaming of others, irritability
- Lacking feelings, indifferent
- Isolation or disconnection from others
- Poor self-care (hygiene)
- Tired, exhausted, or overwhelmed
- Feeling like
  - A failure
  - Nothing you can do will help
  - You are not doing your job well
  - You need alcohol or other drugs to cope

Signs of secondary traumatic stress

- Excessive worry about or fear of something bad happening
- Easily startled or "on guard" all of the time
- Physical signs of stress (e.g., racing heart)
- Nightmares or recurrent thoughts about the traumatic situation
- The feeling that others' trauma is yours

Useful tips for support

- Limit your time working alone by trying to work in teams.
- Get support from team members.

TABLE 6–6.   CDC guidance to prevent and mitigate burnout and secondary traumatic stress (continued)

- Develop a buddy system, in which two responders partner together to support each other and monitor each other's stress, workload, and safety.
  — Get to know each other. Talk about background, interests, hobbies, and family. Identify each other's strengths and weaknesses.
  — Keep an eye on each other. Try to work in the same location if you can.
  — Set up times to check in with each other.
  — Listen carefully and share experiences and feelings. Acknowledge tough situations and recognize accomplishments, even small ones.
  — Offer to help with basic needs, such as sharing supplies and transportation.
  — Monitor each other's workloads. Encourage each other to take breaks. Share opportunities for stress relief (rest, routine sleep, exercise, and deep breathing).
  — Communicate your buddy's basic needs and limits to leadership—make your buddy feel "safe" about speaking up.

Responder self-care techniques
- Limit work to shifts no longer than 12 hours.
- Work in teams and limit the amount of time working alone.
- Write in a journal.
- Talk to family, friends, supervisors, and teammates about your feelings and experiences.
- Practice breathing and relaxation techniques.
- Maintain a healthy diet and get adequate sleep and exercise.
- Know that it is OK to draw boundaries and say "no."
- Avoid or limit caffeine and alcohol.

It is important to remind yourself of the following:
- It is not selfish to take breaks.
- The needs of survivors are not more important than your own needs and well-being.
- Making your best contribution does not mean working all of the time.
- There are other people who can help in the response.
- Responding to disasters can be both rewarding and stressful. Knowing that you have stress and coping with it as you respond will help you stay well, and this will allow you to keep helping those who are affected.

Source.   Centers for Disease Control and Prevention 2018.

TABLE 6–7. Factors contributing to moral injury during the COVID-19 pandemic

Risk of contracting or transmitting COVID-19

Inability to work on the frontlines

Provision of suboptimal care

Care prioritization and resource allocation

Perceived lack of support and unfair treatment by the organization

Stigma, discrimination, and abuse

Note. COVID-19=coronavirus disease 2019.
Source. Xue et al. 2022.

TABLE 6–8. Recommendations for disaster responders returning home from service

To prevent and manage stress, practice the following self-care tips:

- Maintain a healthy diet and get routine exercise and adequate rest.
- Spend time with family and friends.
- Pay attention to health concerns.
- Catch up on neglected personal tasks (e.g., check mail, pay bills, mow the lawn, shop for groceries).
- Reflect on what the experience has meant personally and professionally, for both you and your loved ones.
- Make sure you and your loved ones have a disaster preparedness plan.

Source. Substance Abuse and Mental Health Services Administration 2014a.

Health Services Administration 2014b). Responders who experience depressive symptoms without relief after settling home should seek professional guidance to help readjust to postdisaster life. Those who do not feel physically well should consult their primary care physician for contributing medical factors, including posttravel infectious diseases.

It may be advisable to go back to work for a day or two before taking personal time off to ease anxiety about returning to work. Reconnecting with colleagues and reviewing job responsibilities can be helpful. Because self care is often not ideal during disaster assignments, it is important to focus on basic needs to ensure physical health, which can increase resilience and decrease negative effects of trauma exposure. The Substance Abuse and Mental Health Services Administration has a list of recommendations for returning disaster responders (Table 6–8).

Posttraumatic Growth

Posttraumatic growth refers to the enduring positive psychological change experienced as a result of adversity, trauma, or highly challenging life circumstances (Jayawickreme et al. 2021). Posttraumatic growth can occur for disaster responders and health care workers as well as disaster survivors. Experiencing posttraumatic growth means that people do not just "bounce back" to their pretrauma state but exceed prior psychological functioning (O'Donovan and Burke 2022). Included in posttraumatic growth may be a greater sense of closeness to people in one's life, a recognition of opportunities ahead, a change in direction such as pursuing education or a new job, or an increased sense of meaning and purpose. Some people may begin to believe they are mentally or physically stronger than they had previously perceived themselves to be. Some may experience stronger religious beliefs or a new appreciation of life and the meaning of life (O'Donovan and Burke 2022).

In a study of posttraumatic growth among health care workers on the front lines of the COVID-19 pandemic, a total of 76.8% of frontline health care workers endorsed moderate or greater posttraumatic growth, primarily in the areas of increased appreciation of life, improved relationships, and greater personal strength (Feingold et al. 2022). A study of posttraumatic growth in nurses who worked in frontline departments during COVID-19 found several factors related to nurses' posttraumatic growth. These included being older, being married, having a higher level of education, having a higher professional title, and having more working years. In addition, a higher level of posttraumatic growth was found among those who had participated in previous public health emergencies, received psychological intervention or training during the COVID-19 pandemic, had confidence about performing frontline work, and were aware of the high risk of frontline work (Cui et al. 2021). Also associated with higher levels of posttraumatic growth was the ability to engage in *deliberate rumination*, a constructive cognitive processing of the traumatic events, including reflection on what they learned as a result of their experience, what the experience might mean for their future, and how the experience might have changed their beliefs about the world.

TABLE 6–9.   Teaching points on self-care for disaster responders and health care workers

- Self-care for disaster responders and health care workers is critical to their ability to care for others and to reduce the negative consequences some experience during and after disaster work.

- Individuals who have enormous capacity for feeling and expressing empathy tend to be more at risk of compassion fatigue or secondary traumatic stress disorder.

- Important in self-care are one's awareness of one's emotions and the effects of others' emotions on oneself.

- There is growing knowledge of the cost to caregivers of caring, as well as an increasingly important need to develop social and professional support networks, administrative structures, and policies to support workers in affected caregiving fields.

- Secondary traumatic stress, compassion fatigue, and vicarious victimization—three overlapping concepts—are potential adverse consequences of disaster relief work.

- The recommendation is not to avoid disaster response but rather to engage in it with an adequate plan for self-care.

Conclusion

Much of what has been recommended with regard to the risks and recommendations for disaster responders also applies to health care workers, as the COVID-19 pandemic so poignantly demonstrated. Understanding normal reactions to stress, as well how to prevent or mitigate burnout, compassion fatigue, and secondary trauma, is essential. Despite the risks and precautions described in this chapter, responding to a disaster and providing health care in times of crisis such as the COVID-19 pandemic can be a life-changing and rewarding experience, underscoring the value of camaraderie, strengthening peer bonding, and reminding mission-driven professionals why they chose to do this kind of work in the first place (Cherepanov 2022). Key takeaways are provided in Table 6–9.

References

American Psychiatric Association: COVID-19 Pandemic Guidance Document: Moral Injury During the COVID-19 Pandemic. Washington, DC, APA Committee on the Psychiatric Dimensions of Disaster and COVID-19, 2020. Available at: www.psychiatry.org/File%20Library/Psychiatrists/APA-Guidance-COVID-19-Moral-Injury.pdf. Accessed March 28, 2024.

American Red Cross: Take a Red Cross Course. Washington, DC, American Red
    Cross, 2010. Available at: www.redcross.org/flash/course01v01. Accessed De-
    cember 26, 2010.
Bradberry T, Greaves J: Emotional Intelligence 2.0. New York, TalentSmart, 2009
Campbell RJ: Campbell's Psychiatric Dictionary, 9th Edition. New York, Oxford
    University Press, 2009
Centers for Disease Control and Prevention: Emergency Responders: Tips for Tak-
    ing Care of Yourself. Washington, DC, U.S. Department of Health and Hu-
    man Services, March 19, 2018. Available at: https://emergency.cdc.gov/
    coping/responders.asp. Accessed March 28, 2024.
Centers for Disease Control and Prevention: COVID Data Tracker. Atlanta, GA,
    U.S. Department of Health and Human Services, 2024. Available at: https://
    covid.cdc.gov/covid-data-tracker. Accessed July 4, 2024.
Cherepanov E: Responding to the psychological needs of health workers during
    pandemic: ten lessons from humanitarian work. Disaster Med Public Health
    Prep 16(2):734–740, 2022 32907680
Cui PP, Wang PP, Wang K, et al: Post-traumatic growth and influencing factors
    among frontline nurses fighting against COVID-19. Occup Environ Med
    78(2):129–135, 2021 33060188
D'Ettorre G, Pellicani V, Ceccarelli G, et al: Post-traumatic stress disorder symp-
    toms in heath care workers: a ten year systematic review. Acta Biomed 91(12-
    S):e2020009, 2020 33263341
DePierro J, Marin DB, Sharma V, et al: Developments in the first year of a resil-
    ience-focused program for health care workers. Psychiatry Res 306:114280,
    2021 34800784
Feingold JH, Hurtado A, Feder A, et al: Posttraumatic growth among health care
    workers on the frontlines of the COVID-19 pandemic. J Affect Disord
    296:35–40, 2022 34587547
Figley CR: Compassion fatigue as secondary stress disorder: an overview, in Com-
    passion Fatigue: Coping With Secondary Traumatic Stress Disorder in Those
    Who Treat the Traumatized (Routledge Psychosocial Stress Series). Edited by
    Figley CR. New York, Routledge, 1995, pp 1–20
Figley CR (ed): Treating Compassion Fatigue (Routledge Psychosocial Stress Se-
    ries). New York, Routledge, 2002
Goleman D: Leadership that gets results. Harv Bus Rev (March–April):2–16, 2000
Hall NA, Everson AT, Billingsley MR, et al: Moral injury, mental health and be-
    havioural health outcomes: a systematic review of the literature. Clin Psychol
    Psychother 29(1):92–110, 2022 33931926
International Critical Incident Stress Foundation: Critical incident stress informa-
    tion, in The American College of Emergency Physicians Guide to Coronavirus
    Disease (COVID-19). Edited by Shahid S. Irving, TX, American College of
    Emergency Physicians, July 13, 2021. Available at: www.acep.org/corona/
    covid-19-field-guide/personal-well-being-andresilience/critical-incident-stress-
    information. Accessed July 5, 2024.
Jayawickreme E, Infurna FJ, Alajak K, et al: Post-traumatic growth as positive
    personality change: Challenges, opportunities, and recommendations. J Pers
    89(1):145–165, 2021 32897574
Katz CL: Understanding and helping responders, in Hidden Impact: What You
    Need to Know for the Next Disaster. A Practical Mental Health Guide for Cli-

nicians. Edited by Stoddard FJ, Katz CL, Merlino JP. Sudbury, MA, Jones & Bartlett, 2010, pp 123–130

Li Y, Scherer N, Felix L, et al: Prevalence of depression, anxiety and post-traumatic stress disorder in health care workers during the COVID-19 pandemic: a systematic review and meta-analysis. PLoS One 16(3):e0246454, 2021 33690641

Lluch C, Galiana L, Doménech P, et al: The impact of the COVID-19 pandemic on burnout, compassion fatigue, and compassion satisfaction in healthcare personnel: a systematic review of the literature published during the first year of the pandemic. Healthcare (Basel) 10(2):364, 2022 35206978

Merlino JP: Self-care, in Hidden Impact: What You Need to Know for the Next Disaster: A Practical Mental Health Guide for Clinicians. Edited by Stoddard FJ, Katz CL, Merlino JP. Sudbury, MA, Jones & Bartlett, 2010a, pp 19–26

Merlino JP: Staff support, in Hidden Impact: What You Need to Know for the Next Disaster: A Practical Mental Health Guide for Clinicians. Edited by Stoddard FJ, Katz CL, Merlino JP. Sudbury, MA, Jones and Bartlett, 2010b, pp 171–178

Miller KI, Stiff JB, Ellis BH: Communication and empathy as precursors to burnout among human service workers. Commun Monogr 55:336–341, 1988

Mitchell JT, Bray GP: Emergency Services Stress: Guidelines for Preserving the Health and Careers of Emergency Services Personnel (Continuing Education Series). Upper Saddle River, NJ, Prentice Hall, 1990

O'Donovan R, Burke J: Factors associated with post-traumatic growth in healthcare professionals: a systematic review of the literature. Healthcare (Basel) 10(12):2524, 2022 36554048

Olson KD, Fogelman N, Maturo L, et al: COVID-19 traumatic disaster appraisal and stress symptoms among health care workers: insights from the Yale Stress Self-Assessment. J Occup Environ Med 64(11):934–941, 2022 35959912

Ottisova L, Gillard JA, Wood M, et al: Effectiveness of psychosocial interventions in mitigating adverse mental health outcomes among disaster-exposed health care workers: a systematic review. J Trauma Stress 35(2):746–758, 2022 35182077

Saragih ID, Tonapa SI, Saragih IS, et al: Global prevalence of mental health problems among healthcare workers during the Covid-19 pandemic: a systematic review and meta-analysis. Int J Nurs Stud 121:104002, 2021 34271460

Stamm BH (ed): Secondary Traumatic Stress: Self-Care Issues for Clinicians, Researchers, and Educators, 2nd Edition. Lutherville, MD, Sidran Press, 1999

Substance Abuse and Mental Health Services Administration: Tips for Disaster Responders: Preventing and Managing Stress (HHS Publ No SMA-14-4873). Washington, DC, Substance Abuse and Mental Health Services Administration, 2014a

Substance Abuse and Mental Health Services Administration: Tips for Disaster Responders: Returning to Work (HHS Publ No SMA-14-4870). Washington, DC, Substance Abuse and Mental Health Services Administration, 2014b

Substance Abuse and Mental Health Services Administration: A Guide to Managing Stress for Disaster Responders and First Responders. Publ No PEP22-01-01-003. MD, Rockville, MD, Center for Mental Health Services, Substance Abuse and Mental Health Services Administration, 2022

Vibrant Emotional Health; Group for the Advancement of Psychiatry; Decision Point Systems: Model for Adaptive Response to Complex Cyclical Disasters: A

Community Context-Sensitive Approach to Promoting Adaptive Disaster Response. New York, Vibrant Emotional Health, 2022

Xue Y, Lopes J, Ritchie K, et al: Potential circumstances associated with moral injury and moral distress in healthcare workers and public safety personnel across the globe during COVID-19: a scoping review. Front Psychiatry 13:863232, 2022 35770054

Yassen J: Preventing secondary stress disorder, in Compassion Fatigue: Coping With Secondary Traumatic Stress Disorder in Those Who Treat the Traumatized (Routledge Psychosocial Stress Series). Edited by Figley CR. New York, Routledge, 1995, pp 178–208

7

Engaging in Disaster Response

Preparation, Systems, and Leadership

Giuseppe Raviola, M.D., M.P.H.
Edward M. Kantor, M.D.
David R. Beckert, M.D.
Grant H. Brenner, M.D.

Psychiatrists as Public Health Leaders in Disaster Response

Psychiatry, as a branch of medicine, is focused on the diagnosis, treatment, and prevention of mental, emotional, and behavioral disorders. Psychiatrists serve as leaders and clinical experts, supporting the integration of psychosocial, psychological, and psychiatric interventions in collaboration with other care providers; leveraging expertise in care delivery, supervising, training, and mentoring; and improving care environments and advocating for action on mental health care outside the health system, such as in homes, schools, and workplaces (Kestel 2022). Traditionally, psychiatrists treat complex, comorbid mental health conditions, bringing their knowledge of medicine, neuroscience, psychiatric, medicolegal, ethical, psychological, and social approaches to people living with mental disorders. Given their unique perspective on patients, services, and systems, psychiatrists are well positioned to work as leaders in public health, to support the development of new systems of prevention and mental health promotion. Engaging in disaster response as a psychiatrist brings an opportunity to bring together all of these accumulated skills and experiences in the service of others at times of critical need. It is a calling to which psychiatrists may not feel well prepared but one for which psychiatrists can—in short order—educate themselves and find their place.

The nature and evolving effects of disasters are shifting, the scope of disasters is broadening and their number increasing (see Chapter 10, "Historical, Sociocultural, and Political Considerations"), and all health care workers are increasingly engaged in responding. Therefore, in a sense, all psychiatrists today may be appropriately considered *disaster psychiatrists*. Disaster and preventive psychiatry (see Chapter 2, "Disaster Prevention and Climate Change") is a synthesis of many fields in support of communities and individuals, including emergency psychiatry, community psychiatry, consultation-liaison psychiatry, child and adolescent psychiatry, geriatric psychiatry, addiction psychiatry, trauma-focused psychiatry, forensics, psychotherapy, organizational psychology, global health, and preventive medicine. Fundamentally, disaster psychiatry requires psychiatrists not to lead with their clinical lens and emphasis on diagnosis, but rather to first engage with communities, teams, and systems, with a focus on wellness and prevention, health promotion, and enhancement of individual and collective resilience.

Psychiatrists and allied mental health professionals take on diverse roles in disaster response, ranging from leadership responsibilities to subject matter expertise to direct service provision. As leaders or authorized media contacts, they can share information using good risk communication practices (see Chapter 5, "Communication and Relationships") to inform colleagues, affected persons, the public, policymakers, media, and other stakeholders. They can work to protect the health—mental and physical—of responders, health care workers, and others serving during disaster and crisis response. Furthermore, mental health disaster responders work in a variety of settings, from hospitals and clinical settings to nonclinical settings in the field (e.g., shelters, assistance centers, wellness stations, and related venues), providing services in clinical and public health through expert knowledge and training, working with affected systems, and providing education and offering guidance and support for affected communities. Disaster mental health responders also play a role in building capacity through education, training, planning and equipment procurement, and the development of policies and procedures, with the goal of supporting preparedness, resilience, and recovery (see Morganstein and West 2023, "Module 1: Basic Concepts in Disaster and Preventive Psychiatry").

In this chapter, we seek to integrate knowledge from the past decade and new experience since the coronavirus disease 2019 (COVID-19) pandemic. We also include recent guidance from the American Psychiatric Association (APA) through an online course, "Disaster and Preventive Psychiatry: Protecting Health and Fostering Community Resilience," developed by the APA Committee on Psychiatric Dimensions of Disaster (Morganstein and West 2023). Topics to cover for mental health professionals, including psychiatrists, working in crisis situations include preparedness, educating stakeholders about public health, monitoring for clinically significant problems among affected groups, prevention and early intervention, and leadership roles and responsibility. Disaster mental health efforts across the continuum are based significantly on a public health approach to improving population wellness through prevention whenever possible. It is therefore crucial that education include messaging and interventions that have proven to be effective (see Morganstein and West 2023, "Module 4: Public Health Approaches to Interventions and Disasters").

In disaster preparedness, as in other disciplines, preparedness is ongoing, and good planning improves efficiency of response and conserves resources. Preparation can be simple; for example, having basic supplies on hand, such as backup food and water, saves lives. Preparation not only covers the response phase but also includes readiness to transition from response to recovery and growth, with the potential to not only return to baseline for affected communities but to "build back better" because underlying risk factors such as insufficient local resources can be identified and ameliorated for the next time (see Morganstein and West 2023, Module 4).

Collaboration and communication are key aspects of disaster preparedness and response. They are covered in detail in Chapter 5. Generally, it is important to practice *cultural humility* (Nakintu 2021; Tervalon and Murray-Garcia 1998; Wells 2000), which includes cultural competence as well as the objective recognition that everyone has important expertise and experience to consider when facing crises. Communication starts with listening and is impeded when external groups proceed without understanding where other parties are coming from and what they already know.

Personal Considerations for Engagement in Disaster Response

Chapter 6, "Rescuing Ourselves," is about self-care and how the individual orients to the work of disaster response. Working in disasters stirs up personal history, which can be understood through four key considerations: affiliation, knowledge, purpose, and function (Table 7–1).

It is strongly recommended that volunteers work with an established group as part of a coordinated effort. Unaffiliated volunteers often become part of the problem and get frustrated during disaster events, not to mention having increased individual safety concerns and liability risks. Professionals interested in working in disaster and crisis environments are referred to Chapter 1, "Disaster Psychiatry Education," for recommended training programs and organizational affiliations. In spite of overlap with areas of mental health care and psychiatry, disaster mental health response is considerably different from conventional settings. Responders are advised to differentiate between day-to-day work and crisis-specific roles (also addressed in Chapter 1) and to engage in formal training. Formal training includes longer certifications and frequent just-in-time training. Precredentialing via a variety of potential avenues is key for disaster response (see Chapter 9, "Legal and Ethical Considerations") so that responders are able to operate in areas where they may not be formally licensed or credentialed and cleared with regard to malpractice.

There are many other ways for psychiatrists and mental health care providers to affiliate as volunteers in disaster work. Finding the organization that fits one's interests, personality, and skill set is very important. Some local and state medical and specialty societies have disaster committees and offer training opportunities. They recommend that instead of responding independently, members connect with their local response organizations to ensure that the overall response structure is respected. In major disasters, however, the groups might call for additional volunteers, as happened after Hurricane Katrina, when local stakeholders passed available volunteers' contact information to the federal agencies.

Preparation

Psychiatrists responding to disasters benefit from having a broader perspective on the psychological and psychosocial aspects and phases of disaster. Every disaster is defined by unique characteristics. In pandemics, for example, the epidemiological process is mirrored in the realm of psychology; fear, anger, and a sense of desperation are normal reactions, and they rise with the disease curve in the community. Quarantine, with its

TABLE 7–1. Four major personal considerations for responders to disasters

Affiliation: Join a recognized organization with permission and resources to support the mission

Knowledge: Keep up to date with appropriate interventions and be aware of major issues impacting individuals affected by disasters

Purpose: Participate for the right reasons and understand one's own motivation for responding

Function: Be in good health to operate in a variety of austere circumstances and do not add to the local response burden by becoming a victim

Source.   Adapted from Kantor 2009.

prolonged separation and isolation, is a necessary public health intervention, yet it has its own downstream effects on mental health. Neuropsychiatric sequelae occur among survivors. There is significant mental health burden on health workers, given the risk of infection, with psychological trauma and moral distress.

Culture must also be factored into planning responses tailored to specific communities. Infectious diseases and mental health problems are both highly stigmatized conditions. A diverse range of mental health and psychosocial needs (psychosocial, grief, trauma, stigma, disability) in the short and long term need to be anticipated for all affected (Huremovic 2019). Each disaster or crisis is different, and caution is warranted against broad generalizations. However, a general concept of psychological and psychosocial phases of disasters is necessary for planning.

DeWolfe (2000, p. 15) aptly describes the overarching features of disaster and crisis: "A survivor's reactions to and recovery from a disaster are influenced by a number of factors, some inherent and some malleable." These factors are depicted in Figure 7–1, and as shown, contribute to recovery outcomes. DeWolfe (2000) notes:

> The disaster event itself has characteristics, such as speed of onset or geographic scope, which generates somewhat predict-able survivor responses. Each survivor has a combination of personal assets and vulnerabilities that either mitigate or exacerbate disaster stress. The disaster-affected community may or may not have pre-existing structures for social support and resources for recovery. Disaster relief efforts that effectively engage with survivors and the overall community promote recovery.... The term "psychosocial" is often used to capture the breadth of effects of disaster on survivors. As shown in the diagram below, disasters unavoidably impact survivors both psychologically and socially. Disaster mental health

program planners, administrators, and providers can more easily assess their own communities and design effective interventions when they have an appreciation for this "macro" view of interacting factors.

Since World War II, emergency management has focused primarily on preparedness. Often, this has involved preparing for enemy attack. Community preparedness for all disasters requires identifying resources and expertise in advance and planning how they can be used in a disaster. One of the earliest models of disaster response describes the following phases (Raphael 1986): warning, impact, "honeymoon," and disillusionment, with outcomes ranging from enhanced community and individual adaptation to previous level of equilibrium, to "second disaster," anticipating the cyclical and recurrent nature of disasters at present.

However, preparedness is only one phase of emergency management. Current thinking defines four phases of emergency management: mitigation, preparedness, response, and recovery (see Chapter 8, "Model for Adaptive Response to Complex Cyclical Disasters," Figure 8–1). There are entire courses on each of these phases. *Mitigation* involves preventing future emergencies or minimizing their effects both before and after emergencies. *Preparedness* activities take place before an emergency occurs and include plans or preparations made to save lives and to help response and rescue operations. *Response* includes actions taken to save lives and prevent further property damage in an emergency situation, ideally putting preparedness plans into action. *Recovery* from an emergency includes actions taken to return to a normal or an even safer situation following an emergency (U.S. Department of Health and Human Services 2023).

Many models of disaster response have emerged since this emergency management model was adopted broadly. The most familiar in the United States is the model in Figure 7–1, which depicts a linear sequence from *predisaster* to *reconstruction*. As we discuss in more detail in Chapter 8, it is also useful to include additional elements to 1) capture the uniquely complex and nonlinear quality of multiple concurrent disasters and 2) define actions according to phase of disaster and stakeholder group in order to scaffold effective responses. In Chapter 8, we review prior disaster models and present the recently developed Model for Adaptive Response to Complex Cyclical Disasters (MARCCD). The MARCCD aggregates existing materials into a unifying model. It is intended to present a broad and flexible framework for conceptualizing the complex factors that attend multiple overlapping disasters occurring on different time courses, as well as to provide an organizing scheme to make it straightforward for various stakeholders to access actionable information at various disaster phases.

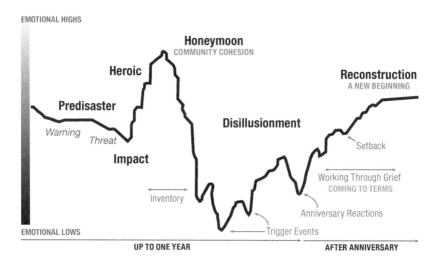

FIGURE 7–1. **Standard model and Chronic Cyclical Disasters Model.**

Source. DeWolfe 2000.

The Centers for Disease Control and Prevention (CDC) Crisis and Emergency Risk Communication (CERC) approach offers robust resources and training for effective communicating and messaging during disasters (Centers for Disease Control and Prevention 2018). With CERC, planning begins in the preparedness phase. CERC crisis communication plans encourage responders to take specific steps in communication and coordination during 1) pre-crisis; 2) the initial phase of a crisis; 3) a maintenance phase that begins when most or all of the direct harm is contained and the intensity of the crisis begins to subside; 4) a resolution phase as the crisis continues to wind down; and 5) an evaluation period to assess the performance of the communication plan, document lessons learned, and determine specific actions to improve crisis systems or the crisis plan (see Chapter 5 for additional information on risk communication).

The CDC's CERC Manual is based on psychological and communication sciences, studies in issues management, and practical lessons learned from emergency responses (Centers for Disease Control and Prevention 2018). The CERC Manual is intended for public health response officials and communicators who have a basic knowledge of public health communication, working with the media and social media, and local and national response structures. The CERC Manual promotes six core principles of effective emergency and risk communication: be first, be right, be credible, express empathy, promote action, and show respect (Centers for Disease Control and Prevention 2018).

The CERC manual describes five pitfalls to avoid: mixed messages from multiple experts, releasing information late, paternalistic attitudes, not countering rumors and myths in real time, and public power struggles and confusion. Effective communication with communities uses common language, demonstrates that the community's concerns have been heard, indicates what is being done to address concerns, and states when additional information will be provided. The use of empathy, avoiding medical jargon, and taking concrete action, as well as indicating exactly when more information will be shared, all help to lower distress and build trust. Recommendations should be based on solid public health information and messaged clearly as such; if they are not based on clear science, they should be reconsidered before asking the public to make sacrifices as a community (American Psychiatric Association 2023, "Module 6: Risk and Crisis Communication").

Response Systems

To be effective, disaster psychiatrists need to be aware of the roles of different systems and organizations active in disaster response. In this section, we review some of the most important organizations and help psychiatrists understand their role within the context of a larger response.

Understanding the hierarchy in disaster response can be very helpful to psychiatrists and other practitioners who either are exposed to a disaster or choose to volunteer in a clinical capacity. Because every disaster is unique, responders on the ground orient to the key players involved both in predeployment debriefings and in real-time assessment while responding. Some aspects of this hierarchy are intuitive and can be navigated easily. Others require learning the structure and terminology used to facilitate coordination among the complex array of players in crisis situations (see Chapter 5). Identifying who the primary decision-makers are in any given response and reporting to them to ensure smooth integration are key.

Local Response

Barring certain military, federal, and aviation emergencies, the initial response to any emergency, including disaster, is the responsibility of local government. Additional resources from other organizations are requested only when necessary or clearly anticipated. Most local and all state government plans include emergency management officials, who are generally the primary decision-makers responsible for establishing an emergency opera-

TABLE 7–2. Major duties and responsibilities during a disaster

1. Interagency coordination
2. Information sharing and education
3. Resource and financial management
4. Site safety regarding hazardous materials
5. Search and rescue
6. Triage, tracking, transport, and evacuation
7. Management of volunteers
8. Dealing with disruption of utilities
9. Medical and mental health support
10. Food and shelter for victims and personnel

Source. Disaster Psychiatry Outreach 2008; Federal Emergency Management Agency 2010b; Kantor 2010.

tions center (EOC) and coordinating the community-wide response in disaster situations. Examples of the major duties are outlined in Table 7–2.

During the acute or impact and early adaptation phases of a disaster, emergency management officials and first responders focus on rescue operations, such as extinguishing fires, locating and extricating injured persons, providing on-site medical treatment, managing hazardous materials and protecting responders, ensuring public safety by saving or restoring major infrastructure elements, and generally attending to basic needs. This includes organizing care for victims and displaced persons, providing resources such as shelter, food, and potable water. In addition to basic physical needs, emotional and psychological support is important early on. Psychological First Aid is a common framework in many responses (see Chapter 16, "Psychological First Aid").

National Response

In the United States, the National Incident Management System (NIMS) is the federal infrastructure set up to navigate interagency and interjurisdictional cooperation during a disaster event. It is designed to be flexible and responsive regardless of the type of disaster and therefore is often referred to as *all-hazards* disaster planning and response. In the wake of lessons learned from canonical disasters, an effort to further minimize coordination problems between agencies and levels of government has grown into a new modified response structure called the National Response Framework (NRF). Examples of response systems in countries other than the United States are discussed throughout this book.

Emergency management was institutionalized in the United States in 1979 with the creation of the Federal Emergency Management Agency (FEMA). Five federal agencies that dealt with many types of emergencies consolidated to form FEMA. Since that time, many state and local organizations have changed the names of their organizations to include the words *emergency management.* Disasters do not just appear one day—they exist over time and have a life cycle of occurrence. The National Preparedness Goal (Federal Emergency Management Agency 2023) highlights the importance of a robust systemic response: "A secure and resilient nation with the capabilities required across the whole community to prevent, protect against, mitigate, respond to, and recover from the threats and hazards that pose the greatest risk." There are five mission areas: prevention, protection, mitigation, response and recovery.

Incident Command System

The U.S. Incident Command System (ICS; Federal Emergency Management Agency 2010a) is the most basic administrative and operational structure in all emergency responses. It facilitates cooperation and operational closures among the various responding agencies, jurisdictions, and individuals. Federal disaster support monies require that localities and institutions orient staff to the ICS and NIMS and that they participate in local response planning and training efforts.

Under the ICS, each incident has an incident commander who is responsible for the entire event. Typically, the incident commander comes from the agency that first responded or that has primary responsibility for the type of event. For example, during a fire, the incident commander is typically a fire chief. If the fire is the result of a crime or terrorist event, the command may pass to the police or a federal law enforcement agency. Figure 7–2 illustrates the overarching ICS organization chart, which is applied across response agencies to ensure that everyone "speaks the same language." It is important to understand ICS both for responses in the United States and as an informative example of how an organizational chart depicting roles and responsibilities in disasters can be crucial to frame response. ICS sets a standardized approach to leadership and management during crisis response, ideally to be used by all stakeholders in any given response. For example, the incident commander will be in the leadership position for the entire response, delegating key responsibilities according to the schema. Operations, planning, logistics, finance, safety, public information, and related subfunctions are laid out clearly. Often,

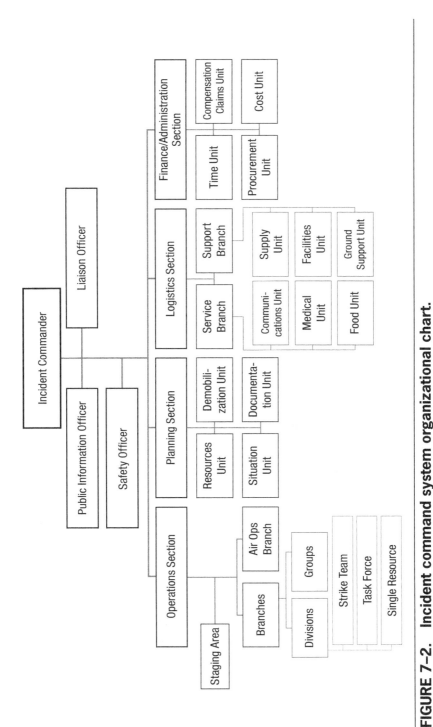

FIGURE 7–2. Incident command system organizational chart.

Source. Federal Emergency Management Agency 2018.

disaster responders have worked together and benefit from preexisting relationships, which facilitates teamwork. ICS allows individuals and teams both familiar and unfamiliar with one another to have a common language and structure to guide coordination and identification of key stakeholders and decision-makers. It is critical for mental health responders to be familiar with any such systems used in disaster and crisis response, regardless of the location, as well as to understand the informal authority relations and organizational structures that also define stricken communities (Morganstein and West 2023, Module 4).

When an emergency is likely to tax the regular response system or requires resources beyond the capabilities of the jurisdiction where it occurred, government officials can declare a disaster and request state and/or federal assistance. Such assistance includes additional personnel, specialized expertise, and potential funding sources to support the communities and finance recovery operations. When resources are needed across state lines, they are available through an agreement known as an emergency management assistance compact. Resources assigned this way often retain both legal authority to function and limited liability protection, depending on the activity and the states involved. Hurricane Katrina in 2005 is an excellent example of a disaster that overwhelmed the local infrastructure and required recovery operations that depended on personnel support and resources from other jurisdictions.

Major Agencies and Response Groups

Since 2002, increased efforts have been made to include mental health needs in disaster planning at the federal level. When it appears that a disaster might overwhelm local resources, assistance is requested by the incident commander through the local EOC. FEMA, now part of the U.S. Department of Homeland Security, is the lead federal agency for disaster planning, mitigation, coordination, and recovery, although many others offer various types of technical assistance and support.

Disaster Medical Assistance Teams (DMATs), established under the National Disaster Management System, operate similarly to mobile military hospital units—fully functional mobile medical teams with specialized equipment that can be taken to a disaster site. A DMAT can be deployed across the country. Several teams specialize in mental health, and others support veterinary, mortuary, and pharmacy activities.

The American Red Cross (ARC), a nongovernmental organization, is charged with providing shelters, family assistance centers, social support, health screening, and basic mental health care during disasters. The ARC is organized by regions and divided into local chapters, each of which is responsible for a particular geographic area; all chapters are coordinated through the national office (American Red Cross 2010). Two prominent volunteer programs to note, among many, are the community emergency response teams and the civilian Medical Reserve Corps, which are different from both the U.S. Public Health Service Commissioned Corps (a branch of the U.S. Uniformed Services) and the military reserve programs (Kantor 2010).

Each mental health care provider should become familiar with and stay up to date on the specific response structure and protocols in their own community because each locale is somewhat different, even though all basically adhere to the NRF in the United States. The disaster medical resources and the expected response can vary greatly by community, and each is heavily influenced by local traditions and the presence of specialized resources such as hospitals, National Guard units, and even medical schools (Kantor 2010). Professional organizations may have both national and local groups supporting disaster responders. For instance, the American Psychiatric Association has both a national Committee on the Psychiatric Dimensions of Disasters and local District Branch representatives to this committee. In addition, emerging interdisciplinary groups such as the Crisis Emotional Care Team of Vibrant Emotional Health provide a national platform for clinicians from diverse professional backgrounds for interdisciplinary collaboration in crisis and disaster preparedness and response.

Global Risk Reduction and Response Frameworks

Adopted in 2015, the Sendai Framework for Disaster Risk Reduction 2015–2030 outlines seven clear targets and four priorities for action to prevent new and reduce existing disaster risks. This effort includes understanding disaster risk; strengthening disaster risk governance to manage disaster risk; investing in disaster reduction for resilience; and enhancing disaster preparedness for effective response and to "Build Back Better" in recovery, rehabilitation, and reconstruction (United Nations Office for Disaster Risk Reduction 2015).

During disasters, the United Nations (UN) Office for the Coordination of Humanitarian Affairs (OCHA) manages several tools to facilitate coordination of multiple actors and resources through the UN Cluster approach, a forum of the most experienced relief agencies. The most recent iteration of these tools can be found at ReliefWeb Response (https://response.reliefweb.int), a specialized digital service of OCHA. RW Response was established to ensure that during a humanitarian emergency, relevant information is available to facilitate situational understanding and decision-making. The UN Cluster

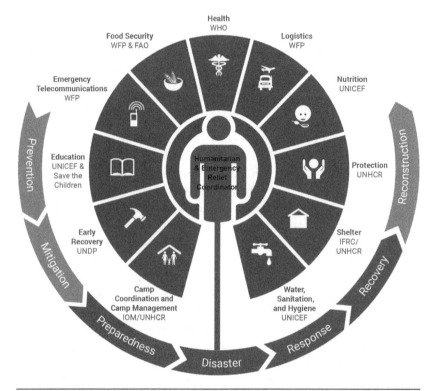

FIGURE 7–3.   UN Cluster approach to disasters and humanitarian response.

Note.   FAO = Food and Agriculture Organization; IFRC = International Federation of Red Cross and Red Crescent Societies; IOM = International Organization for Migration; UNDP = United Nations Development Programme; UNHCR = United Nations High Commissioner for Refugees; WFP = World Food Programme; WHO = World Health Organization.
Source.   United Nations High Commissioner for Refugees 2024.

approach organizes groups of humanitarian organizations, both UN and non-UN, in each of the main sectors of humanitarian action (e.g., water, health, logistics) (Figure 7–3). The sectors are designated by the Inter-Agency Standing Committee and have clear responsibilities for coordination.

Globally, the emergency relief coordinator is the most senior UN official dealing with humanitarian affairs and is mandated by the UN General Assembly to coordinate international humanitarian assistance during emergency response, whether carried out by governmental, intergovernmental, or nongovernmental organizations. The emergence relief coordinator reports directly to the UN Secretary-General and is specifically responsible

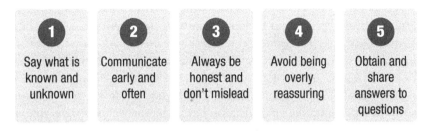

FIGURE 7–4. Essential elements of leader communication.

Source. United Nations Office for the Coordination of Humanitarian Affairs 2023.

for processing members states' requests, coordinating humanitarian assistance, ensuring information management and sharing to support early warning and response, facilitating access to emergency areas, organizing needs assessments, preparing joint appeals, mobilizing resources to support humanitarian response, and supporting a smooth transition from relief to recovery operations (United Nations Office for the Coordination of Humanitarian Affairs 2023).

Leadership

Leadership is a critical function in crisis and disaster mental health response to ensure optimal community resilience and response for acute and ongoing response, supporting effective communication practices (Figure 7–4), as well as for prevention and preparation in relation to future disasters (Morganstein and West 2023). There are several key leadership functions for psychiatrists to bear in mind both in terms of understanding systemic responses and for providing direct support. Leadership functions are numerous and include providing direction to groups and communities; triaging areas of greatest need and overseeing resource allocation; supporting the process of grieving, or "grief leadership"; and supporting recovery after the acute crisis has begun to abate.

Leadership Consultation

Psychiatrists may take on several roles in relation to leadership, including being in direct leadership positions, especially when it comes to mental health clinical response. In addition to clinical roles, psychiatrists provide consultation to leaders across different systemic levels, often in the form of working directly with leadership teams in a variety of different capacities. For example, a team of psychiatrists deployed to work with people evacuated to U.S. military bases following the collapse of a foreign government after a prolonged period of war were deployed to consult onsite with military and governmental leadership teams. In addition to providing individual leadership consultation, the team shared critical information on resilience, Psychological First Aid, risk communication, and other topics that were deployed immediately with good effect. The psychiatrists spoke with staff on the ground as well as with evacuees and were able to identify systems and culturally bound issues, providing direct feedback to leadership to alleviate ongoing practical problems and deescalate tension.

Influence, Vision, and Recovery

Psychiatrists should be aware that leaders are present not just for the big picture but also at intermediate levels, from managers to religious leaders, community pillars and local government officials, as well as first responders. Likewise, it is incumbent on clinicians to recognize that there are three areas critical to crisis leadership: *influence*, *vision*, and *recovery*:

> Influence leading during crisis involves influencing others to maximize their efforts in order to accomplish a mission within an environment of confusion, ambiguity, and extremes of stress. Vision leadership involves a leader remaining aware of what is happening in the present, while holding a vision of where we need to get to, even when all those around them are losing their ability to see beyond the moment. Recovery leadership reflects the ways in which decisions leaders make during a crisis affect how, when and the degree to which a community ultimately recovers. (Morganstein and West 2023)

Leadership Through Walking Around

As in the example from work with evacuees in which speaking directly with various stakeholder groups on the ground was pivotal, *leadership through walking around* means taking time to move among various groups, foster relationships, and practice active listening to learn what people's true concerns are. By doing so, leaders can avoid the common leadership pitfall of being disconnected from those they serve. "Going to where people work and being shoulder-to-shoulder with them communicates respect and value sends the message that leaders are willing to be 'in the trenches' with others, and helps people feel that leaders truly appreciate their challenges and concerns" (Morganstein and West 2023). In addition to cultivating relationships, gathering critical information they would not otherwise fully appreciate, and building trust, being out and about gives leaders the opportunity to demonstrate the skills and capacities they seek to instill in others through modeling rather than only direction.

Leader Communication

Hand in hand with walking around, leader communication is critical. It requires training, practice, and experience. As discussed in Chapter 5, it is essential for leaders to learn and use the principles of risk communication, which are designed to foster the key crisis communication goal of establishing a trusting, credible relationship as the foundation for effective crisis response. Useful leadership behaviors include "communicating regularly; providing resources; normalizing reactions; promoting peer support; role modeling; addressing grief; and thinking forward" (Morganstein and West 2023). The use of rituals and symbols, such as in memorialization following grief, is an essential element of communication, best when integrated with community participation and leadership.

Leader Skills

Role-Model Self-Care

Self-care and related behaviors are important for leaders to model. These behaviors are discussed in more detail in Chapter 6 and include sleep, nutrition and rest, and seeking support. Leaders should model strategies for stress management, including specific coping strategies (e.g., minimizing how much disaster- or trauma-related media is consumed) and avoiding maladaptive coping (e.g., overworking, using alcohol or other substances to manage difficult emotional states). An additional useful strategy is to have a *disaster buddy*, ensuring that there is always another person available to serve as a sounding board and to help leaders know if they are experiencing negative reactions to the high levels of stress they often bear.

Foster a Sense of Purpose and Support Emotion Regulation

Leadership communication also scaffolds key functions, including fostering a sense of purpose and supporting emotion regulation. These two factors contribute to team and community resilience, providing meaning and goal orientation. Mash et al. (2024) reported that

> Research conducted during the COVID-19 [pandemic] with approximately 4,000 National Guard service members revealed that personnel whose leaders reminded them of the purpose and value of their work reported: better physical health, better mental health, improved sleep, decreased use of alcohol, stronger unit cohesion.

> Likewise, whereas emotion dysregulation undermines proper function and well-being and erodes team effectiveness through contagion, when leaders support emotion regulation, function improves for both individuals

and the group. It not uncommon for people to feel there is something wrong with them for having certain emotions, such as sadness, shame, or grief. Leaders can support emotion regulation through careful self-disclosure. For example, a leader can share similar feelings by simply saying, "I feel angry too." Having leaders share that they have the same feelings normalizes the experience and help people feel calmer and more connected. The acronym APC is a useful mnemonic for emotion regulation: *acceptance* ("What can you control vs. what is better to accept?"); *perspective* ("Will this frustration really matter in a week? A month? A year?"); *compartmentalize* ("Is now the time, or should you 'put it away' for a while?") (Morganstein and West 2023).

Grief Leadership

Finally, bereavement is ubiquitous in disasters. It is critical for leaders to practice *grief leadership*: "Communicate directly and continually with the community; acknowledge openly the losses and their impact; honor losses using community-conceived and implemented activities; encourage ways to make meaning of the events that happened; and help people look hopefully to the future" (Morganstein and West 2023; see also Mash et al. 2024). Survivors of disaster face many challenges, and leaders play an important role in tracking which reactions are normal and which require more specialized attention. Psychiatrists can play both consultative and direct roles in assessing the severity of reactions, bearing in mind that formal referral is rare and most reactions to disasters are normal and expected. Psychiatrists can provide leaders with psychoeducation and consultation to determine if a more significant problem is present and counsel leaders to provide support short of medical referral.

Ultimately, leaders guide communities through difficult times, often holding hope and providing support when hope seems absent and encouraging recovery and restoration of hope when hopelessness, despair, and suffering begin to transition from the acute response.

> [L]eaders seek to create a mental toughness and rhythm that allow their communities to go about the work of addressing the problems of today. Leaders remind their communities that eventually the disaster will end and the vast majority of people, even those who have difficulties, will ultimately be okay. (Morganstein and West 2023)

Conclusion

Psychiatrists can serve as leaders in disaster response, taking a public health approach to fostering community and workplace resilience, among other roles and responsibilities. The commonly accepted phases of disaster response include preparedness, response, recovery, and mitigation. Preparation for engagement in disaster response by the psychiatrist includes having an appreciation and understanding of the psychological and psychosocial phases of disaster, as well as familiarity with multiple models. However, disasters are diverse in the ways they occur, and flexibility in applying models is helpful. In contemplating engagement in disaster response, psychiatrists must consider personal factors and preferences, as well as have an understanding of potential roles in disaster response. A broad knowledge and understanding of response systems, both United States and global, is essential. Leadership during disasters and other crisis events is a difficult and complex task, and psychiatrists should appreciate the differences between leadership consultation, leadership through walking around and being present, leader communication, leader skills, and grief leadership.

References

American Psychiatric Association: Disaster and Preventive Psychiatry: Protecting Health and Fostering Community Resilience. Washington, DC, American Psychiatric Association, May 19, 2023. Available at: https://education.psychiatry.org/Listing/Disaster-and-Preventive-Psychiatry-Protecting-Health-and-Fostering-Community-Resilience-6019. Accessed July 4, 2023.

American Red Cross: Become a Volunteer. Washington, DC, American Red Cross, 2010. Available at: www.redcross.org/en/volunteer. Accessed January 3, 2011.

Center for the Study of Traumatic Stress: Grief leadership: leadership in the wake of tragedy. Bethesda, MD, Uniformed Services University, 2024. Available at: www.cstsonline.org/assets/media/documents/CSTS_FS_Grief_Leadership_in_theWake_of_Tragedy.pdf. Accessed July 21, 2024.

Centers for Disease Control and Prevention: Interim results: state-specific seasonal influenza vaccination coverage—United States, August 2009–January 2010. MMWR Morb Mortal Wkly Rep 59(16):477–484, 2010 20431523

Centers for Disease Control and Prevention: CERC Manual. Atlanta, GA, Centers for Disease Control and Prevention, 2018. Available at: https://emergency.cdc.gov/cerc/manual/index.asp. Accessed July 9, 2024.

DeWolfe DJ: Training Manual for Mental Health and Human Service Workers in Major Disasters, 2nd Edition (HHS Publ No ADM 90-538). Rockville, MD, U.S. Department of Health and Human Services, Substance Abuse and Mental Health Services Administration, Center for Mental Health Services, 2000

Disaster Psychiatry Outreach: The Essentials of Disaster Psychiatry: A Training Course for Mental Health Professionals (Course Syllabus). New York, Disaster Psychiatry Outreach, 2008

Federal Emergency Management Agency: ICS Resource Center. Washington, DC, Federal Emergency Management Agency, 2010a. Available at: https://training.fema.gov/emiweb/is/icsresource. Accessed July 9, 2023.

Federal Emergency Management Agency: National Incident Management System (NIMS). Washington, DC, Federal Emergency Management Agency, 2010b. Available at: https://training.fema.gov/nims. Accessed July 8, 2024.

Federal Emergency Management Agency: IIS-100.C: Introduction to the Incident Command System, ICS 100. Washington, DC, Federal Emergency Management Agency, 2018. Available at: https://training.fema.gov/is/courseoverview.aspx?code=IS-100.c&lang=en. Accessed July 8, 2024.

Federal Emergency Management Agency: National Preparedness Goal. Washington, DC, Federal Emergency Management Agency, March 2023. Available at: www.fema.gov/emergency-managers/national-preparedness/goal. Accessed July 9, 2024.

Huremovic D (ed): Psychiatry of Pandemics: A Mental Health Response to Infection Outbreak. Cham, Switzerland, Springer Nature, 2019

Kantor EM: Guidance for potential disaster health and mental health volunteers, in Haiti Updates. New York, Disaster Psychiatry Outreach, 2009

Kantor EM: The disaster response system in the United States, in Hidden Impact: What You Need to Know for the Next Disaster. A Practical Mental Health Guide for Clinicians. Edited by Stoddard FJ, Katz CL, Merlino JP. Sudbury, MA, Jones & Bartlett, 2010, pp 11–18

Kestel D: Transforming mental health for all: a critical role for specialists. World Psychiatry 21(3):333–334, 2022 36073690

Mash HBH, Fullerton CS, Adler AB, et al: National Guard deployment in support of COVID-19: psychological and behavioral health. Mil Med, 189(1–2):e127–e135, 2024 37209168

Morganstein JC, West JC: Disaster and Preventive Psychiatry: Protecting Health and Fostering Community Resilience. Washington, DC, American Psychiatric Association, May 19, 2023. Available at: https://education.psychiatry.org/Listing/Disaster-and-Preventive-Psychiatry-Protecting-Health-and-Fostering-Community-Resilience-6019. Accessed July 4, 2023.

Nakintu S: Diversity, equity and inclusion: key terms and definitions. Washington, DC, National Association of Counties, November 29, 2021. Available at: www.naco.org/sites/default/files/documents/2022-DEI_KeyTerms_V11.pdf. Accessed July 12, 2024.

Raphael B: When Disaster Strikes: How Individuals and Communities Cope with Catastrophe. Basic Books, 1986

Tervalon M, Murray-Garcia J: Cultural humility versus cultural competence: a critical distinction in defining physician training outcomes in multicultural education. J Health Care Poor Underserved 9(2):117–125, 1998 10073197

United Nations High Commissioner for Refugees: Cluster approach, in Emergency Handbook. Geneva, Switzerland, United Nations High Commissioner for Refugees, 2024. Available at: https://emergency.unhcr.org/coordination-and-communication/cluster-system/cluster-approach#:~:text=Clusters%20are%20groups%20of%20humanitarian,to%20fill%20a%20temporary%20gap. Accessed July 9, 2024.

United Nations Office for the Coordination of Humanitarian Affairs: IV. International coordination mechanisms, in Disaster Response in Asia and the Pacific: A Guide to International Tools and Services. Bangkok, Regional Office for Asia and the Pacific, 2023, pp 42–56. Available at: https://asiadisasterguide.unocha.org/IV-international-coordination.html. Accessed August 22, 2023.

United Nations Office for Disaster Risk Reduction: Sendai Framework for Disaster Risk Reduction 2015–2030. Geneva, Switzerland, United Nations, 2015. Available at: www.undrr.org/publication/sendai-framework-disaster-risk-reduction-2015-2030. Accessed August 22, 2023.

U.S. Department of Health and Human Services: Overview of MSCC, emergency management, and the incident command system, in Medical Surge Capacity and Capabilities (MSCC) Handbook. Washington, DC, U.S. Department of Health and Human Services, 2023. Available at: https://aspr.hhs.gov/HealthCareReadiness/guidance/MSCC/Pages/Chapter1-Overview.aspx. Accessed July 9, 2024.

Wells MI: Beyond cultural competence: a model for individual and institutional cultural development. J Community Health Nurs 17(4):189–199, 2000 11126891

8

Model for Adaptive Response to Complex Cyclical Disasters

Grant H. Brenner, M.D.
Kathleen A. Clegg, M.D.
Sander Koyfman, M.D., M.B.A.

Planned Spontaneity and Emerging Disaster Conceptualization

If we do not have a concept of something—a sufficient model for understanding an object, event or phenomenon—we cannot fully make sense of whatever it is. Thomas Kuhn (1962) coined the term *paradigm shift* to designate what happens when a new understanding of reality precipitously emerges, often flying in the face of convention. "Normal" science defines the dominant way of seeing the world, but as anomalies build up, a pattern suddenly emerges and blossoms into a new and useful way of understanding the object of study. Disaster response is humbling, showing us the limitations of our knowledge, understanding and impact. According to Francis Bacon, as Kuhn emphatically reminds us, "Truth emerges more readily from error than from confusion" (Kuhn 1962, p. 18).

A paradigm shift is sorely needed in disaster and crisis response. Although the Model for Adaptive Response to Complex Cyclical Disasters

(MARCCD) does not represent such a paradigm shift, we intend for it to collate several relevant standard elements of disaster response models and introduce new tools to facilitate disaster and crisis response. We understand that although disasters share certain features, including overwhelmed community resources and high levels of threat, destruction, disruption, and loss, our capacity for preparation and response is limited. We understand that compassion and collaboration rise steeply following a disaster—the *post-disaster utopia*—but human behavior typically returns to baseline within a few months. That baseline is often not characterized by long-term planning and thoughtful allocation of resources in the most effective ways; with some exceptions, it is more likely to be about short-term gains and looking out for one's immediate group rather than wisdom-based communal thinking. Only at a later day, with some challenging accounting and flaws of human recollection, do communities make an effort to rebuild better and create solutions— but often only to the *past* disaster, not the *next* one.

This is a very human problem, which transcends but defines disaster response and preparation. Rather than eliminate nuclear weapons, we are wired to build up force multilaterally in order to ensure a fragile safety based on mutually assured destruction. In the words of Nobel laureate Albert Szent-Györgyi, author of *The Crazy Ape*,

> We are forced to face this situation with our caveman's brain, a brain that has not changed much since it was formed. We face it with our outdated thinking, institutions and methods, with political leaders who have their roots in the old, prescientific world and think the only way to solve these formidable problems is by trickery and double talk, by increasing our atomic arsenal—which is already sufficiently stocked to kill every single living individual three times over—by trying to replace the single warhead by multiple ones, creating new missiles and anti- or anti-antimissiles, by spending untold billions on the instruments of death. (Szent-Györgi 1970, p. 17)

Model for Adaptive Response to Complex Cyclical Disasters

Background

Disasters are increasing because of urbanization, extreme weather and climate change, pandemics, wars, rapid population expansion, and geopolitical and socioeconomic transition and perturbation. If sustainable development is a goal, as Alrehaili and colleagues (2022) highlight, we must do a better job at disaster management, including prevention, preparedness and mitigation, and response. As disasters increase in density, we must ask: Are we at a point where disaster planning is increasingly thought of as the norm rather than an exception? If so, the same rules of good housekeeping should apply. We need to understand which resources exist, which may be needed, how quickly they can be expended or shifted to help one's neighbors, and how often some resources can serve us well in times of both peace and disaster, making them even more worthwhile to invest in. However, review of the literature (see Chapter 7, "Engaging in Disaster Response") and experience with disaster response suggest that disaster response models are underused and that more consistent application would improve outcomes—as well as providing an accounting of what has gone into a prior response. It is important to recognize that disasters are complex; linear stages of disaster cannot possibly provide a useful framework for containing a great many crises.

Although disasters and crises are characterized by shared suffering and destruction, and although there are different "types" of disaster—natural and human-made disasters, weather events and earthquakes, terrorist attacks and mass transit events, and so on—it is a mantra among disaster responders that every disaster is unique: "If you've been to one disaster, you've been to one disaster." This highlights the need for flexibility and open-mindedness regardless of best practices. Concerted efforts to capture lessons learned through events such as the symposium "Disaster Preparedness and Response: Building Capacity Through Care Integration" (held in San Juan, Puerto Rico, on August 9, 2018, a year after the devastation of Hurricane Maria) are an exception, not a rule, but models exist. Chapter 7 addresses specific disaster models to date, with an emphasis on operational and logistical elements to spell out the tactical ground game for service delivery in crisis environments, where not only are material resources disrupted, but cognitive and emotional function is also altered, affecting decision-making and behavior for individuals and groups. A consistent approach to capturing learning while remaining nimble is needed.

Genesis

It was with these considerations in mind that a group of disaster psychiatrists from the Committee for Disasters, Trauma, and Global Health of the Group for the Advancement of Psychiatry saw that a new model was needed to try to make sense of the situation we saw emerging as the new global norm. The idea of an updated model for complex cyclical disasters was born one weekend in spring 2020 in Westchester, New York, as the coronavirus disease 2019 (COVID-19) pandemic was picking up speed. At the same time, forest fires were sweeping through California; tornadoes were hitting the Midwest; tsunamis, earthquakes, and radiation events were occurring; and mass shootings remained fresh in our consciousness. All of this occurred against the chronic backdrop of nuclear threat and the more recent recognition of climate crisis.

Over the course of the next several months, a group of disaster mental health experts, not-for-profit partners, Vibrant Emotional Health, and health care information gurus—in consultation with diversity, equity, inclusion, and belonging (DEIB) specialists and a level of cultural consultation—met for several working sessions to derive a "beta version" of the new disaster response framework, the MARCCD. This blueprint, or framework, is necessarily a work in progress—a living model designed to be dynamically responsive and updated on the basis of continuous feedback. For example, although DEIB consultation was sought during the initial design process, subsequent feedback from one of the chapter authors (S.K.) highlighted addressable gaps in cross-cultural applicability. By design, the MARCCD can be iterated and adapted to different groups, particularly in digital format, which allows for real-time adjustment and personalization. Applying a personalized or precision medicine construct to disaster response is appropriate given that individual disasters have both shared and unique qualities.

The MARCCD focuses on high-level constructs, which can be expanded to granular levels and "blown out" to provide as much detail as appropriate, although at this time it remains high level. The model is demonstrably U.S./Westerncentric, and the expectation is that if it is adopted more widely, there will be significant additional development for cross-cultural relevance, including language equity and other forms of equity (Curt et al. 2021).

The elements of the model should be familiar. As of 2018, there are nearly 40 identified existing disaster models, according to a thematic analysis of such models (Nojavan et al. 2018), with types grouped into logical models, integrated models, cause models, combinatorial models, and other models. A meta-model anticipates the emergence of a new way of understanding, communicating, and working together that will unlock more robust and flexible future capability to prevent and limit unnecessary human suffering when disaster and crisis visit. This, of course, requires both increasing resources and refining how they are used, with strong human interdependence.

Overview

The MARCCD is organized into six sections: phases of disaster, stress regulation across disaster phases, faces of disaster, key stress mitigation actions, community stress load threshold, and community balance sheet.

These are based on expert opinion and best practices, integration of prior models, and evidence-based review. The full model (Vibrant Emotional Health 2022) shows how the different sections fit together. Like the many-sided polyhedron, the sections of the MARCCD are different facets of a comprehensive system seen from multiple perspectives. As such, the depicted model uses arrows and colors or texture to show the continuous thread that runs through all aspects of disaster response—the people and communities themselves.

The MARCCD is deliberately very conceptual in order to integrate common factors to encourage a holistic overview while also framing in one place the massive scope of work that needs doing. The goal is to develop a broadly applicable framework that addresses major categories of interest relevant for a comprehensive, flexible, and ongoing disaster response system that covers hazard assessment, risk management, and reasonable action regardless of the situation.

Phases of Disaster

The MARCCD disaster phases are organized into four interconnected and overlapping states: Anticipation, Impact, Adaptation, and Growth and Recovery (Figure 8–1). Each of these can be broken out in more detail tailored for different stakeholder groups, including communities and community leaders, first responders, and disaster-affected persons (survivors). Phases potentially overlap not only within each disaster event but also *among* different disasters (see subsection "Community Balance Sheet and Community Stress Load Threshold"). In addition, the phases can be superimposed on top of systemic factors such as chronic stressors affecting a community (e.g., elevated crime rates) and foundational factors, including factors affecting social determinants of health, recently dubbed *exposomal factors* (Guloksuz et al. 2018).

Following on the Anticipation and Impact phases, the Adaptation phase is intended to capture flexibly a broad range of the disaster response, from early adaptation to more chronic adaptation in the absence of full resolution of the disaster. For example, during the COVID-19 pandemic, early adaptation involved quarantine measures and becoming accustomed to virtual work and school or even to the losses of loved ones and gaps left in their roles in the community. Later on, as vaccines became available and more people had some immunity, adaptation involved various levels of masking and social distancing in public, and quarantine measures were gradually withdrawn. However, the pandemic remained active, if attenuated, with rolling cycles of infection gradually decreasing in amplitude over time. When the pandemic reached an endemic state, public health

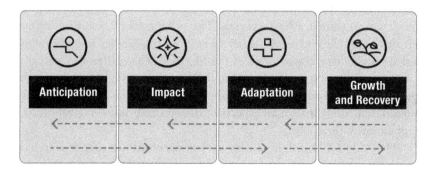

FIGURE 8–1. Phases of disaster.

Source.   Vibrant Emotional Health 2022.

emergencies ended, and life headed toward a new normal, with most near-term adaptations having settled into consistent day-to-day living.

At this point, the Growth and Recovery phase of the disaster applies, with outcomes ranging from return to baseline with restoration of predisaster function, as well as various levels of posttraumatic growth (PTG), defined by Tedeschi and Calhoun (1996) as the "coping process of positive reinterpretation, positive reframing, interpretive control, or reconstrual of events" (p. 466). The relationship between PTSD and PTG is complex, and it is dependent on many factors, including coping style, personality traits, growth actions, resilience, type and degree of trauma, and demographic and related variables (Henson et al. 2021). PTG is not a consequence of trauma but a response of a subset of individuals and communities who have updated their worldview to include and integrate the trauma, including concrete responses such as improved preparation and finding meaning and/or spiritual growth in profound tragedy.

Community Balance Sheet and Community Stress Load Threshold

The Community Balance Sheet (CBS) and Community Stress Load Threshold (CSLT) models (adapted from Chandra et al. 2018) are core elements of the MARCCD, providing different cross-sections of the complex landscape of disaster response framed within a global health context. The CBS (Figure 8–2) visualizes various types of disasters occurring around the same time, partly overlapping and partly distinct. The model can be adapted to represent different scales: temporally from several years to a century or longer and spatially to cover a small community, a region, a nation, or a global framework.

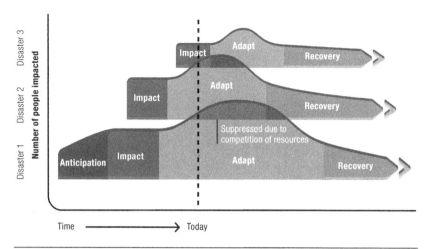

FIGURE 8–2. Community balance sheet.

Source. Vibrant Emotional Health 2022.

The CSLT represents a model of how disasters stack up on top of stressors and foundational issues, showing total load as a function of the horizontal axis (Figure 8–3). This axis can be used to represent time, showing stress fluctuating over the course of events, or it could also be used to represent other variables relevant to stress—for instance, resources from low to high. Right now, what matters is understanding that it is a tool to organize how we understand the impact of stress on various aspects of functioning in order ultimately to efficiently distribute resources to areas of need in a changing environment. As depicted here, the CSLT is used to show how community stress hypothetically varies with disaster phase. Actual use would entail using data from specific events. Such data, with recognition of the needed advocacy and effort to obtain them, would be incorporated into services rendered for the displaced members of the community by relief organizations and established care providers, social resources, and so much more.

Faces of Disaster

The MARCCD is organized around people and communities, including survivors, community leaders, and first responders as core affected persons (Figure 8–4). At the same time, the model is designed to be flexible to accommodate other groups, including policymakers, individuals involved in governance, and media representatives. Survivors are the primary persons affected by disasters as communities, families, individuals, and var-

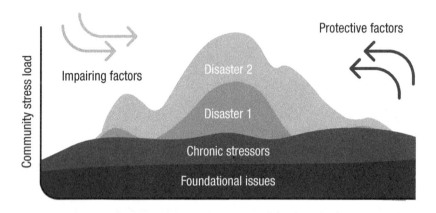

FIGURE 8–3.   Mitigating the cumulative stress load in a community.

Source.   Vibrant Emotional Health 2022.

ious affinity groups. The specific needs of survivors are addressed in detail in relevant chapters. Working with leaders is important because they can provide access and collaboration for assessment and intervention, inform responders about cultural norms to facilitate communication and cultural competency (in addition to predeployment preparation), and provide crucial information about available resources and communication practices (see Chapter 5, "Communication and Relationships," and Chapter 7). Responders are the third group highlighted here (see Chapter 6, "Rescuing Ourselves"). They are integral to response effectiveness, and if they are part of the disaster-affected community, they may be primarily affected as well as affected in the course of responding.

Regulating Stress Throughout Disaster Phases

Stress regulation is critical for all involved in crisis situations, from the smallest local emergency to the largest mass-scale disaster. The MARCCD uses a *homeorhesis* model (Waddington 1957), meaning it depicts optimal stress regulation as keeping within a healthy target zone between regions of overregulation and underregulation (Figure 8–5). This type of model is distinct from the more familiar concept of homeostasis, which aims for a fixed, static state.

The autonomic nervous system governs stress response. The sympathetic division of the autonomic nervous system uses the stress hormone cortisol and related biological responses such as norepinephrine secretion, which leads to increased activation; heightened attention; increased blood

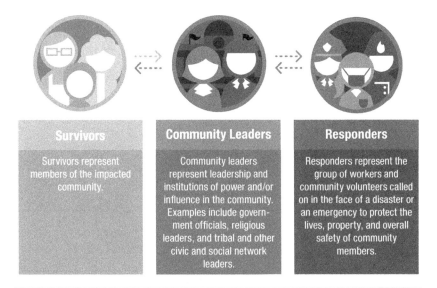

FIGURE 8–4. Faces of disaster.

Source. Vibrant Emotional Health 2022.

flow to organs involved in action; and a relative shutdown of restorative processes, including decreased appetite and sleep. The parasympathetic division of the autonomic nervous system helps the body and mind return to baseline after being activated and recuperate from stress, whether short-term or prolonged. Chronic stress reactions become unsustainable when the body's resources are depleted without time to recharge. It is important for individuals to maintain a state of health and stamina, for example, via good self-care, regular exercise, and a nutritious diet, so that the person can meet the increased physical demands during a crisis: ramping up, sustaining, and monitoring output. For people affected by disasters, self-care and community support are imperative to allow for sustained levels of autonomic activation in the context of ongoing work with limited resources, often for indeterminate durations.

Key Actions by Phase and Stakeholder Group

Finally, the MARCCD focuses on evidence-based and best-practices actions that key stakeholders can take at different stages of disaster (Figure 8–6). The actions presented in the figure are not meant to be comprehensive, but they do depict some key considerations for survivors, community leaders, and responders at each disaster phase. In practice, this section of the MARCCD is intended to be expanded to provide additional informa-

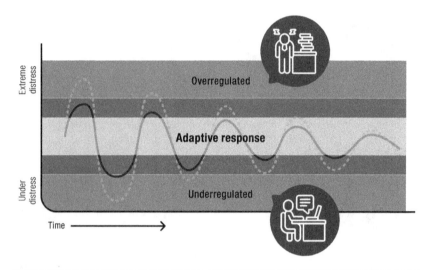

FIGURE 8–5.   Regulating stress throughout disaster and crisis response.

Source.   Vibrant Emotional Health 2022.

tion. For example, in a digital version, scrolling over or clicking on each box would reveal additional resources, such as Psychological First Aid (Brymer et al. 2006) and Skills for Psychological Recovery (Berkowitz et al. 2010; National Child Traumatic Stress Network 2020).

Conclusion

Given the COVID-19 pandemic and escalating disasters credibly linked to climate change, against the backdrop of geopolitical tumult, rising mass human displacement, and conventional disasters both natural and human-made, a need arises for a comprehensive, action-oriented disaster mental health framework. Models must address robust preparedness and response and recovery for single events, as well as disaster prevention (see Chapter 2, "Disaster Prevention and Climate Change") and chronic, overlapping disasters of varying duration and rhythmicity. The COVID-19 pandemic was the first event in this generation characterized by rolling waves of infection, straining the health care system past the breaking point and leaving in its wake an untold swath of grief and stress we have yet to fully recognize. As we were emerging from the pandemic, the Russian invasion of Ukraine supervened, resetting the process of recovery and potential growth for untold numbers of communities worldwide.

Survivors	Identify and promote survivors who have adapted well in prior similar experiences to work within their community Engage in actions to help channel anxious energy, such as calming thoughts, exercise, meditation, and other spiritual practices	Give survivors room to share memories, experiences, and coping skills Share access to correct and credible information	Participate in culturally attuned memorials for collective remembering and grieving Get involved in local projects that are planning for the postdisaster future	Integrate disaster experience Seek treatment for persistent mental health concerns
Community leaders	Clearly message quality information on risk communication Provide anticipated needed resources	Leverage just-in-time partnerships to address the most immediate needs Promote actionable information from trusted resources	Evaluate and restore basic functions (e.g., schools) with appropriate modifications Build resources and resilience for middle- and low-income areas and high-risk subgroups and conduct planning to avoid returning to predisaster neglect	Encourage restoration of productive relationships between subgroups Address competition and resentment between subgroups that has persisted or evolved
Responders	In planning, capture lessons learned from other communities (if initial onset) or from earlier cycles (if this is a new cycle) Address existing or anticipated compassion fatigue and burnout	Focus on training and community building to increase capacity for locals to respond and provide sustainable longer-term supports Address responders' needs to keep own families safe by offering co-sheltering and shared resources	Advise and support responders to feel empowered to continue the work without the influx of outside help Enlist disaster mental health experts to support responders at risk of burnout	Integrate lessons learned into future preparation, training, and response Monitor and seek help for consistent and severe stress or distress

FIGURE 8–6. Key actions for adaptive mitigation of stress.

Source. Vibrant Emotional Health 2022.

The MARCCD—which invites ongoing feedback and revision as a "living" model—provides an early framework designed to enable multiple stakeholder groups to conceptualize the complex global emerging landscape of disaster response on macro levels as well as to zoom in more granularly to support effective response at various stages of disasters for multiple stakeholder groups, across different disasters, in different locations.

The following vignette presents an example of how the MARCDD can be used in the aftermath of recent disasters.

Vignette

You have been asked to support a group of first responders—firefighters, emergency medical services personnel, paramedics, and police officers—in a small, rural town that was recently hit by tornadoes. Many citizens lost their homes, and the fire department was damaged by a tornado. On the ground, you discover that prior to the tornadoes, the first responders were dealing with a spike in opioid overdose cases, which is still going on as they try to recover from the tornadoes.

1. The Faces of Disaster section of the MARCCD highlights that the needs of survivors, responders, and community leaders may differ, but they also may overlap. Responders and community leaders also may be survivors. In this small, rural community, those lost to the opioid crisis may have been known by many of the town's people. Community and fire department leaders will be a key point of contact for responders to gain trust and develop access in order to offer effective assistance.

2. The Phases of Disaster portion of the tool can be used to determine which phase of each disaster the first responders and survivors are in. With regard to the tornadoes, they are likely in the impact and early adaptation phases, whereas with regard to the opioid crisis, they are experiencing a cyclical pattern of impact, early adaptation, and anticipation of the next spike in cases and deaths. This community may have survived other tornadoes, and it is important for disaster responders to tap into potential areas of knowledge and resilience from these prior events.

3. The Regulating Stress portion of the model can be used to evaluate individual and community responses. For example, disorganization and chaos at the community level would suggest an underregulated stress response. Immobilization and inability to respond would suggest an overregulated stress response. If community members have pulled together to take effective action, they may be functioning within the healthy stress regulation window.

4. The Key Actions to Adaptive Mitigation of Stress can be provided to various groups to help them anticipate what may come next for them as well as for others. For instance, during the Impact phase, community leaders could begin planning for actions that survi-

vors will need to take during the Adaptation phase, including creating opportunities for individual and collective memorialization. Community leaders can also begin to plan for the resources needed to address the burnout, compassion fatigue, and vicarious trauma that responders may experience, thereby supporting growth and recovery.

5. The Community Stress Load Threshold section encourages the evaluation of the foundational issues and chronic stressors that exist in the affected community. The presence of foundational issues and chronic stressors in a community increases the amplitude of the disaster, given that disaster response will strain already sparse resources. Many different factors may impair responsiveness to a disaster, such as responders having been personally impacted by the disaster and being less able to function in their roles as responders. Protective factors could include a community that is close knit and has a history and culture of pitching in to help neighbors. Because inequity in disaster response often occurs, marginalized community members may experience greater impacts yet receive fewer resources.

6. The Community Balance Sheet can be used to take stock of an array of resources that are relevant for individuals, families, and stricken communities. After the timelines of the multiple disasters are mapped out, this balance sheet can help individuals and communities to better answer the questions "Where am I/are we?," "What is coming next?," and "What can I/we do to most adaptively manage the stress?"

The MARCCD is presented as an evolving model designed to frame multiple aspects of disaster prevention, preparedness, and response, setting the stage for a future in which disasters are woven into the fabric of our day-to-day lives rather than being seen as departures from the norm.

References

Alrehaili NR, Almutairi TN, Alghamdi HM, et al: A structural review on disaster management models and their contributions. International Journal of Disaster Management 5(2):93–108, 2022

Berkowitz S, Bryant R, Brymer M, et al: Skills for Psychological Recovery: Field Operations Guide. Washington, DC, National Center for PTSD; Los Angeles, CA, National Child Traumatic Stress Network, 2010. Available at: www.ptsd.va.gov/professional/treat/type/skills_psych_recovery_manual.asp#:~:text=Skills%20for%20Psychological%20Recovery%20(SPR,post%2Ddisaster%20stress%20and%20adversity. Accessed July 6, 2024.

Brymer M, Jacobs A, Layne C, et al: Psychological First Aid: Field Operations Guide, 2nd Edition. July, 2006. Los Angeles, CA, National Child Traumatic Stress Network; Washington, DC, National Center for PTSD. Available at: www.nctsn.org/resources/psychological-first-aid-pfa-field-operations-guide-2nd-edition. Accessed July 6, 2024.

Chandra A, Cahill ME, Yeung D, Ross R: Toward an initial conceptual framework to assess community allostatic load: early themes from literature review and community analysis on the role of cumulative community stress. Santa Monica, CA, Rand, June 29, 2018. Available at: www.rand.org/pubs/research_reports/RR2559.html. Accessed August 8, 2024

Curt AM, Kanak MM, Fleegler EW, et al: Increasing inclusivity in patient centered research begins with language. Prev Med 149:106621, 2021 33992655

Guloksuz S, van Os J, Rutten BPF: The exposome paradigm and the complexities of environmental research in psychiatry. JAMA Psychiatry 75(10):985–986, 2018 29874362

Henson C, Truchot D, Canevello A: What promotes post traumatic growth? A systematic review.Eur J Trauma Dissociation 5(4):100195, 2021

Kuhn T: The Structure of Scientific Revolutions. Chicago, IL, University of Chicago Press, 1962

National Child Traumatic Stress Network: Skills for Psychological Recovery. Los Angeles, CA, 2020

Nojavan M, Salehi E, Omidvar B: Conceptual change of disaster management models: a thematic analysis. Jamba 10(1):451, 2018 29955258

Szent-Györgi A: The Crazy Ape. New York, The Philosophical Library, 1970

Tedeschi RG, Calhoun LG: The Posttraumatic Growth Inventory: measuring the positive legacy of trauma. J Trauma Stress 9(3):455–471, 1996 8827649

Vibrant Emotional Health: Model for Adaptive Response to Complex Cyclical Disasters (MARCCD), New York, Vibrant Emotional Health, 2022. Available at https://marccd.info. Accessed May 6, 2024.

Waddington HC: The Strategy of the Genes: A Discussion of Some Aspects of Theoretical Biology. London, George Allen & Unwin, 1957

PART II

EVALUATION

Craig L. Katz, M.D.
Section Editor

9

Legal and Ethical Considerations

Jacob M. Appel, M.D., J.D., M.P.H.

Many of the legal and ethical issues that arise in disaster psychiatry will prove similar to those that arise in the practice of general psychiatry and of medicine more broadly. All physicians should be aware of the relevant laws of the jurisdiction in which they are offering care, the ethical guidelines of their specialty, and where to turn for guidance on challenging ethical and medicolegal issues that arise during the course of service. However, the practice of psychiatry in the setting of disasters also raises a distinct set of considerations that may differ—often greatly—from those that arise in general practice. Sometimes, rules in disaster settings and those in ordinary practice are highly divergent. The legal and ethical rules governing disaster psychiatry differ from those governing emergency psychiatry and also those applicable when rendering assistance as a bystander. For example, state Good Samaritan laws that may protect a physician offering care at the scene of an automobile accident may not offer the same protections to a physician who travels across the country with the intent of offering mental health services to the survivors of an airplane crash. Although lawsuits against mental health professionals providing disaster relief remain relatively rare, psychiatrists would make a serious error in concluding that their risk of liability is negligible. The following fictionalized case may shed light on some of the potential sources of legal and ethical concern:

Vignette

On June 23, 2016, 10 inches of rain fell within 12 hours in portions of West Virginia, resulting in one of the worst flash floods in that state's history. The Elk River crested at an all-time high, breaking a record that had stood since 1888. Rural Greenbrier County was particularly hard hit and witnessed 15 flood-related deaths. Media accounts described the situation on the ground as "complete chaos" (Stanglin and Rice 2016) and "a war zone" (Van Cleave 2016). On that same day, Dr. Tertius Lydgate was driving home from his Park Avenue office in New York City, where he ran a highly successful fee-for-service psychiatric practice in which he specialized in the pharmacological management of depression and anxiety disorders. Dr. Lydgate was born and raised in Greenbrier County, although he had not returned since the deaths of his parents many years earlier. Yet over the past few years, as he approached his 60th birthday, he found himself reflecting that maybe he should have done more to give back to the community of his youth. So when he heard of the flooding on his car radio, he immediately canceled his appointments for the following week, packed an overnight bag, and drove the 400 miles to his hometown. When he arrived, he introduced himself as a volunteer psychiatrist to a sheriff's deputy at a police barricade, and he soon found himself conducting psychiatric evaluations in the gymnasium of the local high school. He offered supportive therapy, but in several cases also phoned in prescription refills at a pharmacy in a neighboring county for survivors who had lost their medication in the flooding and on two occasions ordered short-term courses of benzodiazepines. Because he did not have access to an electronic medical record (EMR), he documented each encounter on an index card that he stored in the locked glove compartment of his car. Two days later, a disaster mental health team from the Red Cross arrived on site. Dr. Lydgate continued to work alongside the Red Cross for 2 weeks before returning to his practice in New York City. At that time, he handed over his stack of index cards to the Red Cross physician-in-charge.

Although Dr. Lydgate appears to have acted with the best of intentions, his conduct raises a series of challenging questions:

- If he is not licensed to practice in West Virginia, were his actions legal, or is he at risk of prosecution for practicing medicine without a license?
- Even if he were practicing legally, were his actions covered by the state's Good Samaritan law and/or the federal Volunteer Protection Act? At what point did these protections initially take effect? How long did they last?
- Whose malpractice insurance, if any, covers his actions?
- Did his storage and exchange of health care information constitute a violation of confidentiality regulations (such as the Health Insurance Portability and Accountability Act of 1996 [HIPAA]) or a breach of patients' privacy?

- What legal and ethical resources were available to guide him in his decision-making as it evolved and to advise him regarding liability after the fact?

Legal Authority, Licensure, and Liability

Physicians generally must hold a valid license in a jurisdiction in which they render medical services. Certain exceptions do exist during disasters. The Emergency Management Assistance Compact, to which all 50 states now belong, allows for the interstate transfer of medical personnel during states of emergency and permits these providers to practice without in-state licensure or fear of liability. However, the compact applies only to providers acting as agents of states, not to physicians who volunteer care on their own. Individual states may also choose to waive licensing requirements for out-of-state providers during particular disasters, as many did during the coronavirus disease 2019 (COVID-19) pandemic (Mullangi et al. 2021). In the absence of such waivers, a physician traveling across state lines to render care during a disaster may be open to civil and criminal liability, so psychiatrists engaged in disaster medicine should be certain of their legal authority before venturing into the field on their own.

All states do have some form of Good Samaritan law. However, these statutes are designed to offer liability protection for bystanders—both physicians and laypeople—who render assistance during emergencies that arise in their vicinity; they are not intended to apply to medical personnel who travel great distances to render care days or weeks after a tragedy. Similarly, the Aviation Medical Assistance Act of 1998 affords physicians protections for emergency services rendered *during* aircraft flights, not subsequent to aviation disasters. In 1997, Congress enacted the Volunteer Protection Act, which was designed to augment liability protection for volunteer first responders (Volunteer Protection Act 1997). It shields such responders from liability for negligent acts undertaken under the authority of government agencies or nonprofit organizations. This act specifically requires that volunteers be licensed in the state in which they render disaster services in order to receive its protections.

Relief organizations, such as the American Red Cross, do not, as a rule, provide malpractice coverage to volunteers offering specific medical services—although their coverage does include nonprofessional interventions such as Psychological First Aid. Many malpractice insurers view such care as beyond the scope of their policies. Psychiatrists volunteering in disaster response should contact their insurers prior to rendering services, clarify any limitations, and arrange additional coverage as needed *in advance*. Doing so is essential for liability protection, and it is also an

ethical imperative to ensure that victims of potential negligence have an
adequate mechanism available for sufficient future recovery.

Physician-Patient Relationship

Treating a patient in a disaster setting may, depending on the nature of the
interaction, establish a formal physician-patient relationship. The length
and depth of engagement will determine whether such a relationship has
been established, as may specific acts or omissions on the part of the provider. For instance, prescribing medication or conducting multiple sessions
is highly indicative of a formal relationship; in contrast, rendering Psychological First Aid as part of a brief encounter (as described in Chapter 16,
"Psychological First Aid") may well not establish such a relationship.

The establishment of a physician-patient relationship may give rise to
additional legal and ethical obligations. For example, such a relationship
may require overt termination, including arranging for an appropriate
transition of care to another provider. In addition, disaster mental health
professionals may find themselves bound by state regulations and professional canons of ethics regarding boundaries, financial conflicts of interest, and mandatory reporting. These might range from prohibitions from
accepting future gifts of gratitude to having a legal obligation in some
states to report the incidental discovery of intimate partner violence.

The American Medical Association Code of Medical Ethics requires
physicians to take "appropriate advance measures, including acquiring and
maintaining appropriate knowledge and skills to ensure they are able to
provide medical services when needed" (American Medical Association
2024). At the same time, physicians cannot be skilled in all domains, and
providers must be careful to act solely within their scope of practice. Usually, these limits will be apparent: a provider trained in psychiatry would be
on extremely shaky ethical and legal ground if they offered their services as
a trauma surgeon in the field. However, within the field of mental health,
these limitations may be less obvious. For instance, evaluating first responders' fitness for duty is a specialized skill and generally should not be undertaken by the untrained psychiatrist who may not have a full understanding
either of the range of the first responders' expected duties or the mechanisms for testing impairments specific to these duties. A trained forensics
expert should be brought in to conduct such specialized assessments.

Confidentiality

Patients have both an ethical expectation and a legal right to be sure that
their personal health information (PHI) remains confidential. HIPAA does

provide exceptions for the exchange of information between health care providers necessary *for the treatment of patients*, but turning over files to another health care entity or provider in bulk without permission at the conclusion of service likely does not meet this requirement. Other rules, such as federal regulation 42 CFR Part 2 (1981) governing substance use disorders, as well as state laws, impose even stricter obligations. Complicating matters further, securing permission to share PHI—either in writing, or even verbally—can prove challenging during times of crisis.

One particular threat to confidentiality that physicians may encounter during a disaster is the presence of the news media. Psychiatrists may be called on to offer impromptu comments regarding the condition of patients—whether individually or collectively. They will not be able to rely on guidance from the press officers or media relations departments of hospitals, as they do in general practice, so they must be prepared to navigate such queries on their own. Disaster psychiatrists obviously must not speak about individual patients without permission. However, it is also important to avoid making public remarks so specific that the general public can deduce to which patient or small group of patients they apply, a breach of confidentiality that may be unwitting but nonetheless highly deleterious.

Documentation

Documentation of mental health services can prove particularly difficult in disaster settings in which an EMR is not available. Even in a hospital setting, documentation is not a priority during a large-scale emergency, and using the EMR may not be feasible when working by flashlight during a power failure (Zoraster and Burkle 2013). Nevertheless, adequate documentation is essential and may be legally required. In many states, failure to adequately document medical services is considered professional misconduct. Physicians often mistakenly believe that the primary purpose of documentation during disasters is to shield providers from liability, so the only victims of inadequate documentation are themselves. The reality is that such documentation is frequently crucial for disaster victims engaged in litigation against parties responsible for human-made catastrophes, such as dam breaks and chemical spills, and to pursue payouts from insurance companies. Data may also serve valuable public health purposes such as review of emergency measures after the fact to improve future disaster responses. In rare cases, clarifying the basis of medical decisions through documentation provides vital evidence to defend physicians from subsequent criminal prosecution, as was the case in the aftermath of Hurricane Katrina (Zoraster and Burkle 2013). When no formal medical record is available, documenting in a notebook or on a laptop, which is then stored securely, may be a sufficient short-term solution. Such records should then be transferred to the appropriate permanent medium when it becomes available, while ensuring that confidentiality is maintained during this process.

One frequent pitfall that arises in disaster psychiatry is the temptation to document injuries in a manner that exaggerates a victim's disability or suffering. Doing so may result from the positive countertransference often generated by helping survivors in need—especially when the physician anticipates that the victims may pursue litigation against a corporation or government entity responsible for their injuries. Yet doctoring the chart in this manner may have unintended consequences. For instance, such exaggerated documentation of psychiatric impairment might later be used against those same individuals in child custody disputes or used to prevent them from purchasing firearms. Even the most well-intentioned and seemingly benign efforts to exaggerate injuries should be avoided because they can result in unanticipated harms.

International Disaster Relief

Physicians engaged in emergency response outside their own countries, particularly in nations with legal systems and cultural practices with which they are not familiar, may face a distinctive set of challenges. Federal regulations such as HIPAA do not apply in foreign refugee camps, although depending on the circumstances, ethical duties to maintain confidentiality and privacy may be just as important. At the same time, providers must be careful to display cultural humility and to respect local customs, especially when doing so does not challenge the physician's core ethical values (Joshi et al. 2008). For example, some cultures may embrace collective medical decision-making for family members over Western notions of absolute autonomy. Providers should seek guidance from local colleagues with experience and insight. Conducting research during disasters is a particularly fraught matter because potential subjects stand at their most vulnerable. Disaster survivors or others touched by a disaster such as first responders should always be aware if they are participating in a research study or if data regarding their care are being collected for research purposes.

Collaboration with foreign governments and public health authorities is often necessary to render the best care during international crises. Unfortunately, these regimes may be totalitarian in nature or may be engaged in chronic human rights abuses. Providing earthquake relief in a failing state like Haiti, a hybrid regime like Turkey, or an authoritarian dictatorship like Iran may raise distinctive sets of challenges. Providers have traditionally been urged to maintain complete political neutrality under such circumstances, but this approach has faced increasing criticism of late. Appel (2022) has warned against the phenomenon of *whitecoat washing*, in which repressive regimes use their collaboration with Western providers to whitewash ongoing human rights abuses or even genocide. Any individual or organization engaged in international relief work has a moral obligation to "examine the long-term political consequences of their work as well as the short-term humanitarian impact" to ensure that the benefits outweigh any subsequent harm to the affected population (Joshi et al. 2008, p. 177). In some extreme circumstances, requirements imposed by authorities may prevent outsiders from offering care in an ethically acceptable manner.

Equity

The American Medical Association Code of Medical Ethics notes that "the physician workforce is not an unlimited resource" and that "when providing care in a disaster with its inherent dangers, physicians also have an obligation to evaluate the risks of providing care to individual patients versus the need to be available to provide care in the future" (American Medical Association 2024). Because psychiatrists are a scarce resource, they may have an ethical responsibility to consider existing health care inequities and historic patterns of social injustice when deciding where and how to volunteer their services. The case for such judicious deployment appears even stronger in light of increasing data revealing long-standing racial inequities in disaster response in the United States (Connor 2018; Flavelle 2021). Volunteer physicians have historically rushed to some locations in large numbers after major disasters—such as lower Manhattan after 9/11 and Boston after the marathon bombing—but have been less engaged in addressing other disasters, such as the Flint, Michigan, water crisis.

Acute disasters are also not the only circumstances in which psychiatrists can contribute to the public welfare. For instance, a severe shortage of pro bono asylum evaluators continues to plague the United States immigration system (Disla de Jesus and Appel 2022), and trained forensic psychiatrists are in particularly high demand for their services in this work. Both individual volunteers and organizations should be sure to donate their time and resources in a manner that is equitable and takes into consideration victims' underlying access to social capital.

Malingering

Malingering is a significant consideration in any diagnosis of posttraumatic stress disorder (PTSD; Ali et al. 2015). Motivations for feigning symptoms after trauma may include direct financial reward through government disability payments or worker's compensation funds, increased damages in civil litigation claims, and avoidance of future responsibilities such as alimony or child support. In addition, malingering pain symptoms may be used as a mechanism for obtaining prescription narcotics. Following high-profile disasters, opportunists may claim to have been victims to generate publicity or sympathy even when they were far from the scene of the disaster. In one notable case, well-known comedian Steve Rannazzisi apologized for lying about having escaped from the World Trade Center in 9/11 to jump-start his stand-up career (Kim 2015).

However, such deception is not necessarily malingering. Factitious disorder, conversion disorder, and confabulation may also explain some instances of disaster-related deception. The case of Spanish heiress Tania Head, the former president of the World Trade Center Survivors Network, whose story of escaping the South Tower on 9/11 unraveled under scrutiny in 2007 (Kim 2015), is often cited as an example of a nonsurvivor whose deception was not the product of malingering or motivated by secondary gain. Although psychiatrists should be wary of potential malingering, they should not be too quick to question the credibility of trauma victims. Trauma survivors, especially those under considerable pressure, often display symptoms of distress (e.g., avoidance, inability to remember) that may be mistaken for deception. Frank John Ninivaggi (2016) terms this the "non-malingerer's dilemma," and it is of particular concern in disaster settings.

Disaster Research

Disaster medicine as a formal field with institutional structures and professional norms dates back to the 1970s and draws on work done in various settings, ranging from disaster management to public health to emergency services (Kocak et al. 2021). Although the many of the same ethical challenges that arise generally in human subject investigations are also central issues in disaster research, this research also raises many distinct elements, including "how urgency impacts the time available to design, review, and implement projects" and "how the degree of devastation impacts the way participants are recruited" (O'Mathúna 2010, p. 67). Needless to say, informed consent is an expectation of nearly all human subject research, and coercion should be avoided at all costs. Although some potential subjects can be "so traumatized by a disaster that their decision-making capacity is impaired," that does not mean that disaster survivors as a group are incapable of consenting to participate in research (O'Mathúna 2010, p. 68). In fact, many are capable of doing so (Collogan et al. 2004). As a result, disaster survivors have not been formally classified as a "vulnerable" population under the Common Rule (45 CFR 46). Nevertheless, disaster survivors are likely at higher risk of consenting under duress than is the average potential research subject. Studies have consistently demonstrated that a small subset of disaster survivors are indeed retraumatized by study participation, although there is no indication that this phenomenon is widespread (Boscarino et al. 2004). Under the circumstances, disaster survivors should not be used as a population of convenience when conducting research. Rather, research should be conducted in disaster settings only when no other population of study that will generate similar data is available.

Physician Welfare

Disaster relief workers, including mental health providers, "are at risk for compassion fatigue, burnout, and vicarious traumatization" (Math et al. 2015, p. 265). Psychiatrists should not forget their ethical obligation to address personal wellness and maintain their own well-being so they can remain in a position to assist others. Reflecting on one's motives for offering disaster assistance and having realistic expectations of oneself are essential if one is to serve the public well over the long term.

Unfortunately, the pressures of disaster care can lead well-intentioned physicians to engage in ethical breaches (Pandya 2010). For instance, positive countertransference may lead a provider to exaggerate a victim's symptoms when documenting an evaluation. Psychiatrists may be tempted to prescribe scheduled substances such as benzodiazepines and opioids without conducting appropriate due diligence. Boundary crossings that would never occur during regular practice, such as giving a patient one's home telephone number, may then lead to boundary violations.

Psychiatrists providing disaster care should make use of mental health resources for themselves as necessary and should discuss any emotional challenges with colleagues. Isolation is a particularly dangerous phenomenon when providing disaster relief, and effective caregiving requires connectedness with one's own needs and with one's fellow caregivers.

Conclusion

Disaster psychiatry has grown into a distinct field since its origins in the 1970s, and the demand for mental health providers in crisis settings continues to grow. Such work can be among the most fulfilling available to psychiatrists. However, that does not mean that disaster psychiatry is without legal risks and ethical responsibilities. Many of the ethical expectations that disaster psychiatrists confront are similar to those that they face in ordinary practice, including maintaining confidentiality, respecting boundaries, and ensuring continuity of care. Other expectations, such as navigating media inquiries and avoiding unnecessary collaboration with repressive regimes, may be distinct to their role as disaster providers. In any setting in which disaster services are provided, psychiatrists must be careful to define their roles, be certain of their legal authority to provide care, and verify their insurance coverage. At the same time, psychiatrists should be careful not to let unfounded or excessive fears of hypothetical liability deter them from engaging in important work. Key takeaways are provided in Table 9–1.

TABLE 9–1. Teaching points

- Laws and ethical standards governing disaster psychiatry differ from those governing emergency psychiatry, and psychiatrists must be aware of legal and ethical expectations in the jurisdiction in which they are rendering services. They should also be certain of their legal authority to act in the jurisdiction and that they are covered by liability insurance for their services.

- Psychiatrists are bound by federal and state laws regarding confidentiality in disaster settings and must take measures to ensure that personal health information is secure.

- Adequate documentation is an ethical imperative that both protects providers from liability and affords necessary evidence to victims pursuing postdisaster claims.

- In providing international disaster relief, practitioners must be sure to act only on behalf of their patients and strive to avoid collaborations with repressive governments that result in whitecoat washing.

- Disaster psychiatry is a scarce resource, and psychiatrists must take steps to ensure that this resource is allocated equitably, especially in light of historic patterns of discrimination.

- Although disaster subjects are not a "vulnerable" population under federal guidelines and are capable of consent, they nonetheless are at risk of acting under duress and should not be used for research as a population of convenience.

- Burnout raises the risk of ethical breaches during disaster care.

References

Ali S, Jabeen S, Alam F: Multimodal approach to identifying malingered posttraumatic stress disorder: a review. Innov Clin Neurosci 12(1–2):12–20, 2015 25852974

American Medical Association: Opinion 8.3: physicians' responsibilities in disaster response and preparedness, in AMA Code of Medical Ethics. Available at: https://code-medical-ethics.ama-assn.org/ethics-opinions/physicians-responsibilities-disaster-response-preparedness. Accessed April 1, 2024.

Appel JM: Against whitecoat washing: the need for formal human rights assessment in international collaborations. Am J Bioeth 22(10):1–4, 2022 36170066

Boscarino JA, Figley CR, Adams RE, et al: Adverse reactions associated with studying persons recently exposed to mass urban disaster. J Nerv Ment Dis 192(8):515–524, 2004 15387153

Collogan LK, Tuma F, Dolan-Sewell R, et al: Ethical issues pertaining to research in the aftermath of disaster. J Trauma Stress 17(5):363–372, 2004 15633915

Connor M: America's sordid legacy on race and disaster recovery. Washington, DC, Center for American Progress, April 5, 2018. Available at: www.americanprogress.org/issues/race/news/2018/04/05/448999/americas-sordid-legacy-race-disaster-recovery. Accessed April 1, 2024.

Disla de Jesus V, Appel JM: A call for asylum evaluation and advocacy in forensic psychiatry. J Am Acad Psychiatry Law 50(3):342–345, 2022 37824295

Federal Regulation 45 CFR 46: Protection of Human Subjects, 1981

Flavelle C: Why does disaster aid often favor white people? New York Times, June 7, 2021. Available at: www.nytimes.com/2021/06/07/climate/FEMA-race-climate.html. Accessed April 1, 2024.

Health Insurance Portability and Accountability Act of 1996, Pub L No 104-191, 110 Stat. 1936, 1996

Joshi PT, Dalton ME, O'Donnell DA: Ethical issues in local, national, and international disaster psychiatry. Child Adolesc Psychiatr Clin N Am 17(1):165–185, x–xi, 2008 18036485

Kocak H, Kinik K, Caliskan C, et al: The science of disaster medicine: from response to risk reduction. Medeniyet Med J 36(4):333–342, 2021 34939400

Kim J: Why people lie about 9/11. New York Post, September 20, 2015. Available at: https://nypost.com/2015/09/20/a-psychiatrist-on-why-people-lie-about-911. Accessed April 1, 2024.

Math SB, Nirmala MC, Moirangthem S, et al: Disaster management: mental health perspective. Indian J Psychol Med 37(3):261–271, 2015 26664073

Mullangi S, Agrawal M, Schulman K: The COVID-19 pandemic: an opportune time to update medical licensing. JAMA Intern Med 181(3):307–308, 2021 33439224

Ninivaggi FJ: Malingering, in Kaplan and Sadock's Comprehensive Textbook of Psychiatry, 9th Edition, Vol 2. Edited by Sadock BJ, Sadock VA, Ruiz P. Philadelphia, PA, Lippincott Williams & Wilkins, 2016, pp 2479–2490

O'Mathúna DP: Conducting research in the aftermath of disasters: ethical considerations. J Evid Based Med 3(2):65–75, 2010 21349047

Pandya A: Personal accounts: reconsidering the role of a disaster psychiatrist. Psychiatr Serv 61(5):449–450, 2010 20439363

Stanglin D, Rice D: At Least 26 Dead as Historic Floods Sweep West Virginia. USA Today, June 25, 2016. Available at: www.usatoday.com/story/news/2016/06/24/2-dead-floods-sweep-west-virginia/86329316. Accessed April 1, 2024.

Van Cleave K: Trooper: Flood-Damaged West Virginia Looks Like a War Zone. CBS News, June 25, 2016. Available at: www.cbsnews.com/news/flood-damaged-west-virginia-looks-like-a-war-zone. Accessed April 1, 2024.

Volunteer Protection Act of 1997, Pub L 105-19, 42 USC sec 14501, 1997

Zoraster RM, Burkle CM: Disaster documentation for the clinician. Disaster Med Public Health Prep 7(4):354–360, 2013 24229517

10

Historical, Sociocultural, and Political Considerations

Giuseppe Raviola, M.D., M.P.H.
Vinh-Son Nguyen, M.D.
Frederick J. Stoddard Jr., M.D.

Disaster psychiatry has evolved from responses to local community and natural disasters, such as fires and floods, to today addressing a broader range of complex crises. Knowledge and systems to prepare for and respond to disasters were not available until the late twentieth century. Disasters have often resulted in feelings of helplessness as well as lack of medical and psychiatric care for those afflicted. Mental health concerns can often be an afterthought in the planning of responses to disasters and crises. For example, development assistance funding for mental health in global health settings remains very low. There is therefore a need to optimize opportunities, funding, and existing resources to efficiently and effectively prepare for and respond to crises. Although our capacity to respond has improved on the basis of learning from specific events, as well as growth in the study of disasters and disaster response, the nature of the threats has also shifted. Consideration of broad historical, sociocultural, and political dimensions regarding both the contexts within which disasters occur and the populations that are affected stands to inform our abilities as mental health and health professionals to respond to disasters effectively. This understanding can enhance our capacity to use best practices, optimally mobilize available resources, and minimize the risk of unintentional harm.

Given the lack of predictability and the broadening scope of disasters, from a public health perspective, all psychiatrists today might be appropriately considered *disaster psychiatrists*. With regard to existing formal mental health care delivery, all countries are "developing," including high-income countries such as the United States, where clinicians work in the context of inadequate social supports and safety nets for the people they serve. Yet the relative extreme lack of basic resources in lower-income countries has created a false divide in perceptions of need and impact between richer and poorer nations and neighborhoods. The presence of basic resources, including food, shelter, and public safety, as emphasized by the Inter-Agency Standing Committee (IASC), the longest-standing and highest-level humanitarian coordination forum of the United Nations (UN) system, remain critical to mitigating the impacts of disasters on communities across all contexts (Inter-Agency Standing Committee 2023). When disasters happen, psychiatrists more often than not work in a situation of *acute on chronic* need, in terms of crises being overlaid on top of inadequate existing care delivery systems for the broad range of untreated, existing mental health conditions. A summary of some historical, sociocultural, and political perspectives on disaster response is provided here in order to inspire curiosity and engagement with the challenge and to make easier the work of psychiatrists in disaster readiness and response.

Historical Perspectives

The chronological progression of community and worldwide devastations over the past quarter-century requires that the field of psychiatry reflect on the evolving definition and progression of disasters and crises. The evolution of disasters to those caused by climate change and other new threats is altering our understanding of the meanings and scope of disaster psychiatry. In the decade prior to the coronavirus disease 2019 (COVID-19) pandemic, global health was moving past a stage of development assistance into an era of greater global cooperation and increasing focus on fragile states; the poorest communities; and global public goods, including health security and innovation (Pablos-Méndez and Raviglione 2018). COVID-19 caused significant disruptions to various

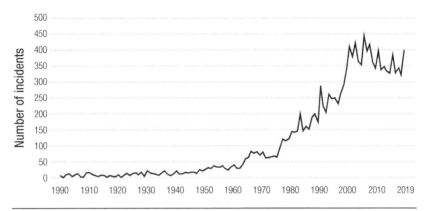

FIGURE 10–1. Trend in number of natural disasters, 1900–2019.

Source. Institute for Economics and Peace 2020, p. 49. Used with permission.

kinds of progress in global health and health care delivery. COVID-19 in the context of evolving climate change continues to present a unique moment for humanity, in which the universal pandemic (and climate) threat has brought a sense of shared experience, transcending national boundaries and identities. Concurrently, a narrative of national threat across all countries during the pandemic legitimized unprecedented political measures of physical distancing and lockdown. This led to a focus on reactive emergency measures and a perpetual cycle of making health a concern of national and local security (Sondermann and Ulbert 2020). By extension, the politicization of disasters and varied government emergency stances on COVID-19 globally have deepened authoritarianism, nationalism, prejudice, and support of antidemocratic political systems (Deason and Dunn 2022).

Regarding disasters in general, over the past century, the trend in number has been upward, with a tenfold increase since 1960 (Figure 10–1). The United States, China, India, and the Philippines have been impacted by the greatest number of *climate-related* disasters over the past 30 years, with floods and storms the most common natural disaster per year, accounting for 71% of the disasters since 1990 (Table 10–1).

With the advancing of climate change, poorer countries bear the greatest burdens in terms of water and food scarcity. This has driven the migration of peoples in historic numbers. Since 2008, displacement of populations directly from acute natural disasters has been greatest in low-income countries, specifically countries in Asia (Table 10–2). The Institute for Economics and Peace estimates that 1.2 billion people live in coun-

TABLE 10–1. Countries with the greatest number of climate disasters, 1990–2019

	Drought	Extreme temperature	Flood	Storm	Wildfire	Total
United States	14	20	145	444	81	704
China	31	13	246	264	6	560
India	7	39	216	110	3	375
Philippines	6	0	123	219	1	349
Bangladesh	1	22	65	108	0	196
Indonesia	3	0	170	5	11	189
Vietnam	6	0	85	90	1	182
Mexico	5	14	52	87	3	161
Australia	5	7	45	66	28	151
Japan	0	16	27	103	1	147
Russia	5	21	66	21	24	137
Brazil	10	4	95	10	4	123
France	2	18	41	56	6	123
Pakistan	2	15	84	20	0	121
Thailand	12	2	68	33	1	116
Afghanistan	5	7	85	9	1	107
Haiti	5	0	45	34	0	84
Canada	0	4	33	28	17	82
Argentina	4	7	48	16	4	79
Colombia	2	0	68	5	3	78

Source. Institute for Economics and Peace 2020, p. 50.

tries, particularly in sub-Saharan Africa, the Middle East and North Africa, and South and Central Asia, where societal resilience is insufficient to withstand the impact of ecological threats between now and 2050, placing them at immediate risk of displacement (Figure 10–2).

The definition of disasters has broadened over time to encompass natural disasters (e.g., earthquakes, floods, fires, hurricanes, tsunamis); major disease outbreaks, (e.g., pandemics and epidemics, including outbreaks of animal diseases passing to humans); mass violence (e.g., confrontation, conflict, warfare, child soldiers, peacekeeping, terrorism and threats of terrorism, active shooter incidents, riots); human-made disasters (e.g., climate change leading to natural disasters); technological disasters (e.g., failed systems; equipment and engineering failures); and chemical, biologi-

TABLE 10–2. Countries with the largest number of displacements by acute disaster event, 2008–2019

	Year	Disaster type	Displacements
China	2010	Flood	15,200,000
China	2008	Earthquake	15,000,000
Pakistan	2010	Flood	11,000,000
India	2012	Flood	6,900,000
Philippines	2013	Typhoon Haiyan	4,095,280
Nigeria	2012	Flood	3,871,063
China	2011	Flood	3,514,000
Philippines	2014	Typhoon Rammasun	2,994,054
India	2019	Flood	2,623,349
Nepal	2015	Earthquake	2,622,733
Cuba	2008	Storm	2,616,000
Philippines	2016	Typhoon Nock-Ten	2,592,251
India	2009	Flood	2,500,000
India	2008	Flood	2,400,000
Philippines	2016	Typhoon Haima	2,376,723
India	2009	Cyclone Aila	2,300,000
Myanmar	2008	Storm	2,250,000
Bangladesh	2019	Cyclone Bulbul	2,106,918
India	2008	Flood	2,100,000
China	2019	Typhoon Lekima	2,097,000
China	2012	Storm	2,079,000
India	2008	Flood	2,055,925
Philippines	2008	Storm	2,039,155
Chile	2010	Earthquake	2,000,000
India	2012	Flood	2,000,000
China	2016	Flood	1,990,000
India	2018	Flood	1,967,258
Philippines	2012	Storm	1,931,970
United States	2008	Storm	1,900,000
Pakistan	2012	Flood	1,856,570
Philippines	2014	Typhoon Hagupit	1,823,176

Source. Institute for Economics and Peace 2020, p. 53.

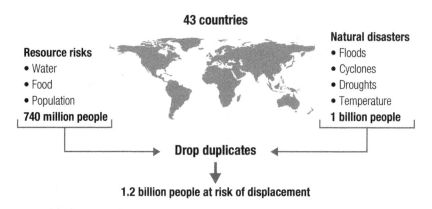

FIGURE 10–2. Current risk of ecological threat and displacement from acute and chronic disaster events.

Source.   Institute for Economics and Peace 2020, p. 8.

cal, radiological, and nuclear disasters across all global contexts. Major disease outbreaks since the twentieth century have included Spanish flu (1918–1920), polio (1920–1955), HIV/AIDS (1981 to present), severe acute respiratory syndrome (SARS; 2002–2004), H1N1 (2009), Ebola (2013–2016), Zika (2015–2016), and COVID-19 (2020–2023). A chronological review of seminal large-scale events over the past 50 years yields stunning impacts on human lives in terms of mortality and morbidity, as well as a remarkable breadth of lived experience, human suffering, and traumatic impacts on the human psyche (Table 10–3). In considering and mourning the nearly 6.9 million people globally who died from COVID-19 within the first 3 years of the pandemic, we gain some perspective by recalling that the Black Death (1347–1351) caused 200 million deaths and that in the twentieth century, 78 million people died in Mao-era China (1949–1976), 72 million people died in World War II (1938–1945), 65 million people died in World War I (1914–1918), and the HIV/AIDS epidemic has taken 40 million lives since 1981.

The 2020–2023 COVID-19 pandemic exacerbated the global challenge of mental health, highlighting preexisting inequities in availability of mental health services for individuals and families with fewer economic resources and raising awareness of the need for functional, accessible systems of care delivery to supplement response to crises and emergencies. The universality of the COVID-19 pandemic experience globally has pointed toward seemingly unprecedented global challenges as well as to our interconnectedness, with implications for how we observe and engage

TABLE 10–3. Chronology of selected disasters over the past half-century

Event	Year(s)	Number of deaths
Mount Saint Helens eruption, Washington State (United States)	1980	57
Iran-Iraq War	1980–88	700,000
Somali Civil War	1981 to present	1,000,000
HIV/AIDS pandemic	1981 to present	40,000,000
Bhopal poison gas leak (India)	1984	20,000
Chernobyl nuclear disaster (Soviet Union)	1986	30
Israel-Palestine conflict since the First Intifada	1987 to present	54,903
Manjil-Rudbar earthquake (Iran)	1990	45,000
Bangladesh cyclone	1991	138,000
Rwanda genocide	1994	1,000,000
U.S. Embassy bombings (Kenya and Tanzania)	1998	224
Tiananmen Square crackdown (China)	1989	5,000
Second Congo War (Democratic Republic of Congo)	1998–2003	3,800,000
Oklahoma City bombing (United States)	1999	168
Columbine High School massacre (United States)	1999	15
September 11 World Trade Center terrorist attack (United States)	2001	2,996
U.S. war in Afghanistan	2001–2021	212,000 (2,448 U.S. deaths)
Iraq War	2003–2011	306,000 (4,400 U.S. deaths)
Indian Ocean tsunami (Sri Lanka, India, Indonesia, Thailand, Maldives)	2004	225,000

TABLE 10–3. Chronology of selected disasters over the past half-century (*continued*)

Event	Year(s)	Number of deaths
Hurricane Katrina, Louisiana (United States)	2005	1,392
Kashmir earthquake (Pakistan)	2005	73,276
Cyclones Sidr and Nargis (Bangladesh, India, Myanmar)	2007–2008	32,500
Sichuan earthquake (China)	2008	87,000
Haiti earthquake	2010	316,000
Russian heat wave and forest fires	2010	50,000
Fukushima tsunami and nuclear disaster (Japan)	2011	18,500 deaths
Syrian Civil War	2011 to present	613,000
Sandy Hook Elementary School shooting (United States)	2012	27
Garment factory collapse (Bangladesh)	2013	1,134
Yemen Civil War	2014 to present	377,000
Ebola outbreaks (Guinea, Liberia, Sierra Leone)	2013–2016	11,323
Hurricane Maria (Puerto Rico, United States)	2017	3,059
Australia wildfire	2019–2020	450
Tigray War (Ethiopia)	2020–2022	800,000
COVID-19 pandemic	2020–2023	6,887,000 (1,117,054 U.S. deaths)
Russian invasion of Ukraine	2022 to present	372,820
European heat waves	2022	20,000
Turkey-Syria earthquake	2023	57,759

Note.　COVID-19=coronavirus disease 2019.

with disasters as they are occurring, in real time. All of these events, and our increasing exposure to them, seem to be raising concern regarding our existential condition as a species and our sense of safety and threat in the world (Spitzenstätter and Schnell 2022). Mental health professionals are in a position to interpret this existential anxiety and to support those suffering from it (Pashak et al. 2022).

The field of disaster psychiatry emerged from the experience of U.S. military psychiatry in the major wars of the twentieth century; the writings of Erich Lindemann, M.D., in seeking to understand within psychiatry the meanings of and responses to the 1942 Cocoanut Grove Fire disaster in Boston (Cobb and Lindemann 1943); the emergence of posttraumatic stress disorder in the *Diagnostic and Statistical Manual of Mental Disorders,* 3rd Edition (DSM-III) as a direct result of the Vietnam War (American Psychiatric Association 1980); and research following major events, including the Oklahoma City bombing (1995), the September 11 attack on the World Trade Center in New York (2001), Hurricane Katrina (2005), and multiple mass shootings from Columbine (1999) to Sandy Hook (2012) to the present.

Research evidence on disasters and resilience collected through these experiences has shown that positive mental health outcomes are related to the finding that most persons are generally resilient and manifest few or no long-term adverse health outcomes. Predictors of psychological resistance or resilience include availability of psychosocial resources and absence of preexisting vulnerabilities, including mental health disorders and genetic risk factors. Risk factors include the level of trauma exposure, and protective factors include exposure to early, brief psychosocial interventions (Boscarino 2015). Mental health policies inclusive of disaster preparedness, informed by better characterization of disaster type and classification and by disaster psychiatry research, are increasingly supporting planned and funded psychiatric readiness, evaluation, and treatment, both nationally and internationally (Below and Wallemacq 2018; Pfefferbaum and North 2020). This includes meeting child and adolescent needs as well. The current moment, however, challenges us to advance research in disaster mental health and psychiatry to meet the complex and rapidly evolving nature of the crises of the future.

Discussions about disasters in the U.S. context invite discussion about our prioritization of additional long-standing public health crises. In the United States in 2021, there were 48,800 gun deaths, 54% of which were suicides (Centers for Disease Control and Prevention 2023). Federal Bureau of Investigation data show a clear increase in casualties from active shooter incidents in the United States over the past 20 years, with a neg-

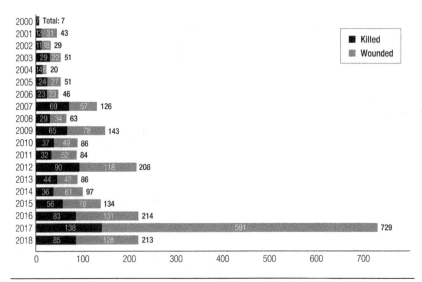

FIGURE 10–3. Active shooter incidents in the United States, 2000–2018.

Source.   Federal Bureau of Investigation 2018.

ative feedback loop between popular fear, gun ownership, and increased frequency and severity of incidents (Figure 10–3). As shown in Figure 10–4, more Americans have died from guns in the United States since 1968 than on battlefields of all the wars in American history (Kristof 2015). This represents a form of community disaster in the United States that requires its own specific public health and policy approach.

Another example of a grinding, longitudinal community disaster in the United States is the neglect, abuse, chronic disease, untreated mental illness, and premature deaths of the homeless population, all of which were recently exacerbated by COVID-19 (Koh and Gorman 2023). These concerns provoke additional questions with regard to our prioritization and collective urgency regarding ongoing public health and community crises, disasters, and emergencies.

With regard to the growing burden of mental disorders, which doubled globally in the quarter-century before the pandemic, COVID-19 increased the prevalence of major depressive disorder and anxiety disorders, which disproportionally affected young people and women (Santomauro et al. 2021). Increased levels of intimate partner violence, substance abuse, and complication of medical and psychiatric problems in the context of COVID-19 contributed to the emergence of the notion of *pandemics within the pandemic*. Delayed medical care, lower life expectancy, deaths from

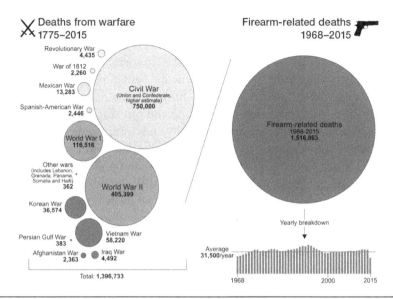

FIGURE 10–4. Comparison of U.S. mortality from warfare (1775–2015) and firearm deaths (1968–2015).

Source. Grandjean 2016.

overdoses of medications, and additional economic impacts on families have all challenged our definition of *disaster* in the postpandemic period.

It can be argued that today, COVID-19; health inequities; climate change; structural racism; and other concurrent health, economic, and social crises are intersecting as a set of epidemics to constitute an ongoing synergistic epidemic. Questions remain as to whether humanity has entered a new era of *polycrisis* with cascading global challenges spanning pandemics, climate, migration, conflict over resources, and political extremism (Lawrence et al. 2022). *Syndemic* theory, drawn from the study of the intersection of HIV/AIDS and poverty, argues that whereas all individuals experience stress, how stress is internalized and articulated is culturally indicative of context-specific causes and local, lived experiences (Mendenhall et al. 2022; Workman 2022). A syndemic approach to mental health disaster preparedness for the post-COVID future encourages organizations to take into consideration social determinants and their impact on marginalized groups more directly and aggressively, as well as to prioritize the embedding of preventive mental health programs and interventions across sectors (an *in-all-policies public health approach to mental health*) (Kienzler 2019).

Sociocultural Perspectives

The ways in which disasters and emergencies are framed, not only historically but also in terms of their relationship to social and cultural experiences, carries significant relevance to how the field of psychiatry positions itself to address the challenges of the future with a person-centered approach. The conceptualization of trauma and our reactions to stress, for example, are to a significant degree socially and culturally determined. The description and definition of disasters as they relate to human traumatic experience are embedded within sociocultural and political contexts and reflect a variety of discourses that are applicable to these concepts, as well as to our individual and collective responses to them. As we engage with the populations most vulnerable to ongoing disasters—people living in low-income regions of the world and economically disadvantaged populations in high-income countries—the place of culture and local context takes on more immediate relevance in designing responses and in supporting and enhancing community resilience. Attending to discrimination and long-standing gaps in equitable access to services and resources in less advantaged communities requires greater collective action. The American Psychiatric Association's *Clinical Manual of Cultural Psychiatry*, 2nd Edition (Lim 2015) provides foundational guidance on assessment of culturally diverse individuals and cultural formulation that are relevant in the context of responding to disasters.

A *social medicine* perspective enriches our understanding of disaster response and mental health by emphasizing the ways in which social and cultural factors can influence the suffering and lived experience of others, as well as the interventions that are developed to address crises and disasters (Trout and Kleinman 2020). Kleinman (2010) has described four social theories for global health:

1. *The unintended consequences of purposive (or social) action*—This theory is often applicable in the context of mental health and psychosocial response when describing how the humanitarian apparatus frames response and victimhood and the political economy of humanitarian action in the context of crises and disasters (e.g., international organizations profiting financially from claiming expertise in the support of specific, vulnerable populations).
2. *The social construction of reality*—This theory includes the ways in which we choose to describe psychological distress as "either-or" and categorically, such as through diagnosis using DSM-5-TR (American Psychiatric Association 2022) or the ICD-10, rather than dimension-

ally and transdiagnostically, that is, a solely clinical approach rather than blending public health and clinical approaches.

3. *Social suffering*—Suffering can be caused by the illness experience, emergencies and crises, or slower socioeconomic and sociopolitical forces and the experience of poverty. It also can be informed by the ways in which institutions and health care delivery systems that are developed to respond to suffering can potentially make suffering worse.

4. *Biopower*—Biopower can be described as the many ways in which political and economic governance exert control over populations.

These theories offer a guidepost in considering each crisis, individually and in context, and how to most effectively mobilize available resources while minimizing the risk of unintentional harm to individuals and communities.

The term *trauma* has most commonly been used to refer to an event or events where an individual witnessed or was directly exposed to actual or threatened death or harm, with acute and chronic variables. Today, the term is used increasingly to describe collective as well as individual experiences of suffering in response to events. The biological approach to trauma has been driven largely by psychological research, emphasizing the physiological threat response (fight or flight) and "the complex debilitation of adaptive abilities—emotional, cognitive, physical, spiritual and social—following an event that was perceived by our nervous system as life-threatening to oneself or others (especially loved ones)" (Kraybill 2019). This includes dimensions that are emotional (e.g., feelings of fear, anger, hopelessness, shame, guilt, foreshortened sense of future), cognitive (compromising thought processing, memory, and judgment), physical (having a broad range of effects, including neurological, muscular, metabolic, sleep, and immune system), spiritual (impacts on worldview such as the world being unsafe, questioning the meaning of life), and social (affecting relationships with loved ones and friends such as a sense of separation or isolation as well as strangers, such as lack of trust) (Kraybill 2019).

The tendency of the field of psychiatry toward binary diagnostic systems as opposed to dimensional, transdiagnostic interpretations of suffering that blend clinical and public health approaches can lead to the overmedicalization of disasters and public health crises. The psychiatric approach to trauma has tended to emphasize illness over resilience and a biopsychosocial perspective, with an emphasis on mental disorders as treatable entities. The binary worldview, with its emphasis on "caseness" and illness, has also had implications for access and funding of services. In humanitarian settings, for example, an overemphasis on traumatic illness and diagnosis by clinical experts in the field has fed a political economy of trauma and "trauma portfolios" by organizations seeking to raise funds for their efforts, to financially benefit a growing humanitarian market (James 2010, p. 33). This can be reinforced by the pharmaceutical industry and its influence, which can continue to draw resources away from building human resource capacity to deliver needed evidence-based psychological interventions predisaster and postdisaster for task-shared, nonspecialist-delivered psychosocial interventions and for needed social support (Clark 2014).

Culturally, there has been an expansion of accepted definitions of trauma and crisis. *Community crisis* refers to any event leading to an unstable and dangerous situation affecting a community, with implications for physiological stress response and the development of mental disorders. *Intersectionality*, a more recent concept, describes the social, personal, and political contexts in which trauma is experienced and the ways that various forms of discrimination overlap, especially in the experiences of marginalized individuals and groups (Ezell et al. 2021). According to Ezell et al., the psychosocial marginalization of individuals across various overlapping axes of identity, including race, ethnicity, gender, nativity status, religion, sexual orientation, mental health status, first language, immigration status, disability status, neurodivergence, and body size, can be described with the term *intersectional trauma*.

The intersectionality of trauma requires interdisciplinary, collaborative action by psychiatrists and other mental health professionals as leaders, across local and global contexts. Today, the concepts of collective and intergenerational trauma—and resilience—have also evolved (Hirschberger 2018; Matoba 2023; Mokline and Ben Abdallah 2022). *Collective trauma* refers to events that are cataclysmic with regard to loss of life but also cause a crisis of meaning and in the social construction of meaning (Hirschberger 2018). *Intergenerational trauma* refers to the effects of serious untreated trauma that has been experienced by one or more members of a family, group, or community and has been passed down from one generation to the next through epigenetic factors. In Rwanda, for example, there is now evidence of genomic impact of violence exposure not only in survivors of the 1994 genocide of the Tutsi but also in their children due to violence exposure during the perinatal period (Musanabaganwa et al. 2022). *Collective resilience* refers to the adaptability of social behavior and the evolution of a sense of collective continuity as a source of social motivation in times of crisis (Mokline and Ben Abdallah 2022).

The field of global health offers another relevant area of discourse. *Global health* prioritizes improving health and achieving health equity for people around the globe (Koplan et al. 2009). The field of *global mental health* has focused on reducing mental health disparities between and within nations and seeking innovative community-based, systemic solutions to increase access to care (Patel and Prince 2010). It is increasingly acknowledged that global health is a field grounded in and ideally responsive to the history of colonialism (Abimbola and Pai 2020). Acknowledging the legacies of the history of colonialism and genocide on Indigenous peoples worldwide, as well as the ongoing impacts of these histories, leads to actions to correct the structures that continue to perpetuate them; to seek to make reparation for these past wrongs; and, at a minimum, to learn how to not reenact them.

The fields of global health and disaster mental health have advanced the concepts of *mental health and psychosocial support* (MHPSS). The UN High Commission for Refugees describes MHPSS activity as any type of local or outside support that seeks to protect or promote psychosocial well-being and to prevent or treat mental disorders in the context of emergency responses (United Nations High Commission for Refugees 2023). The concept of leadership to enhance societal resilience in the face of new threats has included incorporating practices drawn from the field of global health, including *task sharing* of a wide range of counseling and preventive approaches that can be modified and delivered by clergy, community health workers, teachers, peers, parents, and other community members, with coaching and support from mental health clinicians (Belkin 2020). From a historical perspective, this also represents a shift in who is being engaged formally as responders as civilians across all settings are increasingly impacted by disasters and now engaged in providing response and support.

As disasters and disaster response become increasingly transnational in scope, efforts are being made to respond to crises with specific attention to the historical and cultural context of affected groups. This context includes the following (Tankink et al. 2023):

- The history of politics and prior conflicts
- Ethnicity and diversity
- Identity and sociocultural context
- The constitution of family and community
- The self and the concept of the person
- Cultural conceptualization of the life cycle and becoming an adult
- Death and burial
- Gender roles and gender relations
- Manifestations of psychosocial distress in context, including somatic manifestations, cultural concepts of mental illness, and idioms of distress

- Cultural manifestations of communal distress
- Cultural conceptualization of severe (psychotic) mental health concerns and emotional distress, including overwhelming sadness and grief, which can lead to local forms of depression and anxiety

Religion and spirituality are factors that must also be considered contextually as they relate to mental health during disasters because of the overwhelming presence of religious and spiritual beliefs and practices around the world, as well as the capacity for religious and spiritual beliefs to support individuals and families in making meaning of the events impacting their lives (Sen et al. 2022).

Political Perspectives

Effectively mobilizing mental health and psychiatric responses to the increasing frequency of disasters of various kinds requires direct and urgent political engagement and action. Psychiatrists and other mental health professionals in the public realm serve as effective leaders and communicators with patients, allied health professionals, politicians, and the public (Koh et al. 2021). An understanding of major political commitments, global and domestic, and of the political governance and frameworks that surround responses to disasters can be useful. When disasters occur, social safety nets established by governments can mitigate some of the longer-term impacts and serve as a key to recovery. As an example, Germany, France, Britain, Canada, and some other high-income countries provide social insurance or universal health care, whereas in the United States, persons receiving mental health care through Medicare, Medicaid, and private insurers represent about 90% of the population, leaving about 30 million people uninsured, varying by state (U.S. Census Bureau 2022). Working to bolster social supports in between disasters and crises is an important area for political action by psychiatrists.

Several international and national organizations and documents have shaped disaster response. The UN Office of the High Commissioner for Human Rights is mandated to protect all human rights for all people. The UN Universal Declaration of Human Rights, with 30 articles approved in 1948, was a powerful statement after the devastation of World War II and remains so today (United Nations 1948). Article 25, adopted in the wake of that war, states:

1. Everyone has the right to a standard of living adequate for the health and well-being of himself and his family, including food, clothing, housing, and medical care and necessary social services,

and the right to security in the event of unemployment, sickness, disability, widowhood, old age or other lack of livelihood in circumstances beyond his control.
2. Motherhood and childhood are entitled to special care and assistance. All children, whether born in or out of wedlock, shall enjoy the same amount of protection.

Disaster psychiatry aims to address and seek to aid afflicted populations in accord with UN human rights doctrine and the aims of the World Health Organization, the International Red Cross, and (in the United States), the Federal Emergency Management Agency (FEMA). The UN Office for the Coordination of Humanitarian Affairs (OCHA) was created in 1998 to assist governments in mobilizing international assistance when the scale of a disaster exceeds national capacity. OCHA manages several tools to facilitate coordination of multiple actors and resources through the UN Cluster approach (see Chapter 7, "Engaging in Disaster Response"), a forum of the most experienced relief agencies. Its aim is to strengthen partnerships and ensure more predictability and accountability in international responses to humanitarian emergencies by clarifying the division of labor among organizations and to better define their roles and responsibilities within the key sectors of the response.

Initiated in 1997, Sphere (https://spherestandards.org/about) is a worldwide community—a collaboration with leading nongovernmental organizations, interested donor governments, and UN agencies—that brings together and empowers practitioners to improve the quality and accountability of humanitarian assistance. Sphere describes a set of minimum standards to be attained in disaster assistance in each of five key sectors: water supply and sanitation, nutrition, food aid, shelter, and health services. Sphere also includes indicators for mental and social aspects of health (United Nations High Commission for Refugees 2011).

The IASC, created in 1992 by the UN, has served as an interagency forum for coordination, policy development, and decision-making involving key UN and non-UN humanitarian partners. The IASC MHPSS Reference Group was established in 2007, with a main purpose to support and advocate for the implementation of the 2007 IASC Guidelines. The Reference Group consists of more than 30 members and fosters a unique collaboration between nongovernmental organizations, the UN, and international agencies and academics, promoting best practices in MHPSS (Inter-Agency Standing Committee 2023).

Additional international guidance has been developed to support the implementation of effective and consistent practices in disaster mental health response. Given the high need of mental health services after disasters and the limited availability of mental health practitioners, a strategic stepped model of care called the Psychosocial Care for People Affected by Disasters and Major Incidents, developed in 2008, has been adopted as nonbinding guidance by North Atlantic Treaty Organization (NATO) countries (North Atlantic Treaty Organization 2008). The Royal College of Psychiatrists in the United Kingdom subsequently brought together work undertaken in Europe with the World Health Organization, NATO Guidance, and the IASC Guidelines to produce a set of basic principles for disaster and major incident psychosocial care, informed by the best evidence available at the time (McFarlane and Williams 2012; Williams et al. 2014). This guidance identified four basic levels of interventions to address the psychosocial needs of people after a disaster (Table 10–4). It details the target population for each level, examples of possible interventions, and who should conduct each intervention, ultimately stratifying appropriate care from generally everyone affected by a disaster to people with sustained distress and functional impairment (McFarlane and Williams 2012). Schools are vital for community development after large-scale events because they offer stability, safety, mental health support, continuity in education, and a hub for resource distribution and community cohesion. Children need a sense of consistency and normalcy to acclimate after a disaster, which school can provide.

Since the NATO guidance was adopted, there have been ongoing efforts to translate lessons learned through research and best practice experience in integrated ways into policy at four levels, with cultural and ethical values permeating each level of policy and planning: 1) government policies, 2) strategic policies for service design, 3) service delivery policies, and 4) policies for good clinical practice (McFarlane and Williams 2012). It is increasingly understood that for implementation of best practices in societies, government policies should set the aims and objectives for psychosocial and mental health care responses, specifying the requirements for services to be designed, developed, and delivered, offering mental health care that is integrated into all disaster response plans, adapting knowledge to the society, cultures, and risk profiles of populations (Williams et al. 2014). Mental health services for moderate- and large-scale emergencies should be well integrated with humanitarian aid, welfare, and psychosocial care in disaster response plans.

Beyond the concept of a collaborative stepped-care approach that bridges services and support both outside and within the health sector (and across all sectors) during crises lies an increasing commitment to *building back better*. Ten key lessons learned over the past several decades of responding to disasters should be taken as opportunities to strengthen health systems (Epping-Jordan et al. 2015). These lessons are as follows:

TABLE 10–4. Summary of recommended interventions in the aftermath of disasters based on WHO, NATO, and IASC guidance

Level	Intervention	Target population	Examples of interventions	Who should conduct interventions
1	Psychological First Aid	Most of the people who are affected	• Restoring immediate safety • Restoring contact with loved ones	All responders and aid workers
2	Community development	Communities after large-scale events	• Schools, sports, and meetings • Newsletters to unite groups of people	All responders and aid workers
3	Skills for Psychosocial Recovery	People whose distress is sustained by bereavement or secondary stressors	• Brief needs assessment • Problem-solving • Social support	Health care practitioners and workers trained in the skills
4	Psychosocial interventions for medium- and long-term problems	People whose distress is sustained and associated with functional impairment	• Trauma-focused cognitive-behavioral therapy	Staff of mental health care facilities

Note. IASC=Inter-Agency Standing Committee; NATO=North Atlantic Treaty Organization; WHO=World Health Organization.
Source. McFarlane and Williams 2012.

1. Mental health reform should be supported through planning for long-term sustainability from the outset.
2. The broad mental health needs of the emergency-affected population must be addressed.
3. The government's central role should be respected.
4. National professionals play a key role.
5. Coordination across agencies is crucial.
6. Mental health reform involves review and revision of national policies and plans.
7. The mental health system should be considered and strengthened as a whole.
8. Health workers need to be reorganized and trained.
9. Demonstration projects offer proof of concept and attract further support and funds for mental health reform.
10. Advocacy helps to maintain momentum for change.

At a global policy level, a 2020 report from the Pan American Health Organization during the height of the COVID-19 response made a number of health policy recommendations for strengthening societal mental health responses out of that crisis (Tausch et al. 2022):

1. Scale up emergency MHPSS programming to address population needs; integrate these needs into primary care, education, social services, and community support systems; and train frontline workers in WHO's Mental Health Gap Programme Intervention Guide (mhGAP-IG), mhGAP Humanitarian Intervention Guide (mhGAP-HIG), and other psychosocial interventions such as Psychological First Aid (World Health Organization 2011, 2015, 2016).
2. Improve and scale up telemental health, including infrastructure, development of policy frameworks and legislation, linked to facilitation of relevant workforce training while striving to minimize inequities.
3. Reach populations shown to be in greater need of mental health support, including frontline and health care workers, children and adolescents, women, people with preexisting mental health conditions, racial and ethnic minorities, and Indigenous peoples.
4. Increase social protections, including economic support, food and housing assistance, livelihood protection, and childcare as essential to minimize risk factors for mental health conditions for groups in situations of vulnerability.
5. Develop communication materials to promote psychosocial well-being and connect people to appropriate MHPSS services that are adapted to reach at-risk groups.

6. Implement the strategies recommended by the 2018 Lancet Commission on Global Mental Health and Sustainable Development (Patel et al. 2018), including prioritizing mental health care as an essential component of universal health coverage, strengthening public awareness and engagement of people with mental disorders, enhancing investments, guiding innovation and implementation through research, and strengthening monitoring and accountability for global mental health.

7. Advance the transition from mental health care in psychiatric hospitals to community-based care, reducing the number of long-stay beds in psychiatric institutions.

8. Implement a whole-of-society approach to MHPSS with multisectoral responses that include not only health care but collaboration with other sectors, including education, employment, housing, and social welfare, to tackle mental health risk factors exacerbated by emergencies.

9. Actively work to incorporate MHPSS into all existing and future national emergency and disaster plans, in all emergency phases (preparedness, response, and recovery) (Tausch et al. 2022).

Significant future initiatives to prevent disasters must continue to mobilize against international conflicts and climate change, as well as to support vulnerable groups in process of migration. The annual UN Framework Conventions on Climate Change (UNFCCC) serve as the formal meeting of the UNFCCC parties, or conference of the parties (COP), to assess progress in addressing climate change and to negotiate obligations for developed countries to reduce their greenhouse gas emissions. The last COP was in Glasgow, Scotland, in 2022. Progress is occurring, but not all nations, including the United States, have agreed to the climate goals set by the COP.

In response to climate change and COVID-19, seven countries in the Asia-Pacific region (Australia, Japan, China, Nepal, Sri Lanka, India, and the United States) created a collaborative platform for rigorous research, evidence-based practice, and tailored policies among disaster-affected communities known as the Asia Pacific Disaster Mental Health Network. Established in 2020, this group aimed to foster advancements and coordination of psychosocial supports and mental health service delivery, policy development, and collaborative research in the region, which has historically had the highest frequency of hazards and greatest number of people affected by disasters annually. The network set an agenda that prioritizes strengthened community engagement and improved capacity for mental health and community services to respond to the needs of disaster-affected populations as well as to integrate emerging technologies, seeking to address the impacts of climate change and to support high-risk groups. Through multidisciplinary regional partnerships, the network will contribute to effective and culturally secure intervention design and delivery, translation of evidence to support community preparedness and response, and collection of high-quality data to inform knowledge, policy, and practice specific to the Asia-Pacific region and relevant across the globe (Newnham et al. 2020).

Conclusion

We live in an era of rapid converging social and ecological change (Shultz et al. 2017). Disasters are increasing in frequency and, despite improved health and mental health resources and disaster management capabilities, often leave devastated peoples in their wake. Stepwise local and societal interventions, including in the political sphere, are necessary to address the mental health needs of populations during and after disasters while maximizing the limited availability of mental health care providers. We must prioritize a focus on vulnerable populations whose thriving is hindered by historical legacies, structural barriers, and economic disadvantage. In tandem, policies need to be developed to address multiple levels of social support from government to appropriate care from health systems, and the public needs to be mobilized to enhance community-based resilience. Evolving and improving disaster mental health research, education, and training promise to continue to inform improved mental health disaster responses. The key to unlocking this promise includes substantial collaborations across countries and agencies. Global and regional entities such as the IASC Reference Group on MHPSS in Emergency Settings and the Asia Pacific Disaster Mental Health Network serve as channels to coordinate the integration of research advancements, policy developments, and innovative models of mental health and psychosocial support, adapted to the type of crisis and context.

References

Abimbola S, Pai M: Will global health survive its decolonisation? Lancet 396(10263):1627–1628, 2020 33220735

American Psychiatric Association: Diagnostic and Statistical Manual of Mental Disorders, 3rd Edition. Washington, DC, American Psychiatric Association, 1980

American Psychiatric Association: Diagnostic and Statistical Manual of Mental Disorders, 5th Edition, Text Revision. Washington, DC, American Psychiatric Association, 2022

Belkin G: Leadership for the social climate. N Engl J Med 382(21):1975–1977, 2020 32433837

Below R, Wallemacq P: Annual Disaster Statistical Review 2017. Brussels, Centre for Research on the Epidemiology of Disasters, 2018. Available at: https://cred.be/annual-disaster-statistical-review-2017. Accessed May 5, 2023.

Boscarino JA: Community disasters, psychological trauma, and crisis intervention. Int J Emerg Ment Health 17(1):369–371, 2015 25983663

Centers for Disease Control and Prevention: All injuries. Atlanta, GA, Centers for Disease Control and Prevention, 2023. Available at: www.cdc.gov/nchs/fastats/injury.htm. Accessed May 5, 2023.

Clark J: Medicalization of global health 2: the medicalization of global mental health. Glob Health Action 7:24000, 2014 24848660

Cobb S, Lindemann E: Neuropsychiatric observations. Ann Surg 117(6):814–824, 1943 17858228

Deason G, Dunn K: Authoritarianism and perceived threat from the novel coronavirus. Int J Psychol 57(3):341–351, 2022 35118658

Epping-Jordan JE, van Ommeren M, Ashour HN, et al: Beyond the crisis: building back better mental health care in 10 emergency-affected areas using a longer-term perspective. Int J Ment Health Syst 9:15, 2015 25904981

Ezell JM, Salari S, Rooker C, et al: Intersectional trauma: COVID-19, the psychosocial contract, and America's racialized public health lineage. Traumatology (Tallahass Fla) 27(1):78–85, 2021

Federal Bureau of Investigation: Quick Look: 277 active shooter incidents in the United States from 2000 to 2018. Washington, DC, Federal Bureau of Investigation, 2018. Available at: www.fbi.gov/how-we-can-help-you/safety-resources/active-shooter-safety-resources/active-shooter-incidents-graphics. Accessed April 17, 2023.

Grandjean M: More Americans killed by guns since 1968 than in all U.S. wars. Martin Grandjean, 2016. Available at: www.martingrandjean.ch/united-states-guns-and-wars. Accessed April 17, 2023.

Hirschberger G: Collective trauma and the social construction of meaning. Front Psychol 9:1441, 2018 30147669

Institute for Economics and Peace: Ecological Threat Register 2020: Understanding Ecological Threats, Resilience and Peace. 2020. Available at: https://reliefweb.int/attachments/973d79e1-3a71-3d43-9f39-2d65abab77f7/ETR_2020_web-1.pdf. Accessed April 17, 2023.

Inter-Agency Standing Committee: IASC Reference Group on Mental Health and Psychosocial Support in Emergency Settings. Washington, DC, Inter-Agency Standing Committee, 2023. Available at: https://interagencystandingcommittee.org/iasc-reference-group-on-mental-health-and-psychosocial-support-in-emergency-settings. Accessed April 17, 2023.

James EC: Democratic Insecurities: Violence, Trauma, and Intervention in Haiti. Oakland, University of California Press, 2010, p 33

Kleinman A: Four social theories for global health. Lancet 375(9725):1518–1519, 2010 20440871

Kienzler H: Mental health in all policies in contexts of war and conflict. Lancet Public Health 4(11):e547–e548, 2019 31677773

Koh KA, Gorman BL: Reimagining institutionalization and a continuum of care for people experiencing homelessness and mental illness. JAMA 329(17):1449–1450, 2023 37036729

Koh KA, Raviola G, Stoddard FJ Jr: Psychiatry and crisis communication during COVID-19: a view from the trenches. Psychiatr Serv 72(5):615, 2021 33950743

Koplan JP, Bond TC, Merson MH, et al: Towards a common definition of global health. Lancet 373(9679):1993–1995, 2009 19493564

Kraybill O: What is trauma? Psychology Today. January 31, 2019. Available at: www.psychologytoday.com/us/blog/expressive-trauma-integration/201901/what-is-trauma. Accessed April 17, 2023.

Kristof N: Lessons from the murders of TV journalists in the Virginia shooting. New York Times, August 27, 2015. Available at: www.nytimes.com/2015/08/27/opinion/lessons-from-the-murders-of-tv-journalists-in-the-virginia-shooting.html. Accessed April 17, 2023.

Lawrence M, Janzwood S, Homer-Dixon T: What Is a Global Polycrisis? And How Is It Different From a Systemic Risk? Cascade Institute Discussion Paper No 2022-4. Victoria, BC, Canada, Cascade Institute, September 2022. Available at: https://cascadeinstitute.org/technical-paper/what-is-a-global-polycrisis. Accessed April 17, 2023.

Lim RF: Clinical Manual of Cultural Psychiatry, 2nd Edition. Washington, DC, American Psychiatric Association Publishing, 2015

Matoba K: "Measuring" collective trauma: a quantum social science approach. Integr Psychol Behav Sci 57(2):412–431, 2023 35488141

McFarlane AC, Williams R: Mental health services required after disasters: learning from the lasting effects of disasters. Depress Res Treat 2012:970194, 2012 22811897

Mendenhall E, Kim AW, Panasci A, et al: A mixed-methods, population-based study of a syndemic in Soweto, South Africa. Nat Hum Behav 6(1):64–73, 2022 34949783

Mokline B, Ben Abdallah MA: The mechanisms of collective resilience in a crisis context: the case of the "COVID-19" crisis. Global J Flex Syst Manag 23(1):151–163, 2022 37519339

Musanabaganwa C, Wani AH, Donglasan J, et al: Leukocyte methylomic imprints of exposure to the genocide against the Tutsi in Rwanda: a pilot epigenome-wide analysis. Epigenomics 14(1):11–25, 2022 34875875

Newnham EA, Dzidic PL, Mergelsberg ELP, et al: The Asia Pacific Disaster Mental Health Network: setting a mental health agenda for the region. Int J Environ Res Public Health 17(17):6144, 2020 32847057

North Atlantic Treaty Organization: Psychosocial Care for People Affected by Disasters and Major Incidents. Brussels, North Atlantic Treaty Organization, 2008. Available at: www.coe.int/t/dg4/majorhazards/ressources/virtuallibrary/materials/Others/NATO_Guidance_Psychosocial_Care_for_People_Affected_by_Disasters_and_Major_Incidents.pdf. Accessed April 17, 2023.

Pablos-Méndez A, Raviglione MC: A new world health era. Glob Health Sci Pract 6(1):8–16, 2018 29540441

Pashak TJ, Nelson OM, Tunstull MD, et al: Embrace subjectivity: existentially informed clinical psychological science, practice, and teaching. Clin Psychol 27(1):4–21, 2022

Patel V, Prince M: Global mental health: a new global health field comes of age. JAMA 303(19):1976–1977, 2010 20483977

Patel V, Saxena S, Lund C, et al: The Lancet Commission on global mental health and sustainable development. Lancet 392(10157):1553–1598, 2018 30314863

Pfefferbaum B, North CS: The association between parent-reported child disaster reactions and posttraumatic stress disorder in parent survivors of disasters and terrorism. Ann Clin Psychiatry 32(4):256–265, 2020 33125449

Santomauro DF, Herrera AMM, Shadid J, et al: Global prevalence and burden of depressive and anxiety disorders in 204 countries and territories in 2020 due to the COVID-19 pandemic. Lancet 398(10312):1700–1712, 2021 34634250

Sen HE, Colucci L, Browne DT: Keeping the faith: religion, positive coping, and mental health of caregivers during COVID-19. Front Psychol 12:805019, 2022 35126256

Shultz JM, Galea S, Espinel Z, et al: Disaster ecology, in Textbook of Disaster Psychiatry, 2nd Edition. Edited by Ursano RJ, Fullerton CS, Weisaeth L, Raphael B. New York, Cambridge University Press, 2017, pp 44–59

Sondermann E, Ulbert C: The threat of thinking in threats: reframing global health during and after COVID-19. Zeitschrift fur Friedens und Konfliktforschung 9(3):309–320, 2020

Spitzenstätter D, Schnell T: The existential dimension of the pandemic: death attitudes, personal worldview, and coronavirus anxiety. Death Stud 46(5):1031–1041, 2022 33357041

Tankink M, Belay HT, Mukasa MB, et al.: Culture, Context, and Mental Health and Psychosocial Well-Being of Refugees and Internally Displaced Persons from South Sudan. Geneva, Switzerland, United Nations High Commissioner for Refugees, 2023

Tausch A, E Souza RO, Viciana CM, et al: Strengthening mental health responses to COVID-19 in the Americas: a health policy analysis and recommendations. Lancet Reg Health Am 5:100118, 2022 35098200

Trout LJ, Kleinman A: Covid-19 requires a social medicine response. Front Sociol 5:579991, 2020 33869507

United Nations: Universal Declaration of Human Rights. Geneva, Switzerland, United Nations, 1948. Available at: www.un.org/en/about-us/universal-declaration-of-human-rights. Accessed April 17, 2023.

United Nations High Commission for Refugees: The Sphere Project: Humanitarian Charter and Minimum Standards in Disaster Response. Geneva, Switzerland, United Nations, 2011. Available at: www.unhcr.org/media/31692. Accessed April 17, 2023.

United Nations High Commission for Refugees: Mental Health and Psychosocial Support (MHPSS). UNHCR Emergency Handbook. Geneva, Switzerland, United Nations, 2023. Available at: https://emergency.unhcr.org/entry/49304/mental-health-and-psychosocial-support. Accessed April 17, 2023.

U.S. Census Bureau: Health insurance coverage in the United States: 2021. Suitland, MD, U.S. Census Bureau, 2022. Available at: www.census.gov/library/publications/2022/demo/p60-278.html. Accessed April 17, 2023.

Williams R, Bisson J, Kemp V: Principles for responding to people's psychosocial and mental health needs after disasters. Occasional Paper OP94. London, Royal College of Psychiatrists, 2014. Available at: www.apothecaries.org/wp-content/uploads/2019/02/OP94.pdf. Accessed April 17, 2023.

Workman CL: Syndemics and global health. Nat Hum Behav 6(1):25–26, 2022 34949782

World Health Organization: Psychological First Aid: Guide for Field Workers. Geneva, Switzerland, World Health Organization, 2011. Available at: www.who.int/publications/i/item/9789241548205. Accessed April 17. 2023.

World Health Organization: mhGAP Humanitarian Intervention Guide (mhGAP-HIG): Clinical Management of Mental, Neurological, and Substance Use Conditions in Humanitarian Emergencies. Geneva, Switzerland, World Health Organization, 2015. Available at: www.who.int/publications/i/item/9789241548922. Accessed April 17, 2023.

World Health Organization: mhGAP Intervention Guide for Mental, Neurological, and Substance Use Disorders in Nonspecialized Health Settings: Mental Health Gap Action Programme (mhGAP)—Version 2.0. Geneva, Switzerland, World Health Organization, 2016

11

Infant, Child, and Adolescent Psychiatric Evaluation

Linda Chokroverty, M.D.
Kunmi Sobowale, M.D.

In the wake of a disaster, entire families are affected. However, the main focus of attention is usually on adults and the family unit as a whole. The specific concerns for infants, children, and adolescents are often considered to be lower priority, if they are considered at all. However, it is essential to consider the needs of these groups because they are different from those of adults, requiring a perspective that includes childhood development and relationships.

Clinicians evaluating children or adolescents (the term *child* includes all children ≤11 years old, *adolescent* includes those 12–18 years old, and *youth* includes both children and adolescents) should be cognizant of multiple factors. These factors include the cultural context and influence of culture on manifestations of stress and trauma. The role of adolescents in family and society varies, and individualized attention to members of this group may be received with hesitation. Many cultures do not view adolescents as a separate entity from the family. Worldwide, however, contemporary problems of gun violence in communities and schools, human trafficking, and climate change have brought a new focus on adolescent needs. As discussed in Chapter 10 ("Historical, Sociocultural, and Political Considerations"), a cultural formulation can enhance the evaluation.

Psychiatrists and other mental health providers called on to help are accustomed to viewing individuals through a clinical lens. With disasters, however, a public health approach is needed, the goals of which are to promote resilience by preventing further harm and achieving normal or close to normal functioning and to identify those who need services (Pfefferbaum et al. 2013). The disruptions of displacement and loss of home, belongings, and routines are universal stressors incurred by any disaster that will cause temporary distress in most people. This distress may last days or weeks, or in the case of prolonged disaster states such as the coronavirus disease 2019 (COVID-19) pandemic, it may last months or more. Yet most youth will recover from a disaster without requiring clinical interventions. Mental health professionals need not intervene with presumably healthy children and adolescents by seeking to evaluate them; evaluations are usually selective, often at the request of caregivers or other concerned professionals working in a disaster assistance space, and generally brief.

However, screening and triage of more vulnerable groups are needed because they are most likely to have negative mental health outcomes. These groups include those who suffer direct loss of family, sustain disaster-inflicted injuries, or were previously disabled or mentally or physically ill. Other vulnerable youth to screen for are those most proximal to an event, such as those who witnessed it (e.g., were in the space where people were killed). Orienting community leaders or organizers in a disaster recovery space (e.g., shelter, school, family assistance center, social media platform) to these vulnerable groups can prioritize screening and referral of youth and families who may be a risk for more serious mental health symptoms to mental health clinicians (Wessells and Kostelny 2013).

In this chapter, we take a developmental and relational approach for evaluation. First, methods to optimize evaluation are discussed. Then, developmental capacities, presenting symptoms, and evaluation tips are discussed in children and then adolescents.

Methods in Evaluation

Because children and adolescents are at different stages of development, their communicative skills may be immature. Consequently, clinicians will often have to use indirect verbal and nonverbal approaches (drawings, play) during a direct interview. Observing appearance and behavior in the general environment is part of an assessment of children and adolescents. Additionally, as with nonemergencies, obtaining other perspectives, in the form of interviews with other adults in their life such as parents, family members, or teachers, is generally needed to accurately assess individual, peer, and family functioning for youth (King and American Academy of Child and Adolescent Psychiatry 1997). To this end, speaking with adults (e.g., teachers) who are familiar with a youth's earlier development, prior level of functioning, and coping postdisaster is important. Direct interview of youth is also important because adults may underestimate their children's level of distress (Meiser-Stedman et al. 2007). Information on mental health screening and interview assessments is presented in Table 11–1.

It is especially important to obtain permission to conduct any postdisaster evaluation with minors and caregivers because a sense of control over most things may already be lost. Usually, such permission would be assent for children and adolescents and parental or caregiver consent. Although some cultures may overlook individual viewpoints of youth apart from their caregivers, it has been generally agreed that all children have rights, as described in the United Nations Convention on the Rights of the Child, in this case specifically as "respect for children's views," children's rights on "sharing thoughts freely," and their "freedom of thought and religion" (United Nations 1989). Assent or consent under emergency circumstances is often in the form of verbal agreement, although further written permission may be requested if conditions are more stable and written records are maintained for such encounters.

Observation of Parent-Child Interactions

In addition to a direct interview, observation of parent-child interactions (e.g., bonding, rapport) is indicated. Is warmth, tension, fear, or hostility noted between a parent and child? Does the parent respond positively or negatively to the child or vice versa? Is the child clinging to the parent, or are they arguing or screaming at each other? Severe levels of stress may trigger interpersonal violence between parents and children in the form of excessive physical punishment or among adults in the form of domestic violence. Increases in violence against women following many disasters, including Hurricane Katrina, the 2004 Indian Ocean tsunami in Sri Lanka, the 2010 Haitian earthquake, and the early COVID-19 lockdown, have been described (Anastario et al. 2009; Avalos et al. 2023; Kolbe et al. 2010; Leslie and Wilson 2020; Sontag 2010). The rise in abuse against children following disasters is less conclusive, largely due to decreased reporting mechanisms and problems with study design in this population (Cerna-Turoff et al. 2019; Seddighi et al. 2021). Given the serious effects on children and adolescents from exposure to family violence, it is imperative to intervene and not merely observe whether such violence is occurring.

TABLE 11–1. Validated assessments of trauma, depression, and anxiety in children and adolescents

Measure	Age range (years)	Description	Reference
Screenings			
Children's Revised Impact of Event Scale (CRIES)	7–18	Trauma, 8 or 13 items	Perrin et al. 2005
Child PTSD Symptom Scale Self-report for DSM-5 (CPSS-5-SR)	8–18	Trauma, 27 items	Foa et al. 2018
Child and Adolescent Trauma Screen (CATS)	7–17	Trauma, 40 items	Sachser et al. 2017
Revised Child Anxiety and Depression Scales (RCADS-25)	9–18	Depression and anxiety, 25 items	Ebesutani et al. 2012
Interviews			
Child PTSD Symptom Scale—Interview for DSM 5 (CPSS 5-I)	8–18	Trauma, 27 items	Foa et al. 2018
Clinician-Administered PTSD Scale for DSM-5 Children/ Adolescents (CAPS-CA-5)	7–18	Trauma, 30 items; training required	Pynoos et al. 2015

Note.   All measures are freely available and are in multiple languages.
Source.   Ebesutani et al. 2012; Foa et al. 2018; Perrin et al. 2005; Pynoos et al. 2015; Sachser et al. 2017.

Observation of the parent's behavior during the interview about the child(ren) can provide important information about the parent's mental status. Anxious, agitated, or visibly mentally ill caregivers present additional harmful exposures to youth. Parents who are in shock, withdrawn, or detached because of severe trauma or loss may neglect children and cause family risk, as might caregivers who are "high" or appear intoxicated. In such situations, additional referral for assessment, support, and possible treatments of the adults are indicated, while avoiding separation of children from their parents (see also Chapter 19).

Location of Evaluation

For older children and adolescents, private space should be sought for a separate interview away from the parent(s) whenever possible. In the case of younger children, an interview with the parent present and a separate parent interview are likely necessary (King and American Academy of Child and Adolescent Psychiatry 1997). Privacy and time may be limited and possibly prohibitive in chaotic and overcrowded circumstances. In the absence of a separate and private room, a space physically distant from the larger group where individuals can speak freely without being heard must be sought. With the improved capabilities in care afforded by technology, access to individuals needing attention may be greatly expanded through telehealth if connectivity and an appropriate space are available. This has certainly been the case with the clinical care of patients in remote or low-resource settings with pre-existing shortages of specialists or when in-person access is prohibited (e.g., COVID-19 precautions) (American Academy of Child and Adolescent Psychiatry [AACAP] Committee on Telepsychiatry and AACAP Committee on Quality Issues 2017; Myers et al. 2008). Telehealth has been described as a modality to use during disasters for some time (Simmons et al. 2003). However, telehealth with children and youth may be less desirable than in-person assessments because distractibility and lessened engagement is common among this population when in front of a screen.

Timing of Screenings

The evidence to date suggests that most children recover from posttraumatic stress symptoms by 1 year postdisaster (Witt et al. 2024). Screening within the first month postdisaster will likely capture many children experiencing acute stress, of which the majority will recover. Practical guidance, when possible, is to screen all children at 1 month and 3 months, with the expectation that intervention, even if universal in nature (see Chapter 19), will be provided for children with clinically significant symptoms. Children without elevated symptoms by 6 months are unlikely to develop PTSD later on (Witt et al. 2024). Therefore, at later time points (e.g., 12 months), indicated screening of children with prior elevated symptoms is reasonable. Clinicians must use their judgment in the context of the specific disaster. For example, children in higher-risk groups may require earlier or more frequent monitoring.

Higher-Risk Groups

In disaster response, special attention should be given to youth who are at increased risk for negative mental health outcomes. These youth include those with prior mental health disorders or disabilities. Advance planning for resources (e.g., equipment, medications, services, direct care) for emergencies is especially important for this population (Pfefferbaum et al. 2013). Children and adolescents with developmental delays and developmental disabilities, including neurodevelopmental disorders (e.g., intellectual developmental disorder [intellectual disability]), may be especially vulnerable to disruptions created by disasters.

Psychosocial risks include prior adverse childhood events (ACEs) such as abuse or neglect, witnessing violence at home, and exposure to parents with mental illness or substance use (Centers for Disease Control and Prevention 2019). Youth with multiple ACEs are at greater risk for the negative impacts of a disaster compared with those without ACEs (Guo et al. 2020). New problems created by a disaster that put previously well children and adolescents at significant future risk include the sudden death of a primary caregiver, separation from caregivers (brief or extended), high exposure or proximity to an event, and illness or injury sustained by the event. A recent literature review on risk and resilience among youth following disasters found that "female gender, a higher trauma exposure (i.e., suffering injury, perceived life threat), a higher number of life events, less social support, and negative coping" were associated with less favorable posttraumatic stress symptom trajectories (Witt et al. 2024, p. 9).

Minoritized youth, including BIPOC (Black, Indigenous, and people of color) and LGBTQ+ (lesbian, gay, bisexual, transexual, and queer/questioning) youth are at higher risk for ACEs (Bruner 2017; Schnarrs et al. 2019), access mental health services less often (Alegría et al. 2022), and in recent years have attempted suicide more often than white or heterosexual peers do (Centers for Disease Control and Prevention 2019, 2023). Therefore, attention to the added vulnerability of these and other marginalized groups is paramount, especially during emergencies.

Risks among vulnerable youth are important to identify, but resiliency factors that may buffer risks and protect all children and adolescents are equally essential to understand. These include individual, family, and community characteristics (see subsection "Adolescent Mental Health Signs and Symptoms After Disasters" and Chapter 19).

Evaluating Young Children (0–5 Years Old)

Familiarity with typical child development is necessary to understand children's reactions in the context of disaster. Mental health professionals are well-positioned to share information on child development with caregivers. One tenet to share with caregivers is that development is not linear (Brazelton 1992). For children between birth and 5 years, gains, regressions, and plateaus in behaviors are common. For example, an infant who slept through the night now wakes up every few hours. Alternatively, a 4-year-old girl cannot read the word "cat," but just a week later, she reads it with ease. Parents' concerns usually center on regressions. Clinicians can reassure caregivers that as children grow older, these regressions are less likely to occur unless provoked (e.g., by a stressful situation). Further, clinicians can use developmental knowledge to assess whether children are functioning below their expected or baseline level for a prolonged period, indicating they may need more formal psychiatric intervention.

Generally, development is separated into motor, cognitive, language, and socioemotional domains. Using the updated 2022 Centers for Disease Control and Prevention (CDC) developmental milestones, disaster mental health clinicians attending to children should be conversant in the developmental milestones in the first 5 years of life in motor, cognitive, language, and socioemotional domains (Zubler et al. 2022). Starting at 6 months, babies can roll from tummy to back, reach for a desired toy, take turns making sounds, and laugh. At 12 months, we expect babies to pull to a stand, wave bye, put something in a container, and play pat-a-cake. At 18 months, children scribble, play with toys in a simple way (e.g., pushing a toy car), follow one-step directions, and point to show something of interest. By 2 years, most children can run, eat with a spoon, hold something in one hand while using the other hand, say two-word phrases, and notice when others are upset. Most 3-year-olds can partly dress themselves, copy a circle, say their first name when asked, and calm down within 10 minutes of being separated from a primary caregiver (e.g., at childcare). Four-year-old children can usually catch a large ball, name some colors, construct sentences of four or more words, and pretend to be something else (e.g., a superhero) during play. Finally, at 5 years old, most children can hop on one foot, fasten some buttons, count to 10, answer simple questions about a book or story, and take turns during play with others.

We chose the developmental milestones in the examples above because they are easy to assess in disaster settings, but they are not exhaustive. Clinicians and caregivers can view the full list in multiple languages on the CDC website under "Learn the Signs. Act Early" and download the CDC's Milestone Tracker app that makes it easy to track milestones by age using a smartphone (Centers for Disease Control and Prevention 2022a). Videos and pictures of typical developmental milestones are also available at the CDC's website (Centers for Disease Control and Prevention 2022b).

Tips for Evaluating Young Children

When evaluating young children and their caregivers, clinicians should consider the following tenets. First, most caregivers want the best for their children. Caregivers are experts on their children and are often the first to notice behavioral changes. Professionals should leverage the caregivers' concern and curiosity. They can ask caregivers about the meaning or description of the child's behavior. For example, a psychiatrist could ask, "Can you help me understand what you see?" or "How do you feel the hurricane has affected her?" When discussing development, asking caregivers when they expect a development milestone to be reached can help clinicians determine parents' expectations and counsel them in normal development.

Even in the limited time that clinicians have to evaluate children in disasters, they can foster engagement. Clinicians need to be mindful that young children, who are in a heightened arousal state (e.g., hypervigilance), may be wary of talking to an unknown adult. To increase the chance of connection, mental health professionals should first observe the child's behavior. When the opportunity arises, a professional can try to join the child's activity. Alternatively, offering toys or games such as building blocks or checkers can help. Following the child's lead in play supports engagement. Clinicians should sit near or with the child and avoid standing over or crowding them.

It is essential to keep development in mind when interacting with children. Being as specific as possible in questioning can help them better understand the question. Asking too many questions, especially "why" questions, can be off-putting because they can seem like an interrogation. Instead, using open-ended questions such as "how" and "what" questions, as well as summaries and reflective statements, can help. For children who are less willing to talk, having them draw or write out their thoughts and feelings is another approach to consider. Similarly, using pictures or illustrations to explain concepts or ask questions can increase understanding.

Finally, clinicians should be aware of the DSM-5-TR (American Psychiatric Association 2022) age-appropriate alternative algorithm for diagnosing PTSD in children ages 6 years or younger (PTSD-AA), which requires the presence of only one symptom item from either the avoidance or negative alterations in cognitions and mood criteria (Scheeringa et al. 2012). The PTSD-AA is more behaviorally focused and has shown significantly higher prevalence rates of PTSD in young children compared with traditional PTSD criteria (Woolgar et al. 2022).

Evaluating Older Children (6–11 Years Old)

Developmental Considerations

For 6- to 11-year-olds, clinicians should be aware of several unique aspects of development (Dixon and Stein 2006). Cognitively, children have an expanded knowledge base and skills. They have more realistic reasoning and grasp the concept of time and sequential events. For example, children can create coherent narratives to recount past events or tell a story. This ability can potentially lead to new worries in the setting of disaster. For example, most children this age understand the finality of death, but they have difficulty separating fiction from reality. Their understanding, particularly at younger ages, is concrete: they take what they hear literally and rely on what they observe in the physical world around them. Children this age tend to see things as "good" or "bad" without nuance. Children can reason about cause and effect, but they cannot think in the abstract. For example, metaphors and idioms may not be understood by this group.

Socioemotionally, children in this age group become more independent. Connections to parents remain central but shift toward classmates and noncaregiver adults over time. There is a desire for peer acceptance, and self-esteem is often tied to that. Friendships tend to be gender-based (e.g., boys playing together). As children grow older, they are better able to regulate their emotions. Some children, particularly girls, may begin puberty as early as age 8 years. Unfortunately, these early pubertal changes may place children at risk of being sexualized and abused.

Children's Mental Health Signs and Symptoms After Disasters

Clinicians should be aware of the signs and symptoms of stress in children from birth to 11 years old. These signs and symptoms will vary by age. Observed behavior is often more important than self-report for younger children, particularly those with limited verbal ability. Emotionally, be-

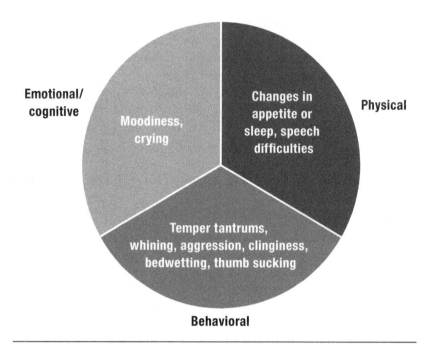

FIGURE 11–1. Child response to stress (0–5 years old).

tween ages 0 and 5 years, stress causes children to be moodier and cry more (Figure 11–1). Infants tend to have two types of cries: a pain cry, which is loud, sudden, and high-pitched, and a basic cry, characterized by a gradual buildup and lower pitch (Lester et al. 1990). Behaviorally, after a disaster, young children can show increased temper tantrums and aggression, which can also be a manifestation of anxiety. Regressive behaviors such as whining, bedwetting, thumb sucking, and clinginess may occur. Physically, there may be changes in appetite or sleep. Sleep is often disturbed, but hypersomnolence can also occur with trauma. Speech difficulties such as mutism can also arise. Infants and toddlers may not understand the dangerousness of the situation, which can sometimes be protective, but caregivers' distress can influence them.

Older children (6–11 years old) are more verbal, leading to a wider range of signs and symptoms after disasters (Figure 11–2). Similar to younger children, they may be moodier and cry. In addition, they can experience more difficulty concentrating or even talk excessively about the disaster. Behaviorally, increased whining, aggression, and clinginess are common. Despite the increased importance of social activities at this age, withdrawal from activities can occur when children are stressed. Prolonged nonparticipation may indicate more serious mental health difficul-

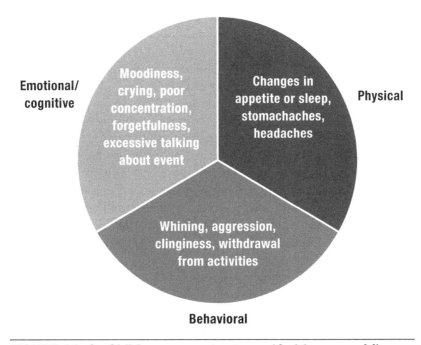

FIGURE 11–2. Child response to stress (6–11 years old).

ties, such as depression or PTSD-related avoidance. Physically, somatic symptoms such as stomachaches and headaches are more likely to occur in school-age children.

Evaluating Adolescents (Ages 12–18 Years)

Developmental Considerations

Younger adolescents between 12 and 14 years are likely in the throes of puberty, with multiple changes in secondary sexual characteristics such as body hair, sweat, growth spurt, voice lowering, and changes in breasts and genitalia. Most girls will have had menarche and will be in the latter stages of puberty, but boys will often be in the earlier stages. These physical changes and the social reaction to them can bring about body image concerns, disordered eating, social anxiety, and depression. Moodiness and difficulty controlling affect are common, and adolescents are often at odds with their parents. They may be self-absorbed and more concerned about relationships with peer rather than with adults. Higher-level thinking and the ability to communicate complex thoughts and feelings are developing at this age, but also anxiety and stress around schoolwork and social issues (Centers for Disease Control and Prevention 2024a). Bullying is most frequently reported in middle school (Centers for Disease Control and Prevention 2024b). Sleep requirement is about 9–11 hours per day for this group. They may have been introduced to drugs and alcohol, and vaping is becoming increasingly common.

Development for older teenagers, ages 14–17, typically includes advancement and completion of puberty, prioritization of social relationships, interest in romantic relationships and sexuality, and concerns around the future. These adolescents are capable of abstract and complex thought and moral reasoning, and they have well-formed opinions. The need to separate further from parents in favor of peers is a major developmental task, and future orientation around work and personal identity are priorities as well. They may have a job and participate in civically oriented activities. Conflicts with parents may exist, but they may also have settled down compared with conflicts during the early teenage years. Sleep requirement at this age is 9–10 hours per day. After puberty, depression increases for boys and girls, but more so for girls; suicides and suicidal behaviors may increase; and risky behaviors such as unprotected sex, substance abuse, and excessive social media use may occur. Impulsivity is common (U.S. Department of Health and Human Services 2021).

Adolescents in the young adult range (18 years old and older) continue to advance in their physical and emotional independence and have complex cognitive abilities and social and political interests. They may also have existential thinking. Although they are adults in the eyes of the law in most societies, their brains are not fully mature until about age 25 or later—especially the frontal lobe, which oversees executive functioning. As a result, they may continue to have impulsivity, poor planning, and bad judgment. Complete independence from parents (*launching*) may or may not have occurred, although some cultures imagine this age group separating from the family only if they are entering marriage and starting their own families. Major mental illnesses such as schizophrenia may emerge, and suicide rates continue to rise in this age period. Sleep requirement at this age is usually 7–8 hours per day. Sexuality and intimate relationships continue to be important, and exposure to intimate partner violence may have occurred by this age.

Adolescent Mental Health Signs and Symptoms After Disasters

As with younger children, adolescents may experience regression under extreme stress, returning to behaviors from a younger age such as separation problems, crying and poor distress tolerance, tantrums, co-sleeping with

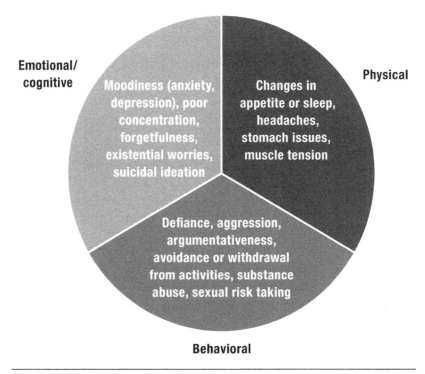

FIGURE 11–3. Adolescent response to stress (age 12–18 years).

parents or siblings, irritability, social withdrawal, and somatic symptoms (e.g., headaches, stomachaches). Hopelessness, loss of faith in authorities, and existential worries may occur. Maladaptive habits such as smoking, drinking, drug use, excessive media use, or sexual risk-taking may arise in response to high stress, as might poor eating and sleep habits, lack of physical activity, and excess caffeine use (Figure 11–3). Youth of all ages with special needs such as autism spectrum disorder, intellectual developmental disorder, or prior mental illness may especially demonstrate regression or a lack of coping as seen in younger children when under duress. During emergencies, autism, in particular, puts affected youth at much higher risk due to communication and behavioral challenges because they are often prone to wandering and elopement, which may result in drowning, injuries, or assaults (National Autism Association 2012, 2017).

As with adults, positive behaviors in reaction to extreme challenges may occur among youth as well, such as social and political activism (e.g., "March for Our Lives," Climate Action), and engagement in community self-help/recovery (see also Chapter 15, "Vulnerability, Resilience, Grief").

TABLE 11–2. Positive childhood experiences

A positive self-image

A predictable home routine

Beliefs that give comfort

A sense of belonging or enjoyment in school

At least one good friend who is supportive

A caring noncaregiver adult

An adult in the home that makes the child feel safe and protected

Opportunities to have a good time

Opportunities to participate in community traditions

Source.   Adapted from Merrick and Narayan 2020.

Assessment for other positive features among children and adolescents is important, as these qualities enable resilience and recovery following difficult events. Table 11–2 provides examples of positive childhood experiences (see also Chapter 19).

Tips for Evaluating Adolescents

Play or drawing may be appropriate for older but emotionally immature adolescents, but in general, these youth are able to engage directly in talking interviews, although they may need additional elements to allow for that. Starting out together with parents, as with younger children, is helpful with adolescents, who may be untrusting of strangers asking questions. Explaining why you were asked to see them and what you will do is helpful in building rapport and putting them more at ease. The parent(s) might be asked about any concerns they have, and then the youth may be able to be seen separately (Cepeda 2000). Activities that can further break the ice include games (cards, board games) or doodling if the adolescent is quiet and it is hard to engage in conversation. Further discussion might happen more easily during the course of game play, when the young person might be more relaxed. The adolescent (and examiner) should be asked to refrain from using an electronic device during the interview because it is a potential distraction unless the device is specifically being used for engagement (e.g., an electronic building game that allows for more than one player). Sitting together with an activity at a table (if available) or on the floor or ground is less intimidating with preadolescents and younger children than sitting face to face in chairs for an interview. The language of the interview should be simple and free of adult psychiatric jargon—for example, "sad" rather than "depressed" and "nervous or worried" rather than anxious (Cepeda 2000). Older teens may be able to engage in an interview in the same way as adults. However, if they seem uncomfortable, methods suitable for younger patients, such as talking during card games, may also be appropriate.

Emergency evaluation of children and adolescents might be required if family members are concerned about safety, as in the case of violent, agitated, or suicidal behavior. Similar guidance applies to younger patients as to adults; for more details on these types of situations, see Chapter 12, "Adult Psychiatric Evaluation." The American Academy of Child and Adolescent Psychiatry (AACAP) Suicide Resource Center has a variety of assessment tools, psychoeducational documents, and clinical materials that may help in the urgent evaluation of suicide in children and adolescents (AACAP Suicide Resource Center 2023). An important aspect of the evaluation of suicide is to assess if the child or adolescent, with the help of their caregivers, can engage in a suicide safety plan. A safety plan is an evidence-based strategy that identifies an individual's warning signs; coping strategies; social, family, and professional supports; and ways to create a safe environment by reducing access to lethal means (Stanley and Brown 2021). The suicide safety plan is often used in emergency settings (Bettis et al. 2020) and can provide guidance on whether a young person can be managed safely in the community rather than in a hospital or clinical setting.

The last stage of evaluation with children and adolescents might include a summary of how the examiner sees the situation for the individual as well as the parent(s), validating and empathic statements, and some interventions that will help with coping (see Chapter 19) such as psychoeducation or other elements of Psychological First Aid.

Conclusion

Children and adolescents are generally very resilient in the face of even the most challenging circumstances, provided they have their families and parent(s) available to them, routines, and activities that are familiar. Short-term reactions to stress will be evident in developmentally specific ways. Parents and adult caregivers of youth are the best sources of information about specific concerns that might need the attention of a mental health practitioner, and their engagement is crucial for any evaluation of their children. Parents' reactions to stress heavily influence those of their children, so adults who are coping poorly need additional evaluation and support themselves. Older children and adolescents need assessment separately from their caregivers for at least part of the evaluation, either after meeting with parents or after meeting with the family together. Using age-appropriate toys, games, and drawing in a comfortable space helps facilitate the engagement and evaluation of children and adolescents. Although evaluating the younger population can be more challenging for practitioners without experience with this group, many resources are available online and via mobile apps for further guidance in assessment, and readers are encouraged to use them.

References

Alegría M, O'Malley IS, DiMarzio K, et al: Framework for understanding and addressing racial and ethnic disparities in children's mental health. Child Adolesc Psychiatr Clin N Am 31(2):179–191, 2022 35361358

American Academy of Child and Adolescent Psychiatry: Suicide Resource Center. Washington, DC, American Academy of Child and Adolescent Psychiatry, 2023. Available at: www.aacap.org/AACAP/Families_and_Youth/Resource_Centers/Suicide_Resource_Center/Home.aspx. Accessed April 16, 2023.

American Academy of Child and Adolescent Psychiatry (AACAP) Committee on Telepsychiatry and AACAP Committee on Quality Issues: Clinical update: telepsychiatry with children and adolescents. J Am Acad Child Adolesc Psychiatry 56(10):875–893, 2017 28942810

American Psychiatric Association: Diagnostic and Statistical Manual of Mental Disorders, 5th Edition, Text Revision. Washington, DC, American Psychiatric Association, 2022

Anastario M, Shehab N, Lawry L: Increased gender-based violence among women internally displaced in Mississippi 2 years post-Hurricane Katrina. Disaster Med Public Health Prep 3(1):18–26, 2009 19293740

Avalos LA, Ray GT, Alexeeff SE, et al: Association of the COVID-19 pandemic with unstable and/or unsafe living situations and intimate partner violence among pregnant individuals. JAMA Netw Open 6(2):e230172, 2023 36811863

Bettis AH, Donise KR, MacPherson HA, et al: Safety planning intervention for adolescents: provider attitudes and response to training in the emergency services setting. Psychiatr Serv 71(11):1136–1142, 2020 32838677

Brazelton TB: Touchpoints: Your Child's Emotional and Behavioral Development. Reading, MA, Addison-Wesley, 1992

Bruner C: ACE, place, race, and poverty: building hope for children. Acad Pediatr 17(7):S123–S129, 2017 28865644

Centers for Disease Control and Prevention: Adverse childhood experiences prevention. Atlanta, GA, Centers for Disease Control and Prevention, 2019. Available at: www.cdc.gov/violenceprevention/pdf/ACEs-Prevention-Resource_508.pdf. Accessed March 2, 2023.

Centers for Disease Control and Prevention: Positive parenting tips: young teens (12–14 years old). Atlanta, GA, Centers for Disease Control and Prevention, September 2, 2024a. Available at: www.cdc.gov/child-development/positive-parenting-tips/young-teens-12-14-years.html. Accessed August 11, 2024.

Centers for Disease Control and Prevention: Positive parenting tips: Adolescence (15–17 years old). Atlanta, GA, Centers for Disease Control and Prevention, September 23, 2024b. www.cdc.gov/child-development/positive-parenting-tips/adolescence-15-17-years.html?CDC_AAref_Val=https://www.cdc.gov/ncbddd/

childdevelopment/positiveparenting/adolescence2.html. Accessed March 2, 2023.

Centers for Disease Control and Prevention: Learn signs: act early. Atlanta, GA, Centers for Disease Control and Prevention, September 19, 2022a. Available at: www.cdc.gov/ncbddd/actearly/index.html. Accessed March 2, 2023.

Centers for Disease Control and Prevention: Milestones in action. Atlanta, GA, Centers for Disease Control and Prevention, December 20, 2022b. Available at: www.cdc.gov/ncbddd/actearly/milestones/milestones-in-action.html. Accessed March 2, 2023.

Centers for Disease Control and Prevention: Youth Risk Behavior Survey Data Summary and Trends Report: 2011–2021. Atlanta, GA, Centers for Disease Control and Prevention, May 5, 2023. Available at: www.cdc.gov/healthyyouth/data/yrbs/pdf/YRBS_Data-Summary-Trends_Report2023_508.pdf. Accessed March 2, 2023.

Cepeda C: Concise Guide to the Psychiatric Interview of Children and Adolescents. Washington, DC, American Psychiatric Press, 2000, pp 41–52

Cerna-Turoff I, Fischer HT, Mayhew S, et al: Violence against children and natural disasters: a systematic review and meta-analysis of quantitative evidence. PLoS One 14(5):e0217719, 2019 31145758

Dixon SD, Stein MT: Encounters With Children. Philadelphia, PA, Mosby, 2006, p 693

Ebesutani C, Reise SP, Chorpita BF, et al: The Revised Child Anxiety and Depression Scale-Short Version: scale reduction via exploratory bifactor modeling of the broad anxiety factor. Psychol Assess 24(4):833–845, 2012 22329531

Foa EB, Asnaani A, Zang Y, et al: Psychometrics of the child PTSD symptom scale for DSM-5 for trauma-exposed children and adolescents. J Clin Child Adolesc Psychol 47(1):38–46, 2018 28820616

Guo J, Fu M, Liu D, et al: Is the psychological impact of exposure to COVID-19 stronger in adolescents with pre-pandemic maltreatment experiences? A survey of rural Chinese adolescents. Child Abuse Negl 110(Pt 2):104667, 2020 32859393

King RA; American Academy of Child and Adolescent Psychiatry: Practice parameters for the psychiatric assessment of children and adolescents. J Am Acad Child Adolesc Psychiatry 36(10)(Suppl):4S–20S, 1997 9606102

Kolbe AR, Hutson RA, Shannon H, et al: Mortality, crime and access to basic needs before and after the Haiti earthquake: a random survey of Port-au-Prince households. Med Confl Surviv 26(4):281–297, 2010 21314081

Leslie E, Wilson R: Sheltering in place and domestic violence: evidence from calls for service during COVID-19. J Public Econ 189:104241, 2020 32834179

Lester BM, Boukydis CZ, Garcia-Coll CT, et al: Colic for developmentalists. Infant Ment Health J 11(4):321–333, 1990

Meiser-Stedman R, Smith P, Glucksman E, et al: Parent and child agreement for acute stress disorder, post-traumatic stress disorder and other psychopathology in a prospective study of children and adolescents exposed to single-event trauma. J Abnorm Child Psychol 35(2):191–201, 2007 17219079

Merrick JS, Narayan AJ: Assessment and screening of positive childhood experiences along with childhood adversity in research, practice, and policy. J Child Poverty 26(2):269–281, 2020

Myers K, Cain S; Work Group on Quality Issues, et al: Practice parameter for telepsychiatry with children and adolescents. J Am Acad Child Adolesc Psychiatry 47(12):1468–1483, 2008 19034191

National Autism Association: Big Red Safety Toolkit. Barrington, RI, National Autism Association, 2012. Available at: https://nationalautismassociation.org/docs/BigRedSafetyToolkit.pdf. Accessed March 2, 2023.

National Autism Association: First Responder Toolkit. Barrington, RI, National Autism Association, 2017. Available at: https://nationalautismassociation.org/docs/BigRedSafetyToolkit-FR.pdf. Accessed March 2, 2023.

Perrin S, Meiser-Stedman R, Smith P: The Children's Revised Impact of Event Scale (CRIES): validity as a screening instrument for PTSD. Behav Cogn Psychother 33(4):487–498, 2005

Pfefferbaum B, Shaw JA; American Academy of Child and Adolescent Psychiatry (AACAP) Committee on Quality Issues (CQI): Practice parameter on disaster preparedness. J Am Acad Child Adolesc Psychiatry 52(11):1224–1238, 2013 24157398

Pynoos RS, Weathers FW, Steinberg AM, et al: Clinician-Administered PTSD Scale for DSM-5—Child/Adolescent Version. Washington DC, National Center for PTSD, 2015. Available at: www.ptsd.va.gov/professional/assessment/child/caps-ca.asp. Accessed April 2, 2024.

Sachser C, Berliner L, Holt T, et al: International development and psychometric properties of the Child and Adolescent Trauma Screen (CATS). J Affect Disord 210:189–195, 2017 28049104

Scheeringa MS, Myers L, Putnam FW, Zeanah CH: Diagnosing PTSD in early childhood: an empirical assessment of four approaches. J Trauma Stress 25(4):359–367, 2012 22806831

Schnarrs PW, Stone AL, Salcido R Jr, et al: Differences in adverse childhood experiences (ACEs) and quality of physical and mental health between transgender and cisgender sexual minorities. J Psychiatr Res 119:1–6, 2019 31518909

Seddighi H, Salmani I, Javadi MH, et al: Child abuse in natural disasters and conflicts: a systematic review. Trauma Violence Abuse 22(1):176–185, 2021 30866745

Simmons SC, Murphy TA, Blanarovich A, et al: Telehealth technologies and applications for terrorism response: a report of the 2002 coastal North Carolina domestic preparedness training exercise. J Am Med Inform Assoc 10(2):166–176, 2003 12595406

Sontag D: Sexual Assaults Add to Miseries of Haiti's Ruins. The New York Times, June 23, 2010. Available at: www.nytimes.com/2010/06/24/world/americas/24haiti.html. Accessed April 1, 2023.

Stanley B, Brown GK: Safety planning intervention: a brief intervention to mitigate suicide risk. Cogn Behav Pract 19(2):256–264, 2021

United Nations: Convention on the Rights of the Child, New York, 20 November 1989. United Nations, Treaty Series, Vol 1577, p 3. 1989. Available at: https://treaties.un.org/Pages/ViewDetails.aspx?src=TREATY&mtdsg_no=IV-11&chapter=4&clang=_en. Accessed February 26, 2023.

U.S. Department of Health and Human Services: Bullying Prevention for Parents of Middle School Students. Washington, DC, U.S. Department of Health and Human Services, November 17, 2021. Available at: www.stopbullying.gov/prevention/middle-school. Accessed August 11, 2024.

Wessells M, Kostelny K: Child friendly spaces: toward a grounded, community-based approach for strengthening child protection practice in humanitarian crises. Natural helpers play a critical role in ensuring children's safety during and in the aftermath of crises. Child Abuse Negl 37(Suppl):29–40, 2013 24268375

Witt A, Sachser C, Fegert JM: Scoping review on trauma and recovery in youth after natural disasters: what Europe can learn from natural disasters around the world. Eur Child Adolesc Psychiatry 33(3):651–665, 2024 35426528

Woolgar F, Garfield H, Dalgleish T, et al: Systematic review and meta-analysis: prevalence of posttraumatic stress disorder in trauma-exposed preschool-aged children. J Am Acad Child Adolesc Psychiatry 61(3):366–377, 2022 34242737

Zubler JM, Wiggins LD, Macias MM, et al: Evidence-informed milestones for developmental surveillance tools. Pediatrics 149(3):e2021052138, 2022 35132439

12

Adult Psychiatric Evaluation

Craig L. Katz, M.D.
Frederick J. Stoddard Jr., M.D.

Mental health assistance to people affected by disasters begins with evaluation, first of the situation and the affected community, as in Chapter 3, "Needs Assessment," and then of the affected people. Acute psychiatric evaluation of disaster survivors is distinguished from postacute evaluations that occur later in conventional psychiatric settings such as clinics or offices. Here, as in most of this book, we define and focus on acute mental health issues, tracing the unique trajectory of survivors' evolving reactions and emerging diagnoses and the clinical and logistical issues that shape it in the immediate aftermath of a disaster.

Time Frame

One of the most helpful factors in guiding clinical assessment in the aftermath of disaster is timing. The determination of whether a reaction represents psychopathology is often dependent on the amount of time that has elapsed since the event. For example, losing sleep for the first few days after an earthquake is normal and possibly even adaptive, in the event of a major aftershock in the middle of the night. However, losing sleep weeks or months after aftershocks subside suggests reason for clinical concern. The persistence of the problem suggests that it is pathological and possibly symptomatic of a larger disorder, such as posttraumatic stress disorder (PTSD) or major depression.

While the chronic care disaster model described in Chapter 8, "Model for Adaptive Response to Complex Cyclical Disasters," undergoes further development and refinement, the basic timeline of disasters portrayed in Figure 12–1 remains sufficient for understanding the phases of disaster from a psychological perspective. The acute phase can be defined, by extrapolation from the definition of acute stress disorder, as approximately the initial month after the event and its immediate impact (American Psychiatric Association 2022). In practice, this definition lends itself less to such quantification, as the coronavirus disease 2019 (COVID-19 pandemic) with its multiple peaks exemplified and recurrent climate crises continue to exemplify. Therefore, the acute phase can also be considered to be the time dating from the impact to days and weeks later and postacute to be from weeks to months to even years later (Katz 2011). The impact encompasses the earliest initial minutes to hours of the event when the dust is literally or figuratively being kicked up. In the acute phase, the dust begins to settle, and the postacute phase begins when the dust has more or less settled.

Acute Psychological Consequences of Disaster

The Institute of Medicine has developed a framework for categorizing the psychological consequences of disaster that continues to be helpful across the decades (Goldfrank et al. 2003). As depicted in Figure 12–2, three broad categories of responses are posited: behavioral change, distress responses, and psychiatric illness. Short of the extreme endpoint of psychiatric illness that belongs to the postacute phase lies a range of reactions that may be variably problematic, if at all. Indeed, one of the unique aspects of acute postdisaster psychiatric work is working in what we might call a *prediagnostic framework*, consisting of symptoms or resilient reactions rather than diagnoses, which take time to manifest (Katz 2021).

Behavioral changes encompass a broad range of how people do things and go about their lives after a disaster. When a community is turned upside down by disaster, people must act differently to adapt and survive. A family who pitches a Red Cross tent so they have shelter following the destruction of their home by an earthquake is adapting well. But survivors who insist that the Red Cross accommodate them in a hotel are behaving maladaptively, especially because the extent of sudden homelessness and

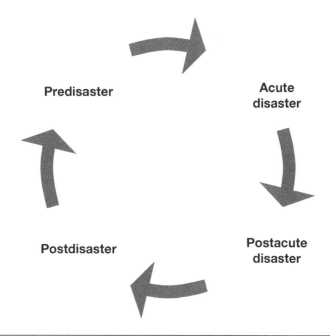

FIGURE 12–1. Time cycle of disasters.

destruction makes such accommodations impossible and potentially unsafe because of aftershocks.

Common maladaptive behaviors include misuse of substances, which we discuss in the next section. On the other hand, adaptive and even prosocial behaviors are often abundant during the acute postdisaster period, such as the 16 college and graduate students who participated in a research study with Meals on Wheels to make impactful "empathy-focused" telephone calls to homebound elderly during the first summer of the COVID-19 pandemic in the United States (Kahlon et al. 2021).

Distress responses include all the ways in which people experience a disaster. Again, these may or may not be abnormal or maladaptive. These responses span cognitive, emotional, and physical reactions (Katz 2011). Insomnia is a very common reaction that probably overlaps behavior and distress, although one should be careful to distinguish it from the impact of disrupted shelter. Cognitive changes can include feeling confused or distracted. A range of thoughts about the event are possible, spanning disbelief to a sense of dependency to a decision to finally change one's career once things are back to normal. Emotional responses are as varied as the people involved but typically include anxiety, fear, grief, and resignation.

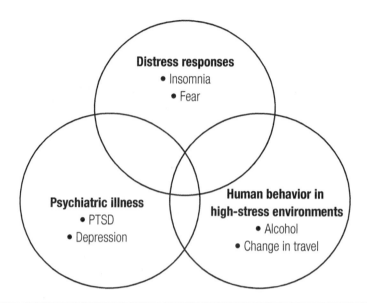

FIGURE 12–2. Psychological consequences of concern from disasters.

Source. Reprinted from Ursano R: "Terrorism and mental health: public health and primary care," in *Status Report: Meeting the Mental Health Needs of the Country in the Wake of September 11, 2001.* Atlanta, GA, The Carter Center, 2002, pp. 64–68. Available at: www.cartercenter.org/documents/1441.pdf. Used with permission.

Positive emotions may also arise, including a heightened sense of community or spirituality.

Many people's reactions to disaster may be fluid and shifting, leading to a frequent experience of feeling that they are on what is often described as an emotional roller coaster. At one moment, survivors may feel inspired by the unity of their community's response to an event, whereas in the next instance they feel overwhelmed and paralyzed by the recovery tasks that lie ahead. Over time, the peaks and oscillations in behaviors or distress will subside for many or most people. If not, the problems begin to coalesce into psychiatric disorders in the postacute phase, the most common of which are PTSD, major depression, and alcohol use disorders (Katz 2021).

Working prediagnostically in the acute phase raises the question of what to call a survivor's distress. One intriguing but yet-to-be-adopted term would be to consider a survivor's distress a *stress injury*, for which the causative stressor is identified as either trauma, fatigue, or grief (Figley and Nash 2007). A more conventional approach would be to use the diagnosis of adjustment disorder from DSM-5-TR, which involves the "development of emotional or behavioral symptoms in response to an identifiable stressor(s) occurring within 3 months of the onset of the stressor(s)" (American Psychiatric Association 2022, p. 286). A third option would be simply to avoid the temptation to diagnose or label and instead to name the symptoms requiring clinical attention.

Substance Use and Substance Use Disorders

In the wake of disasters, evaluation includes substance use disorders (SUDs). In this section, we introduce diagnosis, screening, and treatment strategies for timely interventions prioritizing life-threatening issues such as alcohol withdrawal and deaths from suicide and unintentional overdoses, both of the latter being opioid-related (Bohnert and Ilgen 2019). We introduce screening, consistent with DSM-5-TR diagnoses (American Psychiatric Association 2022). For detailed treatment guidance, see the websites of the National Institute on Alcohol Abuse and Alcoholism (NIAAA) (www.niaaa.nih.gov; U.S. Department of Health and Human Services 2022) and the National Institute on Drug Abuse (NIDA) (https://nida.nih.gov).

Epidemiology of Substance Use After Disasters

In the context of disaster survival, substance misuse and SUDs pose significant risks, including accidents, spread of infectious disease, and drug overdose. Disasters pose a risk for problematic alcohol and substance use consumption, distinct from SUDs, that may not or may persist (Table 12–1). Following a disaster, many more people engage in problematic drinking patterns than meet criteria for an alcohol use disorder. Drinking excessively is associated with many psychiatric and other medical complications and poorer medical-surgical outcomes. The global burden of disease from at-risk drinking is high, and it is often underdiagnosed. Tobacco, sleeping pills, tranquilizers, opioids, and other drugs may also be used.

Epidemiological studies show high prevalence rates of PTSD or other psychiatric disorders and comorbid SUDs, including a study of individuals with COVID-19 (Schieber et al. 2023). PTSD and SUDs, including alcohol use disorder, frequently co-occur after a disaster, as was seen after 9/11 (Vlahov et al. 2004). Rescue workers, such as firefighters, are vulnerable to excessive consumption associated with disaster exposure (North et al. 2002), as are adolescents, individuals who are unmarried, and rescuers

---

TABLE 12–1. Factors that may contribute to the development of alcohol and substance use pathology in the wake of a disaster

---

Presence of major depressive disorder or panic attacks at the time of the disaster

Prior history of alcohol or substance use disorder

Younger age, especially when combined with a disrupted support network

Serving as a rescue worker during the disaster

Perceived loss of considerable resources

---

participating in the recovery of bodies (Green et al. 1985). Some survivors may use opioids in a desperate effort to cope with pain and overwhelming stress (Khantzian et al. 1974). Survivors who experience loss of resources, including homelessness and forced migration (often weather-related), appear to be at greater risk for SUDs and PTSD (Giaconia et al. 2000; Horyniak et al. 2016). Evidence from 9/11 studies suggests that disaster exposure and other variables (see Table 12–1) predict increased alcohol or substance use (North et al. 2013). Surveillance and preventive measures for substance use disorders after a disaster are best applied to reduce relapse, worsening, or complication of predisaster mental disorders and substance use.

Assessment tools such as the CAGE (Cutting down, Annoyance at criticism, Guilty feeling, Eye-openers) questionnaire (Table 12–2) and the Alcohol Use Disorders Identification Test (AUDIT, a World Health Organization–approved instrument; Table 12–3), are useful in determining the severity of an alcohol use disorder (Cook et al. 2005). If the disorder is untreated, withdrawal symptoms may progress to alcoholic hallucinosis within 12–24 hours. The risk of withdrawal seizures (generalized tonic-clonic seizures) is greatest from 24–72 hours postwithdrawal, and the risk of delirium—disorientation, agitation, tachycardia, hypertension, sweating, and visual hallucinations—peaks at 48–72 hours.

In a disaster such as the COVID-19 pandemic, there may high mortality related to opioid use disorders, especially from fentanyl and other synthetic opioids (Garcia et al. 2022). Diagnosing alcohol and opioid dependence may be useful in that early intervention may prevent withdrawal and medical complications and reduce mortality (Table 12–4). Opioid withdrawal symptoms include elevated pulse, sweating, restlessness, constricted pupils, bone or joint aches, runny nose or tearing, abdominal cramping, tremor, yawning, anxiety or irritability, gooseflesh, and hot/cold flashes.

TABLE 12–2. CAGE questionnaire

Two "yes" responses indicate that the respondent should be assessed further.

1. Have you ever felt you needed to Cut down on your drinking?
2. Have people Annoyed you by criticizing your drinking?
3. Have you ever felt Guilty about drinking?
4. Have you ever felt you needed a drink first thing in the morning (Eye-opener) to steady your nerves or to get rid of a hangover?

Source. Ewing 1984.

Even more challenging is the identification of persons with potential SUDs who either have no known prior histories or are not part of a risk group. Sometimes, patients openly bring these concerns to the forefront during the interview or may be observed to be intoxicated. Clinicians may initiate assessment by suggesting that mood, anxiety, irritability, somatic, cognitive, or memory symptoms are common on surviving a disaster and that people sometimes self-medicate with alcohol and drugs. Some patients attempt to treat anxiety, irritability, or insomnia with sedatives, such as alcohol or benzodiazepines, or to treat fatigue with stimulants, such as cocaine or amphetamines. Anxiety and insomnia are common symptoms of sedative or alcohol withdrawal, whereas fatigue occurs while "crashing" from stimulants.

Pharmacological and Treatment Interventions

Because of a likely shortage of addiction specialists in the acute postdisaster period, psychiatrists or other physicians may need to get involved in substance detoxification and can refer to the aforementioned NIDA and NIAAA websites for guidelines. The assessment of a patient at risk for alcohol withdrawal consists of a complete history and physical examination, and laboratory tests are often indicated. Selection of an outpatient or inpatient treatment setting for detoxification, where such choices exist in the postdisaster setting, should be made.

The pharmacological treatment of alcohol withdrawal involves the use of medications that are cross-tolerant with alcohol—typically, the long-acting benzodiazepines diazepam and chlordiazepoxide. The standard treatment often is a fixed schedule with assessments with the Clinical Institute Withdrawal Assessment of Alcohol Scale, Revised (CIWA-Ar; Sullivan et al. 1989). Patients dependent on barbiturates require barbiturate administration to treat withdrawal, which is generally unresponsive to benzodiazepines. Treatment of opioid withdrawal should be conducted

TABLE 12–3. Alcohol Use Disorders Identification Test (AUDIT): Interview Version

Questions	0	1	2	3	4
1. How often do you have a drink containing alcohol? *[Skip to Qs 9–10 if 0 (Never)]*	Never	Monthly or less	2–4 times a month	2–3 times a week	4 or more times a week
2. How many drinks containing alcohol do you have on a typical day when you are drinking?	1 or 2	3 or 4	5 or 6	7–9	10 or more
3. How often do you have 6 or more drinks on one occasion? *[Skip to Qs 9–10 if total score for Qs 2 and 3 is 0]*	Never	Less than monthly	Monthly	Weekly	Daily or almost daily
4. How often during the last year have you found that you were not able to stop drinking once you had started?	Never	Less than monthly	Monthly	Weekly	Daily or almost daily
5. How often during the last year have you failed to do what was normally expected from you because of drinking?	Never	Less than monthly	Monthly	Weekly	Daily or almost daily
6. How often during the last year have you needed a first drink in the morning to get yourself going after a heavy drinking session?	Never	Less than monthly	Monthly	Weekly	Daily or almost daily
7. How often during the last year have you had a feeling of guilt or remorse after drinking?	Never	Less than monthly	Monthly	Weekly	Daily or almost daily

TABLE 12–3. Alcohol Use Disorders Identification Test (AUDIT): Interview Version (continued)

Questions	0	1	2	3	4
8. How often during the last year have you been unable to remember what happened the night before because you had been drinking?	Never	Less than monthly	Monthly	Weekly	Daily or almost daily
9. Have you or someone else been injured as a result of your drinking?	No		Yes, but not in the last year		Yes, during the last year
10. Has a relative, friend, doctor, or other health care worker been concerned about your drinking or suggested that you cut down?	No		Yes, but not in the last year		Yes, during the last year

Note. Read questions as written. Record answers carefully. Begin the AUDIT by saying, "Now I am going to ask you some questions about your use of alcoholic beverages during this past year." Explain what is meant by "alcoholic beverages" by using local examples of beer, wine, vodka, or other beverages. Code answers in terms of "standard drinks." The minimum score (for nondrinkers) is 0, and the maximum possible score is 40. A score of 8 is indicative of hazardous and harmful alcohol use and possibly of alcohol dependence. Scores of 8–15 indicate a medium level, and scores of 16 and above indicate a high level of alcohol problems.

Source. Adapted with permission from Babor TF, Biddle-Higgins JC, Saunders JB, et al.: AUDIT: The Alcohol Use Disorders Identification Test: Guidelines for Use in Primary Health Care (WHO/MSD/MSB/01.6a). Geneva, Switzerland, World Health Organization Department of Mental Health and Substance Dependence, 2001. Copyright © 2001 World Health Organization.

TABLE 12–4. Features of DSM-5-TR substance use disorders

A maladaptive pattern of substance use, leading to clinically significant impairment or distress, as manifested by three (or more) of the following, occurring at any time in the same 12-month period:

Criterion A: Impaired control over substance use

1. The individual may take the substance in larger amounts or over a longer period than was originally intended.

2. The individual may express a persistent desire to cut down or regulate substance use and may report multiple unsuccessful efforts to decrease or discontinue use.

3. The individual may spend a great deal of time obtaining the substance, using the substance, or recovering from its effects.

4. Craving is manifested by an intense desire or urge for the substance that may occur at any time but is more likely when in an environment where the substance previously was obtained or used.

5. More of the substance is needed to get the desired effect (also called tolerance).

Criterion B: Social impairment

6. Recurrent substance use may result in a failure to fulfill major role obligations at work, school, or home.

7. The individual may continue substance use despite having persistent or recurrent social or interpersonal problems caused or exacerbated by the effects of the substance.

8. Important social, occupational, or recreational activities may be given up or reduced because of substance use.

Criterion C: Risky use of the substance

9. Recurrent substance use occurs in situations in which use is physically hazardous.

10. The individual may continue substance use despite knowledge of having a persistent or recurrent physical or psychological problem that is likely to have been caused or exacerbated by the substance.

Criterion D: Pharmacological criteria

11. Tolerance is signaled by requiring a marked increased dose of the substance to achieve the desired effect or a markedly reduced effect when the usual dose is consumed.

12. Withdrawal occurs when blood and tissue concentrations of a substance decline in an individual who had maintained prolonged heavy use of the substance.

Source.   Adapted from *Diagnostic and Statistical Manual of Mental Disorders,* 5th Edition, Text Revision. Washington, DC, American Psychiatric Association, 2022, pp. 483–484. Copyright © 2022, American Psychiatric Association. Used with permission.

TABLE 12–5. Medications useful in treatment of substance withdrawal

Substance	Treatment
Alcohol or sedatives	Diazepam, lorazepam, phenobarbital, carbamazepine, valproic acid, ethanol (disinfectant)
Opioids	Methadone, morphine
Tobacco	Nicotine replacement patches
Codeine	Antidiarrheals
Various substances	Parenteral fluids, antiemetics

Source. World Health Organization 2010.

in accord with standard guidelines (see Mysels et al. 2011). Medications that may be useful in the treatment of alcohol, sedative, or opioid withdrawal are found in the *WHO Model List of Essential Medicines*, 16th Edition (World Health Organization 2010) (Table 12–5).

Treatment of alcohol or opioid withdrawal should be followed by treatment to address drug dependence. Patients completing detoxification should be referred to outpatient treatment. It is important to warn patients that their tolerance is reduced by undergoing opioid detoxification. The risk of postdetoxification overdose is high, and clinicians should inform patients of this risk. Naltrexone and buprenorphine are used for ongoing treatment, and in one study, failure to initiate treatment accounted for almost 100% of relapses and 50% of fatal overdoses (Brady 2021).

Medical Complaints, Injuries, and the Medically Ill

The biological substrates of the mind-body connection are receiving increasing attention. In disaster psychiatry, this is a practical matter in two key areas in triage following mass casualty events such as pandemics and other large-scale events (Morganstein 2022). First, patients with no physical illness who develop fears (e.g., of a toxin or smoke) may present with psychogenic symptoms (medically unexplained physical symptoms [MUPs]) such as shortness of breath, palpitations, or dissociation. Second, injured and medically ill patients may manifest pain syndromes, delirium, alcohol or drug withdrawal, PTSD and other disorders (Rubin and Dickmann 2010), and physical and mental disabilities (Stoddard et al. 2019).

Medically Unexplained Physical Symptoms Following Terrorist or Biological Events

After a terrorist or bioterrorist event, accidental biological exposure, or natural or climate-related disaster, mass panic may ensue, with large numbers of people presenting to the emergency department (ED) seeking evaluation and/or reassurance. These patients are most usefully considered under DSM-5-TR as manifesting functional neurological symptom disorder (conversion disorder) or somatic symptom disorder.

Surge capacity describes the ability of emergency services to deal with this mass panic and resulting surge in ED presentations, whether for medical or psychosomatic symptoms. Rapid triage can reduce the number of low-risk patients arriving at the ED and overwhelming resources. Mental health clinicians serve as educators about medical terminology and reactions to disasters in a language and at a level patients comprehend. To prevent long-term effects, it is essential to collaborate empathically with patients with MUPs to destigmatize their distress and normalize their decision to seek health care.

Triage and Evaluation of Medically Ill Survivors

The disaster mental health clinician may do rapid triage and assessment of patients in the ED and medical or surgical wards. The most vulnerable are usually children; women; older adults; those who have a disability or serious mental illness; and people from minoritized groups, including refugees. The disaster mental health professional may be called on to treat acute delirium and agitation and early symptoms of psychological trauma (Roberts et al. 2010). Patients with serious injuries are usually at higher risk for acute stress disorder, which includes symptoms of insomnia, anxiety, irritability, hypervigilance, and dissociation. Greater levels of early postinjury anxiety, emotional distress, and pain are associated with increased risk of PTSD (Zatzick et al. 2007).

The mental health clinician's evaluation of an injured or medically ill disaster survivor begins with an assessment of the patient's level of consciousness, including brief cognitive evaluation of orientation and level of consciousness to assess for dissociation; delirium; and, where relevant, complications of narcotic analgesics. Next, they should establish a method of communication. Patients who cannot communicate verbally can be asked to write answers on a piece of paper or a whiteboard, although creativity will be required in the case of illiterate survivors who may require the use of images they can point to in order to convey their experience and needs (e.g., a pain scale that uses increasingly unhappy smiley faces). The need to recognize and treat dissociation is highlighted by the fact that dissociation in the peritraumatic periods has been documented by researchers to predict PTSD, including in a study of 715 police officers and other first responders (Marmar et al. 2006).

The disaster mental health clinician may focus on symptoms and elect to treat them individually before waiting for a diagnosable DSM-5-TR disorder to manifest. Particular symptoms of concern are uncontrolled pain, insomnia, agitation, and anxiety. Insomnia can foster derealization and dissociation, preventing full psychological recovery. Screening for suicidal or homicidal ideation (or victimization) is essential, and precautions should be instituted in the medical setting where indicated (see section "Psychological Consequences of Special Concern"). For hospitalized patients, the experience can evoke feelings of loss of control and privacy because of dependence on others for basic tasks such as feeding, toileting, and ambulation. The psychological meanings of illness and injury to patients are important to ascertain because they can vary widely. Finally, and although this may not be relevant to the acute postdisaster period, screening for depression, anxiety, panic, psychosis, mania, acute stress disorder, and PTSD should be considered.

Treatment of Injured Survivors

Trauma and burn injuries have an impact on patients, families, and responders. Patients may be admitted to specialized level 1 burn and trauma centers; psychiatric consultation benefits patient care and reduces morbidity and mortality (Glass et al. 2018). Stoddard et al. (2018) found pain control with morphine important in preventing PTSD in burned children. Similarly, Holbrook et al. (2010) found morphine use after combat injury effective for the secondary prevention of PTSD. Psychological interventions and non-opioid analgesics are preferable when they are effective. Other needs are for higher acute morphine doses for pain relief in persons with opioid use disorder and referral of some patients for prevention or treatment of alcohol use disorder and other SUDs. Social skills interaction training, a variant of cognitive-behavioral therapy involving progressive desensitization, can help injured patients adjust to disfigurement, reducing disability (Partridge et al. 1994).

Psychological Consequences of Special Concern

Suicidality

Concerns about suicidality typically abound in postdisaster settings, at least in the popular imagination. Yet most postdisaster studies of suicidality have detected no increase in suicide rates and have even found decreases. At the very least, data on suicide are conflicting, as borne out by the COVID-19 pandemic. Google searches of terms indicative of suicide techniques found that self-harm was lower than expected during the first month of the pandemic, even though there was an increase in searches related to help-seeking behavior and mental health problems such as depression, anxiety, and loneliness (Halford et al. 2020). However, a nationally representative study of the United States found that 10.7% of adults reported seriously considering suicide in June 2020, more than double the 2018 rate (Czeisler et al. 2020). Reflecting the impact of race, Latinx and Black persons in this same study were among the groups found to have been disproportionately affected by COVID-19-related mental health conditions. Examining rates of suicide, a study in Massachusetts did not find increased suicides during the initial stay-at-home orders from March to May 2020 (Faust et al. 2021). In contrast, and again pointing to the role of race, a Maryland study during a similar lockdown period revealed an increase in suicide among Black residents, whereas the rate among White residents decreased in the same period (Bray et al. 2021).

Given these varied findings, it is probably most accurate to say that with death and destruction literally and figuratively in the air of a disaster-stricken community, questions about the meaning and value of life will naturally arise (Hung 2010). It is natural and expectable that survivors will question how they could go on in life after suffering the loss of loved ones or the destruction of their life as they knew it. But these spiritual and existential questions do not equate with suicidality. On the other hand, even if such questioning is understandable, it does not preclude the presence of suicidality and should not falsely reassure the evaluating clinician. Disaster mental health professionals, especially psychiatrists, should therefore be sure to include a basic suicide assessment in any acute-phase formal psychiatric assessment.

Violence

Prevailing wisdom suggests that harmony and altruism reign in the immediate aftermath of disaster. A small body of research, however, indicates some potential for heightened violence, especially in the postacute period. A study of murder in post–Hurricane Katrina New Orleans revealed that murder rates in 2006 were approximately 50% higher than in 2005 and nearly two-thirds higher than in 2004 (Van Landingham 2007). A recent study of survivors of the 2009 Australian bushfires 3–4 years after the disaster found that women in more highly affected regions experienced greater rates of interpersonal violence compared with women in less affected regions, an outcome associated with the secondary stressor of income loss (Molyneaux et al. 2019). Additional evidence for acute-phase violence comes from reductions in calls to intimate partner violence hotlines in the United States during the COVID-19 pandemic, which was thought to reflect an inability to call due to stay-at-home orders trapping individuals with their abuser (Baidoo et al. 2021; Evans et al. 2020). This includes the possibility of disproportionately increased intimate partner violence in communities of color.

Phua (2008) suggested that the broader umbrella of *postdisaster victimization* may be an overlooked, although still not necessarily common, outcome of disasters. It includes not only violence but also such activities as exploitation of survivors, profiteering, theft and looting, and discrimination. Despite limited research on postdisaster violence, asking whether a survivor has been victimized in any way since (and before) a disaster may provide a significant and potentially even lifesaving glimpse into some of the secondary stresses that may be affecting the individual.

Psychosis

Individuals with psychotic illness are vulnerable to recurrence following a disaster, whereas the likelihood of developing new psychotic illness likely reflects a balance of vulnerability and protective factors (Jing and Katz 2021). This will be discussed in detail in Chapter 14, "Serious Mental Illness."

Clinical Encounter

Considering themselves as a humanitarian before all else, the disaster mental health professional can and should engage in a range of functions that go beyond clinical care to include distribution of blankets, needs assessments, and interagency liaison, especially because these nonpsychological factors have a strong bearing on a survivor's psychological state. Therefore, whereas professional exchanges with individuals always begin with a formal evaluation in the traditional clinical setting, this is not necessarily, or usually, the case in times of disaster. For example, consider the following situation:

> A disaster mental health clinician is assigned to the dining area in a family assistance center following a devastating flood. He winds up talking for 10 minutes over coffee with a firefighter who is aggrieved at the loss of several of his neighbors but eager to get back to the ongoing rescue efforts. The clinician wishes him well, lets the man know where he can find him if ever he wants to talk more, and moves on. The clinician writes a two-sentence note describing the encounter but without the name of the firefighter or other personal information, which he did not collect.

TABLE 12–6. Factors influencing the decision to conduct a full encounter with a disaster survivor

---

How rested, cared for, and nourished the person looks

The degree of organization and focus the person exhibits in their behavior and communication

Any mention of questioning life

Bizarre ideas or dysfunctional levels of denial (e.g., still holding out hope that their loved one survived a month after they disappeared during a flood)

Request from a family member, friend, or coworker

The psychiatrist's "gut feeling"

Availability of resources and time

This so-called brief encounter, which is so named less for the brevity of the interaction and more for its anonymity and superficiality, is nevertheless an important psychiatric encounter. The disaster mental health professional is functioning as humanely as he is professionally, lending a compassionate ear to another person but also looking for indicators that the conversation should be extended into a full encounter, in which a thorough psychiatric evaluation would be conducted with the awareness and consent of the individual of concern. As a rough rule, the need for the transition should come to mind when the clinician decides they need to know the name of the person or, of course, when the person requests a more formal evaluation. The largely heuristic process of deciding when to conduct a formal evaluation can be guided by several factors, as listed in Table 12–6.

Mental health surveys can be used to screen individuals for postdisaster mental health problems (Connor et al. 2006). However, in the acute period, when diagnoses are not the focus, they may have limited utility. On the other hand, resources permitting, it may make sense to identify people at high risk for developing long-term mental health sequelae. Although there is some debate about the predictive utility of risk factors (Howlett and Stein 2016), there are well-known risk factors for developing posttraumatic psychopathology (Katz 2011). O'Donnell et al. (2008) described a helpful framework for identifying and following up with at-risk individuals hospitalized following an acute injury that should lend itself well to the acute disaster setting.

Conclusion

Psychiatric assessment of survivors and others in an affected community during the immediate days and weeks after a disaster differs greatly from conventional mental health care. Rather than zeroing in on diagnosis, care focuses on a wide range of symptoms, reactions, and behaviors, some of which may be adaptive, and others dysfunctional and highly distressing. Consultation to hospitalized patients with injuries or medical illness sustained in a disaster, in some cases related to substance use, requires close collaborative care with medical-surgical colleagues and planned brief psychotherapeutic support and pharmacological interventions to lessen pain, anxiety, depression, or other suffering. The approach to evaluating people during the acute postdisaster phase also often relies on outreach to individuals who did not set out seeking mental health care. Working as a mental health professional in such a setting poses unique challenges but also the unique opportunity to identify and address problems before they coalesce into posttraumatic psychiatric disorders.

References

American Psychiatric Association: Diagnostic and Statistical Manual of Mental Disorders, 5th Edition, Text Revision. Washington, DC, American Psychiatric Association, 2022

Baidoo L, Zakrison TL, Feldmeth G, et al: Domestic violence police reporting and resources during the 2020 COVID-19 stay-at-home order in Chicago, Illinois. JAMA Netw Open 4(9):e2122260, 2021 34473260

Bray MJC, Daneshvari NO, Radhakrishnan I, et al: Racial differences in statewide suicide mortality trends in Maryland during the coronavirus disease 2019 (COVID-19) pandemic. JAMA Psychiatry 78(4):444–447, 2021 33325985

Bohnert ASB, Ilgen MA: Understanding links among opioid use, overdose, and suicide. N Engl J Med 380(1):71–79, 2019 30601750

Brady KT: Optimizing treatment for opioid use disorder (editorial). Am J Psychiatry 178(7):586–587, 2021 34270338

Cherpitel CJ, Borges G: Screening for drug use disorders in the emergency department: performance of the rapid drug problems screen (RDPS). Drug Alcohol Depend 74(2):171–175, 2004 15099660

Connor KM, Foa EB, Davidson JR: Practical assessment and evaluation of mental health problems following a mass disaster. J Clin Psychiatry 67(Suppl 2):26–33, 2006 16602812

Cook RL, Chung T, Kelly TM, et al: Alcohol screening in young persons attending a sexually transmitted disease clinic: comparison of AUDIT, CRAFFT, and CAGE instruments. J Gen Intern Med 20(1):1–6, 2005 15693920

Czeisler MÉ, Lane RI, Petrosky E, et al: Mental health, substance use, and suicidal ideation during the COVID-19 pandemic: United States, June 24–30, 2020. MMWR Morb Mortal Wkly Rep 69(32):1049–1057, 2020 32790653

Evans ML, Lindauer M, Farrell ME: A pandemic within a pandemic: intimate partner violence during Covid-19. N Engl J Med 383(24):2302–2304, 2020 32937063

Ewing JA: Detecting alcoholism: the CAGE questionnaire. JAMA 252(14):1905–1907, 1984 6471323

Faust JS, Shah SB, Du C, et al: Suicide deaths during the COVID-19 stay-at-home advisory in Massachusetts, March to May 2020. JAMA Netw Open 4(1):e2034273, 2021 33475750

Figley CR, Nash WP (eds): Combat Stress Injury: Theory, Research, and Management. New York, Routledge, 2007

Garcia GP, Stringfellow EJ, DiGennaro C, et al: Opioid overdose decedent characteristics during COVID-19. Ann Med 54(1):1081–1088, 2022 35467475

Giaconia RM, Reinherz HZ, Hauz AC, et al: Comorbidity of substance use and post-traumatic stress disorders in a community sample of adolescents. Am J Orthopsychiatry 70(2):253–262, 2000 10826037

Glass S, Nejad SH, Fricchione GL, et al: Burn patients, in Massachusetts General Hospital Handbook of General Hospital Psychiatry, 7th Edition. Edited by Stern TA, Freudenreich O, Smith FA, et al. Philadelphia, PA, Elsevier, 2018, pp 359–370

Goldfrank LR, Bulter AS, Panzer AM: Preparing for the Psychological Consequences of Terrorism: A Public Health Strategy. Washington, DC, National Academies Press, 2003

Green BL, Grace MA, Gleser GC: Identifying survivors at risk: long-term impairment following the Beverly Hills Supper Club fire. J Consult Clin Psychol 53(5):672–678, 1985 4056182

Halford EA, Lake AM, Gould MS: Google searches for suicide and suicide risk factors in the early stages of the COVID-19 pandemic. PLoS One 15(7):e0236777, 2020 32706835

Holbrook TL, Galarneau MR, Dye JL, et al: Morphine use after combat injury in Iraq and post-traumatic stress disorder. N Engl J Med 362(2):110–117, 2010 20071700

Horyniak D, Melo JS, Farrell RM, et al: Epidemiology of substance use among forced migrants: a global systematic review. PLoS One 11(7):e.01590134, 2016 27411086

Howlett JR, Stein MB: Prevention of trauma and stressor-related disorders: a review. Neuropsychopharmacology 41(1):357–369, 2016 26315508

Hung E: Assessment and management of suicide after disasters, in Hidden Impact: What You Need to Know for the Next Disaster. A Practical Mental Health Guide for Clinicians. Edited by Stoddard FJ, Katz CL, Merlino JP. Sudbury, MA, Jones & Bartlett, 2010, pp 53–59

Jing GP, Katz CL: An update on psychotic spectrum disorders and disasters. Curr Opin Psychiatry 34(3):211–215, 2021 33605621

Kahlon MK, Aksan N, Aubrey R, et al: Effect of layperson-delivered, empathy-focused program of telephone calls on loneliness, depression, and anxiety among adults during the COVID-19 pandemic: a randomized clinical trial. JAMA Psychiatry 78(6):616–622, 2021 33620417

Katz CL: Disaster psychiatry: good intentions seeking science and sustainability. Adolesc Psychiatry 1:187–196, 2011

Katz CL: The rewards and challenges of disaster psychiatry. Psychiatria et Neurologia Japonica 123:666–675, 2021

Khantzian EJ, Mack JE, Schatzberg AF: Heroin use as an attempt to cope: clinical observations. Am J Psychiatry 131(2):160–164, 1974 4809043

Marmar CR, McCaslin SE, Metzler TJ, et al: Predictors of posttraumatic stress in police and other first responders. Ann N Y Acad Sci 1071:1–18, 2006 16891557

Molyneaux R, Gibbs L, Bryant RA, et al: Interpersonal violence and mental health outcomes following disaster. BJPsych Open 6(1):e1, 2019 31796146

Morganstein JC: Preparing for the next pandemic to protect public mental health: what have we learned from Covid-19? Psychiatr Clin North Am 45(1):191–210, 2022 35219438

Mysels DJ, Sullivan MA, Dowling FG: Substance abuse, in Disaster Psychiatry: Readiness, Evaluation and Treatment. Edited by Stoddard FL, Pandya A, Katz CL. Washington, DC, American Psychiatric Press, 2011, pp 121–141

North CS, Tivis L, McMillen JC, et al: Psychiatric disorders in rescue workers after the Oklahoma City bombing. Am J Psychiatry 159(5):857–859, 2002 11986143

North CS, Adinoff B, Pollio DE, et al: Alcohol use disorders and drinking among survivors of the 9/11 attacks on the World Trade Center in New York City. Compr Psychiatry 54(7):962–969, 2013 23642636

O'Donnell ML, Bryant RA, Creamer M, et al: Mental health following traumatic injury: toward a health system model of early psychological intervention. Clin Psychol Rev 28(3):387–406, 2008 17707563

Partridge J, Robinson E, Rumsey N: Tissue viability: changing faces: two years on. Nurs Stand 8(34):54–58, 1994 8038078

Phua KL: Post-disaster victimization: how survivors of disasters can continue to suffer after the event is over. New Solut 18(2):221–231, 2008 18511398

Roberts NP, Kitchiner NJ, Kenardy J, et al: Early psychological interventions to treat acute traumatic stress symptoms. Cochrane Database Syst Rev (3):CD007944, 2010 20238359

Rubin GJ, Dickmann P: How to reduce the impact of "low-risk patients" following a bioterrorist incident: lessons from SARS, anthrax, and pneumonic plague. Biosecur Bioterror 8(1):37–43, 2010 20230231

Schieber LZ, Dunphy C, Schieber RA, et al: Hospitalization associated with co-morbid psychiatric and substance use disorders among adults with Covid-19 treated in US emergency departments from April 2020-August 2021. JAMA Psychiatry 80(4):331–341, 2023 36790774

Stoddard FJ, Ursano RJ, Cozza SJ: Population trauma: disasters, in Trauma- and Stressor-Related Disorders. Edited by Stoddard FJ, Benedek DM, Milad, MR, et al. New York, Oxford University Press, 2018, pp 113–130

Stoddard FJ, Simon NM, Pitman RK: Trauma- and stressor-related disorders, in American Psychiatric Publishing Textbook of Psychiatry: DSM-5 Edition. Edited by Roberts L. Washington, DC, American Psychiatric Press, 2019, pp 393–436

Sullivan JT, Sykora K, Schneiderman J, et al: Assessment of alcohol withdrawal: the revised clinical institute withdrawal assessment for alcohol scale (CIWA-Ar). Br J Addict 84(11):1353–1357, 1989 2597811

U.S. Department of Health and Human Services: The healthcare professional's core resource on alcohol. Bethesda, MD, National Institute on Alcohol, Alcohol Abuse, and Alcoholism, May 6, 2022. Available at: www.niaaa.nih.gov/health-professionals-communities/core-resource-on-alcohol. Accessed July 11, 2024.

Van Landingham MJ: Murder rates in New Orleans, La, 2004–2006. Am J Public Health 97(9):1614–1616, 2007 17666685

Vlahov D, Galea S, Ahern J, et al: Consumption of cigarettes, alcohol, and marijuana among New York City residents six months after the September 11 terrorist attacks. Am J Drug Alcohol Abuse 30(2):385–407, 2004 15230082

World Health Organization: WHO Model List of Essential Medicines, 16th Edition (Updated). Geneva, Switzerland, World Health Organization, 2010

Zatzick DF, Rivara FP, Nathens AB, et al: A nationwide US study of post-traumatic stress after hospitalization for physical injury. Psychol Med 37(10):1469–1480, 2007 17559704

13

Specific Needs of Submarginalized Populations

Kathleen A. Clegg, M.D.
Kunmi Sobowale, M.D.

Disasters disproportionately affect certain groups of people. These people who are at higher risk of experiencing disasters and their consequences are called *vulnerable* (Wisner et al. 2004). Traditionally, disaster mental health has considered geographic and demographic or clinical factors (e.g., physical disability, immaturity, psychosis) as markers of vulnerability. However, we must ask why certain groups of people are more vulnerable in the first place.

Marginalized groups are at high risk of vulnerability. Marginalization is the process of pushing groups of people to the periphery of society and limiting their access to power. Policies, social hierarchies, and economic forces shape the conditions where marginalized populations live, work, and play over time. For example, geographic restrictions on housing based on race in the twentieth century in the United States contributed to modern-day racial segregation. Racial segregation, in turn, results in Black people residing in geographic areas that are more disaster-prone, while limiting their ability to migrate because of limited economic opportunities (Bolin and Kurtz 2018). At its root, marginalization is determined by who has power in society and how that power is exercised to support or undermine specific groups of people.

With this lens, clinicians can better appreciate that vulnerability to disaster concerns people's relationship with power rather than the environment (Hsu et al. 2015). Marginalized groups remain disadvantaged even in the absence of disasters, and disasters can exacerbate marginalization. In line with the minority stress theory, marginalization leads to unique additional stress exposures (e.g., discrimination) for certain groups, which is detrimental to mental and physical health (Meyer 2003). Thus, mental health clinicians need to consider these historical, structural, and cultural factors while assessing and treating marginalized populations in disaster contexts.

Many groups can be considered marginalized. Some examples include children, older adults, prisoners, people with intellectual disabilities, and those living in congregate or residential care facilities. In this chapter, we focus on women, LGBTQ+ populations, people with physical disabilities, racial and ethnic groups, and people of low socioeconomic status. Several other groups are covered in other chapters. Although these groups are examined in isolation, clinicians should be mindful that the intersections of these identities can increase or decrease vulnerability.

Women

Although lifetime exposure to traumatic events in general is roughly equal for men and women, the available evidence suggests that women are at higher risk for psychiatric difficulties after a disaster (Norris et al. 2002). This increased risk is relatively consistent across ages and cultures, but there are some differences.

Several factors may account for women's increased risk of psychiatric difficulties after a disaster. In the general population, women have higher rates of depression, anxiety disorders, and posttraumatic stress disorder (PTSD), which are significant risk factors for postdisaster difficulties. Although rates of exposure to trauma may be similar for men and women, the types of trauma and the risk of resulting psychiatric disorders vary. Men are more likely to experience a motor vehicle accident, which has a lower risk, and women experience a significantly higher rate of sexual assault, which has the highest risk of leading to psychiatric difficulties (Frans et al. 2005). Other reasons include greater predisaster traumatic exposure in women, higher prevalence of mental health conditions, and lower socioeconomic status.

The coronavirus disease 2019 (COVID-19) pandemic has had a profound impact on the mental health of women across the life span, exaggerating many existing inequities experienced by women, such as excess responsibilities as primary caretakers for young, old, and infirm family members and overseers of family health care. Women experienced job loss at higher rates than did men during the pandemic, largely because of the type of work that women do. Disproportionate numbers of women work in frontline service positions for which on-site work is mandatory. In addition, school and childcare closures drove more women out of the workforce because of the need to care for children at home. Worldwide, an estimated 70% of the health care workforce is made up of women who are frontline health workers, including a majority of health facility service staff. Therefore, women are more likely than men to work in positions with more exposure to COVID-19 (Berg et al. 2022).

In addition, domestic abuse, including abuse from intimate partners, has disproportionally affected women, and COVID-19 stay-at-home orders, work from home, and loss of employment have amplified family violence (Berg et al. 2022). This mirrors findings from past studies, including of the 2009 bushfires in Victoria, Australia, where a negative change in income predicted 4.68 times higher odds of violence among women residing in high bushfire-affected regions (Molyneaux et al. 2019). These findings highlight the need to consider postdisaster financial stress as a risk factor in postdisaster violence.

In complex humanitarian settings such as war zones, women and girls are particularly vulnerable to gender-based violence (GBV), which is often weaponized during conflict. A systematic review of relevant literature and multiple databases through February 2013 suggested that approximately one in five refugee or displaced women in complex humanitarian settings experienced sexual violence, which may underestimate the true prevalence given the multiple existing barriers to disclosure (Vu et al. 2014). A study of Somali women in a Kenyan refugee camp found that poor mental health was due to both current episodes of intimate partner violence and past experiences of violence during the conflict (Hossain et al. 2020).

GBV is linked to adverse mental health outcomes, such as anxiety, depression, and PTSD, and has been associated with adverse physical and psychosocial outcomes, such as unwanted pregnancy, sexually transmitted infections, discrimination, stigmatization, and ostracism within the family or the community (Hossain et al. 2020). GBV also affects women's ability to secure and undertake employment and participate in recovery efforts and confronts them with obstacles to seeking care for its consequences. In a long-standing refugee camp in Kenya, barriers to seeking GBV care included feeling stigmatized by families or community members, feeling helpless over their situation, fear of future violence, insecurity in the camps, and being denied access to GBV services by guards. Professional staff and refugee community workers were used to overcome these barriers by encouraging service-seeking among GBV survivors and facilitating access to services (Muuo et al. 2020).

The World Health Organization (WHO) has developed clinical and policy guidelines for responding to intimate partner violence and sexual violence against women aimed at health care providers because they are in a unique position to address the health and psychosocial needs of women who have experienced violence (World Health Organization 2013). The recommendations regarding screening women for GBV are included in Table 13–1.

In addition to following the WHO guidelines in addressing the needs of individual women in the aftermath of a disaster, clinicians can also support women by recognizing the unique stressors and needs women have in disaster situations (World Health Organization 2013). Teams responsible for community planning for disasters should include women who are community members, community leaders, and first responders to develop plans that are most responsive to women's needs.

LGBTQ+ People

People with lesbian, gay, bisexual, trans, queer/questioning, and other minority gender and sexual identities (LGBTQ+) face unique vulnerabilities in disaster situations. This diverse group of individuals with varying gender and sexual identities, numbering at least 16 million in the United States, share some similar experiences. Compared with the cisgender population, the LGBTQ+ population is more severely affected by disasters. This vulnerability is due to higher rates of poverty, homelessness, chronic illness, and incarceration, as well as intentional acts of commission and errors of omission in disaster policies and practices (Goldsmith et al. 2022). These inequities increase the risk of poor mental health for this group.

LGBTQ+ people are also overlooked in disaster planning. The Sendai Framework is a global disaster risk reduction policy that omits LGBTQ+ populations when discussing gender inequality (Mills 2015). The Robert T. Stafford Disaster Relief and Emergency Assistance Act is a 1988 U.S. federal law designed to provide assistance to state and local governments in the aftermath of a disaster. The law prohibits discrimination on the basis of many categories but does not provide protections on the basis of gender identity and sexual orientation (Goldsmith et al. 2022).

Acts of commission against LGBTQ+ people also increase disaster vulnerability. The stress theory describes how unique stressors, specifically stigma, prejudice, and discrimination related to marginalized gender and sexual identities, are related to health disparities (Meyer 2003).

TABLE 13–1. World Health Organization recommendations regarding screening women for gender-based violence

Women who disclose any form of violence by an intimate partner (or other family member) or sexual assault by any perpetrator should be offered immediate support. Health care providers should, as a minimum, offer first-line support when a woman discloses violence. First-line support includes the following:

- Ensuring consultation is conducted in private
- Ensuring confidentiality, while informing women of the limits of confidentiality (e.g., when there is mandatory reporting)
- Being nonjudgmental and supportive and validating what the woman is saying
- Providing practical care and support that respond to her concerns but do not intrude
- Asking about her history of violence, listening carefully but not pressuring her to talk; care should be taken when discussing sensitive topics when interpreters are involved
- Helping her access information about resources, including legal and other services that she might think helpful
- Assisting her to increase safety for herself and her children, where needed
- Providing or mobilizing social support

Source. World Health Organization 2013.

The consequences of these errors of omission and acts of commission are numerous. For example, LGBTQ+ family structures such as same-sex partnerships may not be recognized in disaster relief efforts. As a result, LGBTQ+ families may be devalued in resource distribution and reunification efforts after family separation. LGBTQ+ individuals, particularly transgender people, can face housing challenges due to being prohibited from shelters. During the COVID-19 pandemic lockdowns, many LGBTQ+ youth had to live with family members who were unwelcoming or hostile while losing their community supports (Goldberg 2021; Panchal et al. 2021). Faith-based organizations play a significant role in disaster relief, particularly in the short term, and dominant religious beliefs in the United States and abroad are often homophobic and transphobic. Most of the social services provided in the aftermath of Hurricane Katrina came from faith-based organizations (Farrag et al. 2022). Unsurprisingly, some faith-based organizations discriminated against LGBTQ+ communities by not offering this group disaster relief services (Goldsmith et al. 2022).

LGBTQ+ people also experience higher rates of violence, such as verbal, physical, and sexual assault, during disasters (Goldsmith et al. 2022; van Daalen et al. 2022). Marginalization and lack of access to resources in the wake of disasters can place this group at a higher risk of being victimized. The scapegoating of LGBTQ+ people as the cause of disasters because their identities and lifestyle are deemed immoral likely also contributes to violence. In addition, there is a long history of human-made disasters, including mass shootings, targeting this community. Despite all of this, the violence against gender and sexual minorities remains understudied in the disaster literature (van Daalen et al. 2022).

There are a variety of ways for clinicians to support LGBTQ+ people. First, as described in the section "Clinical Pearls and Implications," they should take a culturally humble approach because the LGBTQ+ community is diverse, and some groups have unique challenges, such as transgender individuals experiencing difficulty accessing gender-affirming hormones during disasters. Second, clinicians should take a strengths-based approach and recognize this community's resilience, including community connectedness and belonging, a strong sense of identity, LGBTQ+-serving organizations, and activism during prior disasters such as the AIDS pandemic (Meyer 2015).

Clinicians should familiarize themselves with organizations that serve this community because some will provide disaster relief. The disaster readiness of these organizations vary, which can allow clinicians to partner to provide mental health training to organizations. Awareness of local policies and the stances of local faith-based organizations and shelters is also a way for clinicians to avoid doing harm and to support LGBTQ+-serving organizations and stakeholders' role in disaster planning and response policies and practice.

People With Physical Disabilities

People with physical disabilities suffer disproportionately during and after a disaster. They are two to four times more likely to die or be injured in disasters and are more likely to be left behind in emergency responses and miss out on crucial humanitarian services because of a range of environmental, physical, and social barriers. These barriers include discriminatory triage practices, inadequate medical treatment in institutional settings, gaps in the availability of public health information, and inability to access regular health and rehabilitation services and supports, often preventing individuals with physical disabilities from being able to live independently. The consequences of compromised access are most acute in contexts where health and social systems are less responsive to the specific needs of people with disabilities, notably low- and middle-income countries, where it is estimated that 80% of the 1 billion people in the world who experience a disability live (Hillgrove et al. 2021).

The disparate impact of disasters on persons with disabilities is not limited to low- and middle-income countries. A study of residents in Houston, Texas, after Hurricane Harvey in 2017 found that having a disability that interfered with evacuation was associated with a 219% increase in the odds of going without postdisaster health care (Flores et al. 2020). The 2006 National Council on Disability report summarized the impacts of Hurricanes Katrina and Rita on persons with disabilities. These impacts included persons with sensory disabilities not being able to receive emergency alerts or evacuation instructions when no visual display of communication was employed. Cell phone service was unreliable when service was lost because of 160-mile-per-hour winds. Evacuation plans failed to include necessary transportation and shelters that would accept people with disabilities (Freidan 2006).

Persons with disabilities have been disproportionately affected by the COVID-19 pandemic. They commonly experienced increased risks of contracting COVID-19, more severe disease or death, and new or worsening health conditions. These risks arose from a range of barriers in the health sector, including physical barriers that prevent access to health facilities, informational barriers that prevent access to health information and reduce health literacy, and attitudinal barriers that give rise to stigma and exclusion (Pearce et al. 2022). Isolation due to physical distancing and movement restrictions has exacerbated the risk of violence against persons with disabilities, especially women, girls, and transgender and nonbinary persons with disabilities (Pearce et al. 2022). Guidance on allocating scarce resources during the COVID-19 pandemic, such as that offered by Emanuel et al. (2020), received criticism for failing to discuss bias, discrimination, or disability. The primary recommendation in the guidance was to maximize benefit by shifting resources to patients with better prognoses and focus on life-years saved, thereby demanding a judgment call by heath care providers that was subject to discrimination against disabled, poor, and minority persons (Brown and Goodwin 2020).

Of all the medical care rationed, the most problematic was mechanical ventilation because of the scarcity of ventilators and the life-or-death nature of the decision to initiate or terminate mechanical ventilation. Recommendations about rationing included the use of a triage officer or committee not involved in the clinical care of patients, the application of exclusion criteria such as irreversible shock, the use of a standardized tool to assess mortality risk, and repeat assessments over time to determine when ventilation should be removed (Truog et al. 2020).

Issues with disability inclusion in the COVID-19 pandemic have informed three priority areas for strengthening health systems: 1) data collection and analysis of health inequalities among persons with disabilities, 2) equitable access to new modalities and innovations such as telehealth, and 3) inclusive decision-making processes. Examples of these approaches include ensuring that disability is one of many variables considered in health emergency data collection; upscaling efforts to address the "digital divide" faced by different groups, including persons with disabilities and their family members; and including support services and health care providers in health emergency planning (Pearce et al. 2022).

The Reference Group on Inclusion of Persons with Disabilities, in consultation with the Inter-Agency Standing Committee (IASC), published guidance on applying the IASC guidelines on the inclusion of persons with disabilities in humanitarian action to the pandemic (Inter-Agency Standing Committee 2020). These recommendations, which can also be extrapolated to future public health emergencies, included engaging persons with disabilities in developing COVID-19 outbreak preparedness and response plans; addressing the multiple barriers to implementing preventive measures, accessing distribution of food and other needed items such as personal protective equipment, ensuring that information is available in multiple accessible formats, training on standards regarding working with persons with disabilities, and data collection and monitoring that take the needs of persons with disabilities into account.

Clinicians can support persons with physical vulnerabilities by assisting them with getting necessary medication and medical equipment in postdisaster situations. Clinicians can also advocate for the needs of persons with physical disabilities to be considered in the disaster planning of hospitals and health care institutions and communities, where individuals with physical disabilities and their caregivers should also have a voice.

Race and Ethnicity

The terms race and ethnicity are often used interchangeably, but they are quite different. Race refers to physical characteristics that are used to divide people into groups. Ethnicity is a broader term based on commonalities such as culture, language, heritage, religion, and customs. It is important to remember that race and ethnicity are social constructs and cannot capture groups perfectly, which leads to underinclusivity or overinclusivity. For example, the U.S. Census classifies Indigenous people as a race, but they may be better considered to be a political entity (UCLA Equity, Diversity, and Inclusion 2020).

Terminology aside, ethnoracially marginalized groups experience disaster-related health disparities, with higher mortality and morbidity and worse mental health outcomes (Sharpe and Wolkin 2022). Black and Indigenous youth were more likely to lose a parent or caregiver to COVID-19 infection than were non-Hispanic white children. Meanwhile, these same communities remain less likely to receive mental health care (Thomeer et al. 2023). Hispanic and Latino/Latina people reported a significantly elevated rate of depressive symptoms early in the COVID-19 pandemic (Saltzman et al. 2021). Additionally, Chinese American families faced COVID-19-related racism, resulting in worse mental health (Cheah et al. 2020). Other Asian American groups were subjected to discrimination as well, contributing to mental health challenges within these communities (Wu et al. 2021).

A historical lens is needed to consider why these groups are vulnerable to disasters such as the COVID-19 pandemic. European colonization of North America decimated Indigenous populations starting in the late sixteenth century. Although the 13th Amendment to the U.S. Constitution emancipated enslaved people in 1865, many subsequent laws, policies, practices, and ideologies discriminated against Black people in the United States. Many factors that render these groups more vulnerable to disasters, such as precarious geographic location or poorer mental health, can be traced to these historical injustices. Ongoing discrimination compounds these foundational issues. For example, COVID-19 outbreaks in carceral settings disproportionately affected Black people because of racist mass incarceration of Black people in the United States. These outbreaks, in turn, resulted in increased use of solitary confinement for infection control, which has adverse effects on the mental health of Black prisoners (Reinhart 2023).

Although the enormity of ethnoracial disparities may seem insurmountable, there are practical steps that disaster mental health clinicians can take. They should learn about, reflect on, and acknowledge the history of ethnoracially marginalized groups in the United States and its impact on vulnerability to disasters. This approach dispels *cultural determinism*, the false belief that differences in ethnic and racial groups are due to cultural factors, and builds cultural humility. Clinicians can partner with trusted local leaders. Doing so can increase access to mental health care, decrease power imbalances between clinicians and people from ethnoracially marginalized groups, and ensure that community voices are represented to advocate for their needs. To this end, a community-led COVID-19 vaccine clinic for Métis Nation, an Indigenous group in Canada, had great success with vaccinators from the community and integration of traditional practices (King et al. 2022).

Ultimately, mental health professionals can proactively effect change for ethnoracially marginalized groups by advocating for policies that improve social determinants of mental health and increase access to mental health care. For example, they can support legislation like the FEMA Equity Act, which aims to document and improve racial disparities in federal assistance for disasters. Clinicians can promote policy change by documenting disparities such as differential access to telemental health. The heroic work of pediatrician Mona Hanna-Attisha using health records to expose the Flint water crisis is an example of the power of using documentation in this fashion (Hanna-Attisha et al. 2016). Finally, clinicians can use their professional pulpit to convince elected officials to support just policies.

Low Socioeconomic Status

Lower socioeconomic status (SES), a term encompassing one's income, educational attainment, and occupational status, strongly predicts poor mental health after disasters. First responders with low education status were more likely to have elevated or worsening PTSD symptoms years after the 9/11 terrorism attacks (Feder et al. 2016). Months after Hurricane Ike struck Texas, adults with lower household income and education were more likely to meet criteria for depression (Tracy et al. 2011). Low household income was likewise associated with persistent elevated depressive symptoms during the COVID-19 pandemic (Ettman et al. 2022).

People with low SES are vulnerable to disasters for multiple reasons. First, they are more likely to live in areas that are disaster-prone and underserved. Hurricane Katrina disproportionately affected people living in low-SES areas who, because of their limited means, were less able to evacuate (Kamel 2012). Second, people with limited resources must deal with acute and chronic stress. The precariousness of financial resources causes a present focus that makes planning for future events such as a disaster more difficult. This lack of future planning, along with the increased number and unpredictability of adverse life events for people with low SES, is stressful. Furthermore, adverse life events and limited financial means to change one's life circumstances can lead to a lack of sense of control over one's life. Third, these stresses can increase maladaptive health behaviors, such as drinking alcohol to deal with stress. Finally, lack of access to quality health care increases vulnerability to postdisaster health and mental health consequences. Fewer clinicians, lower quality of care, and logistical barriers such as lack of access to transportation to attend appointments are among the challenges.

In the aftermath of a disaster, people with low SES face unique challenges. Because of the increased chance of property damage or loss, they are more likely to be displaced from their homes and end up homeless and have less access to loans for rebuilding. In addition, people with limited means experience higher rates of job loss and interruption. Overall, disasters exacerbate existing vulnerabilities, resulting in poorer mental health.

Mental health professionals are integral to supporting this population's mental health in the aftermath of a disaster. Because low-SES populations are more likely than the general population to develop mental illness, clinicians should be especially attentive to screening for these conditions in the months after a disaster. To increase access to care, clinicians can offer sliding-scale payment and encourage uninsured people to enroll in health insurance. Telehealth services are not always accessible in disaster contexts, and people with low SES may not have broadband internet or enough phone data to use telehealth. Clinicians can share information about the Federal Communications Commission's Lifeline Support program, which subsidizes the cost of broadband internet and connected devices for low-income families (Universal Service Administrative Company 2024). Another recommendation is to use the Disaster Distress Helpline, a free crisis counseling service for people experiencing disaster-related emotional distress that can be reached by phone.

Supporting basic needs is one of the most important mental health interventions. During the COVID-19 pandemic, the U.S. government sent cash transfers and expanded the child tax credit. Both interventions decreased material hardships for families, and the expanded child tax credit improved adult mental health (Batra et al. 2023). Unfortunately, both financial interventions were only temporary measures. At the policy level, professionals should advocate for continued financial supports such as the child tax credit to people with low SES.

Clinical Pearls and Implications

Given that the needs of marginalized people are frequently overlooked in disaster planning and that they often have a high burden of co-occurring physical, mental, and substance use disorders; have less access to health information; and have scare resources necessary for recovery, clinicians should support them in making disaster preparedness plans (see Chapter 1, "Disaster Psychiatry Education") and in recovery. In April 2020, the Boston Hope Medical Center designed a system of care to address the needs of homeless individuals, a significantly marginalized and vulnerable population, by applying the principles of Psychological First Aid (PFA).

PFA principles include contact and engagement, safety and comfort, stabilization, information gathering, practical assistance, connection with social supports, coping information, and linkage with collaborative services (see Chapter 16, "Psychological First Aid"). Medical Center organizers concluded that whereas the principles of PFA are often applied on the individual level for interaction with survivors, the same principles can be applied at the systems level to organize a population-wide response.

Although this chapter focuses on specific marginalized groups, no individual is defined by a single identity. Intersectional theory considers how the intersection of multiple marginalized identities can leave certain individuals even more vulnerable to disasters. For example, after a disaster, a middle-class woman's experience will differ from that of a woman with low SES, which will differ from that of a woman with low SES and a physical disability. The theory also highlights how the salience of particular identities changes with time and space. To illustrate, a transgender man may be more conscious of their clothing (i.e., gender expression) at a disaster shelter for men than at home.

How can disaster mental health clinicians respect these multiple identities when providing care? They can learn about the culture of the people they serve. Culture consists of the beliefs, attitudes, values, and behaviors that are passed between people through learning and participation in groups or institutions. It shapes how people make sense of disasters and distress, how distress is expressed, and how people seek help. Learning which aspects of a person's culture are important for their care requires maintaining cultural humility and asking them.

Unlike cultural competency, which assumes that clinicians can achieve mastery-level knowledge about a culture, cultural humility proposes that clinicians demonstrate ongoing curiosity about culture by learning and listening to individuals and the community. Further, it requires a lifelong critical self-reflection and a desire to remedy power imbalances between clinicians and patients and between health systems and underserved communities or groups (Tervalon and Murray-García 1998). The Cultural Formulation Interview is a free standardized, person-centered, skills-based interview guide to inquire about an individual's culture (Aggarwal and Lewis-Fernández 2020; American Psychiatric Association 2022). It contains 16 items that focus on the cultural definition of the problem; cultural explanations of illness, including identity, cultural factors that affect coping, and past help-seeking; and cultural factors that affect current help-seeking.

Finally, disaster mental health clinicians should advocate for social justice efforts that mitigate the vulnerability of marginalized populations to future disasters. A return to the status quo after a disaster is insufficient. To build back better, clinicians can advocate for policies such as reparations for descendants of enslaved people in the United States, gender-affirming practices, and land restoration for Indigenous people. Mental health professionals can empower these populations by recognizing their strengths, such as the strong activism of the LGBTQ+ community or healing practices of Indigenous people and African Americans, and connecting individuals who identify with these groups to existing social networks (e.g., community-based organizations) and resources. Indeed, the United Nations has included Indigenous knowledge in disaster risk reduction (United Nations Office for Disaster Risk Reduction 2022). These groups should be part of disaster planning, not just thought of postdisaster.

Conclusion

As demonstrated in this chapter, the process of marginalization makes certain groups more vulnerable to disasters. By recognizing and responding in various ways to the vulnerability of a range of special populations, disaster mental health professionals can help level the playing field as these populations recover from disaster.

References

Aggarwal NK, Lewis-Fernández R: An introduction to the Cultural Formulation Interview. Focus (Am Psychiatr Publ) 18(1):77–82, 2020 32015732

American Psychiatric Association: Cultural Formulation Interview, in Diagnostic and Statistical Manual of Mental Disorders, 5th Edition, Text Revision. Washington, DC, American Psychiatric Association, 2022, pp 864–871

Batra A, Jackson K, Hamad R: Effects of the 2021 expanded child tax credit on adults' mental health: a quasi-experimental study. Health Aff (Millwood) 42(1):74–82, 2023 36623218

Berg JA, Woods NF, Shaver J, et al: COVID-19 effects on women's home and work life, family violence and mental health from the Women's Health Expert Panel of the American Academy of Nursing. Nurs Outlook 70(4):570–579, 2022 35843755

Bolin B, Kurtz LC: Race, class, ethnicity, and disaster vulnerability, in Handbook of Disaster Research, 2nd Edition. Edited by Rodriguez H, Donner W, Trainor JE. Cham, Switzerland, Springer, 2018, pp 181–203

Brown MJ, Goodwin J: Allocating medical resources in the time of Covid-19. N Engl J Med 382(22):e79, 2020 32343499

Cheah CSL, Wang C, Ren H, et al: COVID-19 racism and mental health in Chinese American families. Pediatrics 146(5):146, 2020 32873719

Emanuel EJ, Persad G, Upshur R, et al: Fair allocation of scarce medical resources in the time of Covid-19. N Engl J Med 382(21):2049–2055, 2020 32202722

Ettman CK, Cohen GH, Abdalla SM, et al: Persistent depressive symptoms during COVID-19: a national, population-representative, longitudinal study of U.S. adults. Lancet Reg Health Am 5:100091, 2022 34635882

Farrag H, Loskota B, Flory R: Faithful Action: Working With Religious Groups in Disaster Planning, Response, and Recovery. Los Angeles, CA, Center for Religion and Civic Culture, University of Southern California, November 2022. Available at: https://crcc.usc.edu/wp-content/uploads/2015/02/FaithfulAction2012.pdf. Accessed April 2, 2024.

Feder A, Mota N, Salim R, et al: Risk, coping and PTSD symptom trajectories in World Trade Center responders. J Psychiatr Res 82:68–79, 2016 27468166

Flores AB, Collins TW, Grineski SE, et al: Disparities in health effects and access to health care among Houston area residents after Hurricane Harvey. Public Health Rep 135(4):511–523, 2020 32539542

Frans O, Rimmö PA, Åberg L, et al: Trauma exposure and post-traumatic stress disorder in the general population. Acta Psychiatr Scand 111(4):291–299, 2005 15740465

Freidan L: The impact of Hurricanes Katrina and Rita on people with disabilities: a look back and remaining challenges. Washington, DC, National Council on Disability, 2006. Available at: www.ncd.gov/assets/uploads/reports/2006/ncd-impact-hurricanes-katrina-rita-2006.pdf. Accessed April 2, 2024.

Goldberg SB: Education in a Pandemic: The Disparate Impacts of COVID-19 on America's Students. Washington, DC, Office for Civil Rights, U.S. Department of Education, 2021. Available at: www2.ed.gov/about/offices/list/ocr/docs/20210608-impacts-of-covid19.pdf. Accessed April 2, 2024.

Goldsmith L, Raditz V, Méndez M: Queer and present danger: understanding the disparate impacts of disasters on LGBTQ+ communities. Disasters 46(4):946–973, 2022 34498778

Hanna-Attisha M, LaChance J, Sadler RC, Champney Schnepp A: Elevated blood lead levels in children associated with the Flint drinking water crisis: a spatial analysis of risk and public health response. Am J Public Health 106(2):283–290, 2016 26691115

Hillgrove T, Blyth J, Kiefel-Johnson F, et al: A synthesis of findings from "rapid assessments" of disability and the COVID-19 pandemic: implications for response and disability-inclusive data collection. Int J Environ Res Public Health 18(18):9701, 2021 34574625

Hossain M, Pearson RJ, McAlpine A, et al: Gender-based violence and its association with mental health among Somali women in a Kenyan refugee camp: a latent class analysis. J Epidemiol Community Health 75(4):327–334, 2020 33148683

Hsu M, Howitt R, Miller F: Procedural vulnerability and institutional capacity deficits in post-disaster recovery and reconstruction: insights from Wutai Rukai experiences of Typhoon Morakot. Hum Organ 74:308–318, 2015

Inter-Agency Standing Committee: COVID-19 Response: Key Messages on Applying the IASC Guidelines on Inclusion of Persons With Disability in Humanitarian Action. Geneva, Switzerland, Inter-Agency Standing Committee, June 2020. Available at: https://interagencystandingcommittee.org/sites/default/files/migrated/2020-11/IASC%20Key%20Messages%20on%20Applying%20IASC%20Guidelines%20on%20Disability%20in%20the%20COVID-19%20Response%20%28final%20version%29.pdf. Accessed April 2, 2024.

Kamel N: Social marginalisation, federal assistance and repopulation patterns in the New Orleans metropolitan area following Hurricane Katrina. Urban Stud 49(14):3211–3231, 2012

King KD, Bartel R, James A, et al: Practice report: an Alberta Métis model for COVID-19 vaccine delivery. Can J Public Health 113(1):81–86, 2022 34988925

Meyer IH: Prejudice, social stress, and mental health in lesbian, gay, and bisexual populations: conceptual issues and research evidence. Psychol Bull 129(5):674–697, 2003 12956539

Meyer IH: Resilience in the study of minority stress and health of sexual and gender minorities. Psychol Sex Orientat Gend Divers 2:209, 2015

Mills E: "Leave No One Behind": Gender, Sexuality, and the Sustainable Development Goals. Brighton, UK, Institute of Developmental Studies, October 16, 2015. Available at: http://archive.ids.ac.uk/spl/files/leave-no-one-behind-gender-sexuality-and-sustainable-development-goals.html. Accessed April 2, 2024.

Molyneaux R, Gibbs L, Bryant RA, et al: Interpersonal violence and mental health outcomes following disaster. BJPsych Open 6(1):e1, 2019 31796146

Muuo S, Muthuri SK, Mutua MK, et al: Barriers and facilitators to care-seeking among survivors of gender-based violence in the Dadaab refugee complex. Sex Reprod Health Matters 28(1):1722404, 2020 32075551

Norris FH, Friedman MJ, Watson PJ, et al: 60,000 disaster victims speak part I: an empirical review of the empirical literature, 1981–2001. Psychiatry 65(3):207–239, 2002 12405079

Panchal N, Kamal R, Cox C, et al: Mental Health and Substance Use Considerations Among Children During the COVID-19 Pandemic. San Francisco, CA, Kaiser Family Foundation, 2021

Pearce E, Kamenov K, Barrett D, et al: Promoting equity in health emergencies through health systems strengthening: lessons learned from disability inclusion in the COVID-19 pandemic. Int J Equity Health 21(Suppl 3):149, 2022 36284335

Reinhart E: Reconstructive justice: public health policy to end mass incarceration. N Engl J Med 388(6):559–564, 2023 36780682

Saltzman LY, Lesen AE, Henry V, et al: COVID-19 mental health disparities. Health Secur 19(S1):S5–S13, 2021 34014118

Sharpe JD, Wolkin AF: The epidemiology and geographic patterns of natural disaster and extreme weather mortality by race and ethnicity, United States, 1999–2018. Public Health Rep 137(6):1118–1125, 2022 34678107

Tervalon M, Murray-García J: Cultural humility versus cultural competence: a critical distinction in defining physician training outcomes in multicultural education. J Health Care Poor Underserved 9(2):117–125, 1998 10073197

Thomeer MB, Moody MD, Yahirun J: Racial and ethnic disparities in mental health and mental health care during the COVID-19 pandemic. J Racial Ethn Health Disparities 10(2):961–976, 2023 35318615

Tracy M, Norris FH, Galea S: Differences in the determinants of posttraumatic stress disorder and depression after a mass traumatic event. Depress Anxiety 28(8):666–675, 2011 21618672

Truog RD, Mitchell C, Daley GQ: The toughest triage: allocating ventilators in a pandemic. N Engl J Med 382(21):1973–1975, 2020 32202721

UCLA Equity, Diversity, and Inclusion: Native American and Indigenous Peoples FAQs. Los Angeles, CA, University of California, Los Angeles, April 14, 2020. Available at: https://equity.ucla.edu/know/resources-on-native-american-and-indigenous-affairs/native-american-and-indigenous-peoples-faqs. Accessed April 2, 2024.

United Nations Office for Disaster Risk Reduction: Words into Action Guidelines: Using Traditional and Indigenous Knowledges for Disaster Risk Reduction. New York, UN Office for Disaster Risk Reduction, 2022. Available at: www.undrr.org/sites/default/files/2022-12/11_Traditional%20Knowledges_2022_2.pdf. Accessed April 2, 2024.

Universal Service Administrative Company: Lifeline Support. Washington, DC, Universal Service Administrative Company, 2004. Available at: www.lifeline-support.org. Accessed July 7, 2024.

van Daalen KR, Kallesøe SS, Davey F, et al: Extreme events and gender-based violence: a mixed-methods systematic review. Lancet Planet Health 6(6):e504–e523, 2022 35709808

Vu A, Adam A, Wirtz A, et al: The prevalence of sexual violence among female refugees in complex humanitarian emergencies: a systematic review and meta-analysis. PLoS Curr 6:6, 2014 24818066

Wisner B, Blaikie PM, Blaikie P, et al: At Risk: Natural Hazards, People's Vulnerability and Disasters. New York, Psychology Press, 2004

World Health Organization: Responding to Intimate Partner Violence and Sexual Violence Against Women: WHO Clinical and Policy Guidelines Executive summary. Geneva, Switzerland, World Health Organization, 2013

Wu C, Qian Y, Wilkes R: Anti-Asian discrimination and the Asian-white mental health gap during COVID-19, in Race and Ethnicity in Pandemic Times. Edited by Solomos J. London, Routledge, 2021, pp 101–117

14

Serious Mental Illness

Sander Koyfman, M.D., M.B.A.
Genevieve Jing, M.D.

In this chapter, the aim is to provide practical guidelines for preparedness work focused on serious mental illness (SMI) and suggestions for postdisaster care, for both individuals with predisaster SMIs and individuals with new diagnoses as a result of the disaster. SMI is defined as a mental, behavioral, or emotional disorder that results in serious functional impairment that substantially interferes with or limits one or more major life activities (National Institute of Mental Health 2022). SMI can include diagnoses such as major depression, schizophrenia, bipolar disorder, obsessive-compulsive disorder, panic disorder, posttraumatic stress disorder (PTSD), and borderline personality disorder.

Do Disasters Cause New-Onset Severe Mental Illness?

In a study after the 1979 Three Mile Island accident in Pennsylvania, researchers reported that psychiatric patients may not be more distressed by a disaster than the general population is (Bromet et al. 1982). However, a body of more recent work supports greater vulnerability after a disaster for individuals with SMI. Disasters are associated with new onset of PTSD as well as other anxiety and depressive disorders (Pandya 2009), but evidence connecting disasters with new-onset psychotic spectrum disorders are conflicting (Jing and Katz 2021). Despite scarce literature suggesting that disasters cause new-onset SMIs, several studies have looked at the impact of disasters on people with preexisting SMI. Although findings have varied, studies suggest that at least some individuals with SMI are at risk for worsening of their symptoms, decompensation, and increase in hospitalizations (Aoki et al. 2012; Staugh 2009; Tseng et al. 2010).

Individuals with SMI may experience additional psychological challenges on top of the same physical risk as the general population. Levels of vulnerability to and preparedness for disaster may also vary on the basis of level of preexisting impairment. For example, patients with SMI and lower socioeconomic status, low literacy levels, and inadequate social support had less knowledge related to coronavirus disease 2019 (COVID-19), and some were completely unaware of the ongoing COVID-19 pandemic (Muruganandam et al. 2020).

As noted in Chapter 12, "Adult Psychiatric Evaluation," PTSD and major depressive disorder are the two most common new-onset diagnoses after a disaster. Aside from having higher rates of PTSD than does the general population, individuals with SMI also have higher rates of some of the risk factors for developing PTSD after a disaster, including high rates of past-year victimization (Teplin et al. 2005), substance-related diagnoses (Jané-Llopis and Matytsina 2006), and lifetime trauma (Mueser et al. 1998). However, PTSD is underdiagnosed in people with SMI (Mueser et al. 1998). Various theories are believed to contribute to the underrecognition and undertreatment of PTSD in this population, including the belief that focusing on trauma conflicts with treatment of other diagnoses that should take precedence (Cusack et al. 2007). However, some of this underdiagnosis may also result from the similarity between some symptoms of PTSD and symptoms of SMI (Pandya and Weiden 2001). For example, signs and symptoms such as hypervigilance and reexperiencing phenomena may be written off simply as psychosis.

Interaction between the postdisaster environment and population risks may also exist. For example, prenatal exposure to earthquakes may have long-term effects on adult schizophrenia. Analysis of the Second China National Sample Survey on Disability gathered in 2006 found that individuals in utero at the time of the Great Tangshan Earthquake in 1976 were at increased odds of developing schizophrenia. Further stratification of data showed that only first-trimester exposure led to higher rates (Guo et al. 2019). These findings likely relate to emerging evidence supporting the role of prenatal maternal stress due to traumatic life events such as infection, warfare, and natural disasters in the etiology of schizophrenia spectrum disorders (Lipner et al. 2019). In addition, a large body of evidence suggests significant morbidity associated with early childhood trauma—adverse childhood experiences—likely associated with postdisaster environments (Felitti et al. 1998).

As an example of such stressors, persistent displacement may carry additional risks. Analysis of refugees' experience in Denmark, Sweden, Norway, and Canada found that being a refugee was an independent risk factor in developing nonaffective psychosis. The relative risk of developing nonaffective psychosis in refugees versus nonrefugee migrants was 1.39; the relative risk for refugees versus the native population was 2.41; and the relative risk for nonrefugee migrants versus the native population was 1.92 (Brandt et al. 2019). However, the generalizability of these findings to non-Scandinavian countries is unclear.

Postdisaster Decompensation

There are several pathways to postdisaster decompensation of patients with serious mental illness, which can include direct exposure to trauma, stress and trauma reactions, disruptions to routine and support systems, and access to care and treatment. Consider the hypothetical case of Ms. J:

Vignette

Ms. J is a 35-year-old woman who has recently completed gender transition and has been receiving medication-assisted treatment (MAT) for opioid use disorder for the past 2 years as well as ongoing care for her severe recurring major depression, currently in remission. She has been taking buprenorphine as prescribed and has not used any other opioids during this time but sometimes struggles to renew her antidepressants, which she gets at a separate clinic. She has a stable job and has been able to rebuild her life after struggling with substance use–related problems for several years. Ms. J lives in a coastal city that is prone to hurricanes.

During the most recent hurricane, Ms. J was forced to evacuate her home and travel to a nearby city to stay with relatives. She was unable to bring her MAT medication with her because of concerns about safe storage of the buprenorphine during evacuation. As a result, Ms. J was unable to take her medication for several days, which led to significant withdrawal symptoms. She experienced intense cravings, sweating, muscle aches, and gastrointestinal distress. She found it difficult to sleep or concentrate, was unable to work or engage in other daily activities, and became nonadherent with her antidepressant medication despite having it on hand.

Despite her efforts to access her medication from a local clinic, Ms. J was told that they did not have any prescribers offering MAT. Ms. J felt helpless and frustrated because she had worked hard to maintain her recovery and now felt that she was back to square one. Distressed, Ms. J called #988 and, after sharing her story, was offered new information about recent changes in the federal law regarding the elimination of the need for special prescribing privileges (X-waiver) and was able to return to the clinic with this new information. The primary care provider on staff was able to rapidly confirm the new information and prescribe buprenorphine.

Ms. J's case highlights the challenges that patients receiving MAT for opioid use disorder can face during a disaster. Loss of access to medication can have significant negative consequences for patients, including withdrawal symptoms and increased risk of relapse as well as exacerbation of well-controlled symptoms of chronic SMI, such as depression. It is important for patients to have access to alternative sources of medication during a disaster, as well as support and resources to help them manage the emotional and psychological impacts of the disruption to their treatment.

After a disaster, individuals with SMI may be at risk for a variety of disruptions that are associated with decompensation. These may include decreased availability of medication; disruption of psychiatric care; and loss of psychosocial support, including natural supports such as friends and family, case management services, and support groups. Furthermore, disorder-specific vulnerabilities may exist, such as individuals with bipolar disorder being especially vulnerable to disruption of sleep cycles, which can lead to decompensation. This disruption can extend beyond the impact phase for individuals with SMI who are placed in shelters or are themselves disaster responders. Providers could consider mitigating these risks in the predisaster setting by using treatment planning tools developed for use in disaster settings because these tools can be beneficial for daily challenges. Such use of disaster-related tools in predisaster treatment planning could conceivably help familiarize both patients and providers with these tools, thus facilitating more effective care in the immediate and postdisaster setting. When patients are confronted with lack of availability of a specific medication used in ongoing treatment, providers should familiarize themselves with conversion tables or advocate effectively for common medications to be stocked in emergency pharmacies (Tables 14–1, 14–2, and 14–3).

Pathways for Preventing Postdisaster Decompensation of Serious Mental Illness

We need to emphasize the importance of striving to meet established nondisaster-setting standards of care, even during disasters. Doing "the usual for the usual" is even more important to help recenter both the caregiver and the individual in need of help.

TABLE 14–1. Dose equivalents for first- and second-generation antipsychotics based on 100 mg of chlorpromazine

Generic formulation	Brand name	Dose equivalent (mg)
First-generation antipsychotics		
Haloperidol	Haldol	2
Fluphenazine	Prolixin	2
Pimozide	Orap	2
Trifluoperazine	Stelazine	2–5
Thiothixene	Navane	4
Perphenazine	Trilafon	8
Loxapine	Loxitane	10
Prochlorperazine	Compazine	15
Thioridazine	Mellaril	100
Second-generation antipsychotics		
Risperidone	Risperdal	1–2
Paliperidone	Invega	1.5–2
Iloperidone	Fanapt	3–6
Asenapine	Saphris	4–5
Olanzapine	Zyprexa	5
Aripiprazole	Abilify	7.5
Lurasidone	Latuda	16–20
Ziprasidone	Geodon	60
Quetiapine	Seroquel	75
Clozapine	Clozaril	50–100

Source. American Association of Psychiatric Pharmacists 2024; Danivas and Venkata-subramanian 2013; Woods 2003.

Lack of access to routine mental health services or crisis services may have impacts on another important area of risk—namely, potential increase in suicidality post disasters. Although the data are mixed on the likelihood of suicidality (see Chapter 12), at the very least it is important to mitigate increased suicide risk in those living with SMI because these individuals may already be at an increased risk of suicide. This can be done through such resources as mobile crisis services and emergent hospitalization. In the United States, #988 and the Disaster Distress Hotline should be advertised, and tools, as well as privacy, should be provided to facilitate use.

**TABLE 14–2. Dose equivalents of benzodiazepines based on
1 mg of lorazepam**

Generic formulation	Brand	Onset (hours)	Action duration	Dose equivalent (mg)
Flurazepam	Dalmane	1	Long	15–30
Chlordiazepoxide	Librium	1.5	Long	10–25
Diazepam	Valium	1	Long	5–10
Clorazepate	Tranxene	1	Long	7.5–15
Clonazepam	Klonopin	1	Long	0.25–0.5
Temazepam	Restoril	0.5	Intermediate	30
Lorazepam	Ativan	2	Intermediate	1
Oxazepam	Serax	3	Short	15–20
Alprazolam	Xanax	1	Short	0.5
Triazolam	Halcion	0.5	Short	0.25–0.5

Source. Guina and Merrill 2018.

**TABLE 14–3. Dose equivalents of opioids based on morphine
milligram equivalents**

Generic formulation	Brand name	Conversion factor
Codeine	—	0.15
Fentanyl transdermal (in µg/hour)	Duragesic	2.4
Hydrocodone	Hysingla, Zohydro ER	1
Hydromorphone	Dilaudid	4
Methadone	Dolophine, Methadose	
1–20 mg/day		4
21–40 mg/day		8
41–60 mg/day		10
≥61–80 mg/day		12
Morphine	Avinza, Morphabond, Oramorph, Roxanol-T	1
Oxycodone	Oxaydo, Xtampza ER	1.5
Oxymorphone	Opana ER	3

Note. ER=extended release.
Source. Centers for Disease Control and Prevention 2023.

Other areas of focus for psychiatrists should include a concerted effort to address physical health vulnerabilities because patients with SMI have additional specific health risks. General health advocacy can be of critical importance. During the COVID-19 response, mental health providers advocated for crucial regulatory changes for contactless medication delivery, changes in telehealth requirements, and priority access to COVID-19 vaccines for patients living with SMI.

The Substance Abuse and Mental Health Services Administration has cited a tiered model of community-wide interventions after disasters. Tier 1 includes universal interventions such as psychoeducation, outreach, public health messaging, and Psychological First Aid (PFA) to meet the needs of those with lowest risk of postdisaster mental illness. Tier 2 includes short-term grief-focused interventions such as cognitive-behavioral therapy for trauma in schools and Skills for Psychological Recovery (SPR). Tier 3 consists of the intensive interventions, including psychiatric services and long-term treatment, most likely indicated for individuals with SMI that they experienced before the disaster or that began after the disaster (Substance Abuse and Mental Health Services Administration 2019). All tiers should be made equally and equitably available to community members independent of their predisaster risks because all may benefit in various degrees at various points in time. In addition, practitioners should suggest supplemental interventions and approaches that may help to forestall progression from Tier 2 to Tier 3 for some—with special attention to those living with SMI as the most vulnerable.

Tier 1: Psychological First Aid

The elements of PFA as they may relate to an individual with SMI are as follows:

- **Contact and engagement**—initiating contact and responding to individuals in a compassionate and helpful manner. Individuals with SMI may often be encountered through gatekeepers of congregate housing; protective family; or, if incarcerated, through law enforcement. As such, the engagement approach may need to be modified, with a focus on understanding the "rules" of a particular system of support.
- **Safety and comfort**—enhancing safety and providing physical and emotional comfort. This may be complicated by overt psychotic or other psychiatric symptoms that may be more difficult for those less familiar with SMI to adopt to when large numbers of individuals may need to be housed together.

- **Stabilization**—calming and orienting emotionally overwhelmed survivors. Psychiatrists are equipped to offer additional support to help tease out preexisting symptoms and disaster-induced short-lived normal reactions to abnormal events.
- **Information gathering**—identifying immediate needs. Identifying needs and providing personalized interventions can be more complex with individuals with SMI. Addressing medications, specific diets, or environmental factors can help significantly reduce distress. Failing to address information on the availability of injectable antipsychotics or MAT or even a substance of choice can precipitate withdrawal, with significant consequences.
- **Practical assistance**—this will vary dramatically. Postdisaster providers may find themselves addressing needs not typically addressed in their practices—from food and clothing to housing to replacement and repair of personal medical equipment (e.g., wheelchairs). Exercising flexibility and asking for help from others will be essential for success and the provider's own resilience. Not all that is necessary will be available.
- **Connecting with social supports**—establishing connections with social supports and community resources (e.g, peer supports and self-help groups focused on specific needs). Patients with psychotic illnesses may need a different tier of overall support for social supports to be most effective.
- **Information on coping**—providing psychoeducation on general stress reactions. This can have particular importance; providers should emphasize the need to return to ongoing care as soon as possible to avoid relapse and symptom exacerbation.
- **Linkage with collaborative services**—connecting to services supporting long-term recovery. This can be helped by advanced treatment planning that may include relevant disaster planning activities. Understanding the ability of the person with SMI to engage with new providers or access telehealth or digital health interventions such as digital therapeutics can significantly ease the burden an individual and their family may experience.

Tier 2: Skills for Psychological Recovery

SPR can play an important role in helping individuals with SMI in the weeks to months after a disaster or traumatic event as well as predisaster to assist with crisis and disaster planning (Berkowitz et al. 2010). SPR refers to specific coping strategies and techniques that can be taught and practiced to help individuals manage stress and trauma, promote resilience, and prevent the development of more severe mental illness while considering their unique experiences and challenges. There is evidence that SPR in mental health training positively benefited the community of Queensland, Australia, after floods and cyclones (Wade et al. 2015). The group subsequently created a registry of trained practitioners for future disasters.

To be effective, predisaster planning should include individuals from the target population (National Council on Disability 2006). Although this planning may seem unrealistic to some people, consumer input has been incorporated into the planning and monitoring of a variety of services for adults with SMI in various states (Aron et al. 2009). This is important because individuals with SMI are less prepared for disasters than the public is, even when sociodemographic variables and general health are accounted for by controls (Anglin et al. 2020; Eisenman et al. 2009).

Where psychiatrists and other behavioral health providers could be helpful and effective while engaging the most vulnerable is building *disaster planning and preparedness* around the already familiar principles of routine *treatment planning*. Tables 14–4 and 14–5 provide examples of two SPR worksheets as applied to Ms. J, who was introduced earlier. Doing so could significantly raise the awareness of the preplanning issues as well as increase survivors' familiarity with what kind of interactions should be expected when dealing with relief workers and responders post disaster.

Tier 3: Individual Evaluation and Treatment

The evaluation of individuals with SMI during the acute phase is essentially the same as that for the general population (see Chapter 12, "Adult Psychiatric Evaluation"). This procedure includes taking a detailed history of the patient's experience during the trauma. Although the clinician must remain attuned to signs that an individual does not want to discuss this issue, it is incorrect to presume that asking about the trauma will lead to a decompensation of the individual's more apparent SMI (Cusack et al. 2007). In addition, an individual in prior treatment may demonstrate familiarity and comfort with the available supports and offer their lived experience—helping all engage in more effective coping.

Addressable Stressors and Corresponding Interventions

Postdisaster environments, including evacuation centers, can pose specific challenges for individuals with SMI. The same discomforts and issues that others may experience as uncomfortable and distressing can prove partic-

TABLE 14–4. Example of social connections worksheet for Ms. J

Skills for Psychological Recovery Social Connections Worksheet	
Section	**Ms. J's response**
1. Develop a Social Connections Map	Mother
	Father
	Neighbor
	Therapist
	Case manager
	Psychiatrist
2A. Review Social Connections Map (Part A)	
• Who are your most important connections right now?	Mother and father
• With whom can you share your experiences and feelings?	Therapist, case manager, and psychiatrist
• From whom can you get advice to help with your recovery?	Psychiatrist, therapist
• Whom do you want to spend time with socially in the next couple of weeks?	Mother and father
• Who might be able to help you with practical tasks (errands, paperwork, homework)?	Mother and father
• Who might need your help or support right now?	Neighbor
2B. Review Social Connections Map (Part B)	

TABLE 14–4. Example of social connections worksheet for Ms. J (continued)

Skills for Psychological Recovery Social Connections Worksheet	
Section	**Ms. J's response**
Write down who or what is missing or needs to be changed in your network.	I would like to have more social connections and friends in the community. I am missing support from people who are my age and enjoy similar activities. I would also like to connect with people who have similar mental health challenges in order to support each other. I would enjoy spending my days in a program with support from building relationships, education, employment, housing, and making daily meals. However, I struggle with opening up to others and would like to figure out how to communicate better.
3. Make a Social Support Plan	• I will work with my case manager to identify clubhouses for people with mental health challenges.
	• I plan to enroll in a program and attend each morning from 8 A.M. to 12 P.M. Through this program, I hope to gain social connections with peers and find support in each other.
	• I would like to have lunch with a different peer each week.

Source.   Berkowitz et al. 2010; www.nctsn.org/sites/default/files/resources/special-resource/spr_complete_english.pdf, pp. 157–164.

TABLE 14–5. Example of problem-solving worksheet for Ms. J

Skills for Psychological Recovery Problem-Solving Worksheet	
Section	**Ms. J's response**
1. Define the problem	Remembering to attend my monthly appointment with my psychiatrist
Ask yourself these questions about the problem:	
A. Is it happening to me? Yes or No	Yes
B. Is it happening between me and someone else? Yes or No	Yes
C. Is it happening to someone else? Yes or No	No
D. Is it happening between two or more other people? Yes or No	No
*If you answered "Yes" to A or B, this is likely a good problem for you to work on. If you circled "Yes" to C or D, this may not be a problem you can fix, but a situation for someone else to work on.	
2. Set the goal	I would want someone to remind me about the appointment. It would be great if someone from the clinic or my family can give me a call the day before my scheduled appointment.
3. Brainstorm	• Ask the clerk at the clinic to call me the day before my appointment • Ask my psychiatrist who I should ask to call me the day before my appointment

TABLE 14–5. Example of problem-solving worksheet for Ms. J (continued)

Skills for Psychological Recovery Problem-Solving Worksheet

Section	Ms. J's response
	• Ask my parents if they can let me know the day before my appointment
	• Create a calendar reminder on my phone
	• Set up a reminder through EMR (e.g., MyChart) notification
4. Choose the best solution	I will first ask my psychiatrist who I should ask to get help for appointment reminders from the clinic. I will then follow up with that person for a reminder. As a backup, I will also set up calendar reminders on my phone for the day before the appointment and on the morning of the appointment.

Note. EMR=electronic medical record.
Source. Berkowitz et al. 2010; www.nctsn.org/sites/default/files/resources/special-resource/spr_complete_english.pdf, pp. 84–92.

ularly challenging for someone with PTSD or bipolar disorder. Environmental challenges can be addressed through application of some of the basic tenets of *universal design*—a set of principles making an environment safe and usable "so that it can be accessed, understood and used to the greatest extent possible by all people regardless of their age, size, ability or disability" (National Disability Authority 2023). Application of these principles may serve as an effective primary prevention intervention, diminishing triggers and avoiding need for specialty Tier 3 interventions.

Basic needs that should be accommodated in an evacuation setting include appropriate food, shelter, sleeping arrangements, safety, security, medical needs, leisure, exercise, access to information, access to social media and family connections, religious services, cultural observances, social connectedness, additional safety measures for those who rely on tight-knit networks such as the LGBTQ+ community, and, ultimately, clear prospects of return to predisaster safety.

Applying these principles to the specific situation of a large evacuation center that was rapidly set up in Brooklyn, New York, in 2012 in response to destruction from Hurricane Sandy highlights their importance. New York had to create a 500-bed shelter in the heart of Brooklyn in a former armory building. The building featured a large space with no provisions for privacy, offering temporary shelter to residents of so-called *adult homes*—congregate settings for individuals with significant degree of social dysfunction and high prevalence of SMI. In the first hours of operation, numerous ambulances brought in hundreds of individuals from several adult homes in quick succession. Many of these homes were built in cheaper, low-lying areas in poor shore-adjacent areas of Brooklyn, Queens, and Staten Island. Many individuals—some with prior difficult encounters with the New York City Police Department and emergency medical services—may have been triggered by the increasingly dense communal environment. Several individuals had to be immediately transported to the nearest emergency departments, only to return shortly after because of lack of symptoms severe enough to warrant hospitalization. Something had to be done to stabilize the environment quickly. Applying an understanding of the interface between pathology and environmental triggers led us to a series of simple interventions.

We created an SMI Square—a space within the space—using improvised barriers made from 12-foot-tall chicken wire dividers covered in blankets. The dividers allowed individuals with SMI to be sequestered on a defunct basketball court. Foot traffic pattern was revised, and a Disaster Psychiatry Outreach (a New York-based nonprofit organization now part of Vibrant Emotional Health) volunteer was given the specific task of addressing the needs of the most vulnerable, along with the necessary authority to do so. The large bracket shape of the square, with access controlled by the volunteer and 20 beds inside for persons exhibiting most acute and visible distress, became an important nexus of care. Creation of the square, along with enforcing dimmed lights at 10 P.M. shelter-wide, drastically reduced the number of 911 calls and the need for individuals to be sent to emergency departments. Staff from other areas now knew where to bring someone in distress. Calm followed.

Making this physical space adjustment was immediately necessary, impactful, and cheap. Borrowing this approach was helpful when implementing nearly the same interventions on a larger scale in the aggregate settings of the Afghan evacuee locations on military bases many years later. Environmental assessment matters for all, and even more so for those who can be triggered by lack of sleep, uniforms, noise, light, and other factors. Making an environment assessment a basic community psychiatric intervention can be powerful and can decrease distress for survivors and responders alike.

Conclusion

Although empirical studies continue to be limited, there is a strong theoretical basis for believing that individuals with SMI are at elevated risk for worsening of their predisaster diagnoses and for developing new diagnoses post disaster. This includes evidence that such individuals are less prepared for disasters and have high rates of predisaster trauma and PTSD. Therefore, psychiatrists and other mental health professionals should be aware of the effect of disasters on the course of SMIs and be prepared to consider the environmental and systems factors that can complicate treatment and stabilization of communities post disaster. Being mentally ready can position behavioral health providers to be important champions post disaster.

References

American Association of Psychiatric Pharmacists: Psychiatric pharmacy essentials: antipsychotic dose equivalents. Lincoln, NE, American Association of Psychiatric Pharmacists, 2024. Available at: https://aapp.org/guideline/essentials/antipsychotic-dose-equivalents. Accessed April 2, 2024.

Anglin DM, Galea S, Bachman P: Going upstream to advance psychosis prevention and improve public health. JAMA Psychiatry 77(7):665–666, 2020 32236511

Aoki A, Aoki Y, Harima H: The impact of the Great East Japan earthquake on mandatory psychiatric emergency hospitalizations in Tokyo: a retrospective observational study. Transl Psychiatry 2(10):e168, 2012 23032944

Aron L, Honberg R, Duckworth K, et al: Grading the States 2009: A Report on America's Health Care System for Adults With Serious Mental Illness. Arlington, VA, National Alliance on Mental Illness, 2009

Berkowitz S, Bryant R, Brymer M, et al: Skills for Psychological Recovery: Field Operations Guide. White River Junction, VT, National Center for PTSD and National Child Traumatic Stress Network, 2010. Available at: www.ptsd.va.gov/professional/treat/type/SPR/SPR_Manual.pdf. Accessed April 3, 2024.

Brandt L, Henssler J, Müller M, et al: Risk of psychosis among refugees: a systematic review and meta-analysis. JAMA Psychiatry 76(11):1133–1140, 2019 31411649

Bromet E, Schulberg HC, Dunn L: Reactions of psychiatric patients to the Three Mile Island nuclear accident. Arch Gen Psychiatry 39(6):725–730, 1982 7092506

Centers for Disease Control and Prevention: Calculating total daily dose of opioids for safer dosage. Available at: https://stacks.cdc.gov/view/cdc/38481. Accessed February 10, 2023.

Cusack KJ, Wells CB, Grubaugh AL, et al: An update on the South Carolina trauma initiative. Psychiatr Serv 58(5):708–710, 2007 17463355

Danivas V, Venkatasubramanian G: Current perspectives on chlorpromazine equivalents: comparing apples and oranges! Indian J Psychiatry 55(2):207–208, 2013 23825865

Eisenman DP, Zhou Q, Ong M, et al: Variations in disaster preparedness by mental health, perceived general health, and disability status. Disaster Med Public Health Prep 3(1):33–41, 2009 19293742

Felitti VJ, Anda RF, Nordenberg D, et al: Relationship of childhood abuse and household dysfunction to many of the leading causes of death in adults: the Adverse Childhood Experiences (ACE) Study. Am J Prev Med 14(4):245–258, 1998 9635069

Guina J, Merrill B: Benzodiazepines II: waking up on sedatives: providing optimal care when inheriting benzodiazepine prescriptions in transfer patients. J Clin Med 7(2):20, 2018 29385766

Guo C, He P, Song X, et al: Long-term effects of prenatal exposure to earthquake on adult schizophrenia. Br J Psychiatry 215(6):730–735, 2019 31113505

Jané-Llopis E, Matytsina I: Mental health and alcohol, drugs and tobacco: a review of the comorbidity between mental disorders and the use of alcohol, tobacco and illicit drugs. Drug Alcohol Rev 25(6):515–536, 2006 17132571

Jing GP, Katz CL: An update on psychotic spectrum disorders and disasters. Curr Opin Psychiatry 34(3):211–215, 2021 33605621

Lipner E, Murphy SK, Ellman LM: Prenatal maternal stress and the cascade of risk to schizophrenia spectrum disorders in offspring. Curr Psychiatry Rep 21(10):99, 2019 31522269

Mueser KT, Goodman LB, Trumbetta SL, et al: Trauma and posttraumatic stress disorder in severe mental illness. J Consult Clin Psychol 66(3):493–499, 1998 9642887

Muruganandam P, Neelamegam S, Menon V, et al: COVID-19 and severe mental illness: impact on patients and its relation with their awareness about COVID-19. Psychiatry Res 291:113265, 2020 32763536

National Council on Disability: The Needs of People With Psychiatric Disabilities During and After Hurricanes Katrina and Rita: Position Paper and Recommendations. Washington, DC, National Council on Disability, 2006

National Disability Authority: About Universal Design. Dublin, Ireland, Centre for Excellence in Universal Design. Available at: https://universaldesign.ie/what-is-universal-design. Accessed March 1, 2023.

National Institute of Mental Health: Mental illness. Washington, DC, National Institute of Mental Health, January 2022. Available at: www.nimh.nih.gov/health/statistics/mental-illness. Accessed March 8, 2023.

Pandya A: Adult disaster psychiatry. Focus (Am Psychiatr Publ) 7(2):155–159, 2009

Pandya A, Weiden PJ: Trauma and disaster in psychiatrically vulnerable populations. J Psychiatr Pract 7(6):426–430, 2001 15990557

Substance Abuse and Mental Health Services Administration: Disasters and people with serious mental illness. Washington, DC, Substance Abuse and Mental Health Services Administration, August 2019. Available at: www.samhsa.gov/sites/default/files/disasters-people-with-serious-mental-illness.pdf. Accessed February 9, 2023.

Staugh LM: The effects of disaster on the mental health of individuals with disabilities, in Mental Health and Disasters. Edited by Neria Y, Galea S, Norris FH. New York, Cambridge University Press, 2009, pp 264–276

Teplin LA, McClelland GM, Abram KM, et al: Crime victimization in adults with severe mental illness: comparison with the National Crime Victimization Survey. Arch Gen Psychiatry 62(8):911–921, 2005 16061769

Tseng K-C, Hemenway D, Kawachi I, et al: The impact of the Chi-Chi earthquake on the incidence of hospitalizations for schizophrenia and on concomitant hospital choice. Community Ment Health J 46(1):93–101, 2010 19898984

Wade D, Crompton D, Howard A, et al: Skills for psychological recovery: evaluation of a post-disaster mental health training program. Disaster Health 2(3–4):138–145, 2015 28229008

Woods SW: Chlorpromazine equivalent doses for the newer atypical antipsychotics. J Clin Psychiatry 64(6):663–667, 2003 12823080

PART III

INTERVENTION

Frederick J. Stoddard Jr., M.D.
Section Editor

15

Vulnerability, Resilience, and Grief

Jonathan M. DePierro, Ph.D.
Alisa R. Gutman, M.D., Ph.D.

Vignette

Zara is a 17-year-old girl with a history of childhood maltreatment by her mother and stepfather and subsequent removal from their home. During a psychiatric evaluation to assess readjustment after placement, she discloses several losses, including the murder of her biological father when she was in grade school. After she was removed from her parents' home, she lived for a time with friends of the family who abused her both verbally and physically for minor transgressions. The evaluation reveals evidence of anxiety after her father's death but no current symptoms that support any active psychiatric diagnosis. When asked about her life now, she lights up and answers, "I think I made a friend," adding that she has been sitting with a new girl at the lunch table at school. As she relates this, her affect shifts from the anxious and dysphoric tone that dominated the rest of the interview to one of brightness and hope.

The reader may wonder how to make sense of Zara's presentation. You may be thinking, surely someone who has been through so much trauma, including personal loss, must have a psychiatric disorder as a result of those experiences. How can someone who has been through so many objectively traumatic experiences still present with a positive affect? Over the course of this chapter, we discuss normative and pathological grief reactions and factors that support resilience, hints of which are present in Zara's story.

What Is Grief?

Loss strikes us all at some point in our lives: we will lose a relative, partner, pet, or, in particularly tragic situations, a child. Rather than being a rare event, wide-scale loss has also been a salient aspect of modern times. In recent years, violent conflict and forced displacement, a viral pandemic, and natural disasters brought on by climate change, to name a few cataclysmic events, have affected a large proportion of the global population and caused millions of excess deaths. Turning on the TV, opening a newspaper, or reading online news or social media provides a venue for a deeply personal experience to become a collective one.

Grief is the complex set of emotional reactions, thoughts, and behaviors that follow loss, although they may also occur in anticipation of a loss. There is no one right way to grieve. Countless self-help books have been written based on Elizabeth Kubler-Ross's five stages of grief (denial, anger, bargaining, depression, and acceptance), which were originally developed to document how people cope with their own terminal illness, not the loss of a loved one. These "stages" may give the false impression that the process of grief is predictable and linear and that if one is not progressing through the stages, one is grieving "wrong" or "pathologically." Rather than presenting the process of grief as a stepwise progression, we review a range of adaptive and maladaptive reactions and processes associated with grief, several psychiatric conditions that could emerge, and supportive and skills-based interventions for the postdisaster setting that have been shown to be effective to support the bereaved.

The process of grief poses a challenge to our ability to process emotional information, and we are often compelled to find meaning in a new reality. Human beings strive to make sense of their world: they seek order, patterns, and predictability. But when someone dies, this creates an internal alarm. Let us take one example. When a parent passes away, the surviving adult child is faced with a daunting task. They must make sense of the loss, incorporating the information that the parent is no longer there and that future connection will be through memories rather than in-person interaction. The mismatch between reality and expectation may cause feelings of sadness, social withdrawal, anger, guilt, and anxiety. One of the authors (J.M.D.) lost his maternal grandfather to lung cancer in the late 1990s. Following the death, his mother struggled with the fact that she missed her father's final moments because she had to wait at a nearby traffic light as she was racing over to his house and experienced distressing rumination and self-blame. Common, too, are regrets at thoughts or feelings seemingly left unexpressed. If the death was a result of a terrorist attack or natural disaster, the surviving family member may be plagued with intensely negative repetitive thoughts of whether they could have done anything different to prevent the outcome.

Many large-scale studies have examined trajectories of coping following potentially traumatic events, including loss. One study of 282 individuals who recently lost a spouse found that 71% of participants had low grief symptoms at 3 months, which remained low at 14- and 25-month follow-up assessments (Bonanno and Malgaroli 2020). Researchers commonly call these individuals *resilient*, from the perspective of seeing resilience as *resistance* to developing a disease process in the presence of exposures. The coronavirus disease 2019 (COVID-19) pandemic, which claimed nearly 7 million lives worldwide as of January 2023, has also shed light on processes of grief and recovery. Later in this chapter, we discuss many other ways to define resilience, including adapting and recovering from setbacks broadly construed. We also discuss recent research on psychological factors and underlying neurobiology associated with resilience.

Reactions to loss are highly informed by culture, geography, social status, religion, gender identity, race and ethnicity, and a variety of other contextual factors. In some South Asian countries, such as Nepal and India, public and pronounced expressions of grief are culturally sanctioned. Within Judaism and some branches of Christianity, gathering rituals such as shivas or wakes bring people together in shows of mutual support for the bereaved family after a loss, although they tend to be subdued occasions. However, larger expressions of emotion and *falling out* (passing out) are not uncommon in funerals within the Black church in the United States. Some culturally sanctioned mourning rituals have emerged following large-scale disasters. Following the 2011 triple disaster in Japan (an earthquake, a tsunami, and nuclear meltdown), more than 18,000 fatalities were documented. Soon after these events, a disconnected telephone booth, called *kaze no denwa* (or "phone of the wind"), was set up in the town of Otsuchi, which is estimated to have lost 10% of its population. In this booth, individuals can have conversations with their deceased loved ones, and they have reported that this brings a strong sense of relief and connection (Saito 2021). Clinicians are advised to educate themselves about the cultural manifestations of grief prior to supporting individuals with intersecting identities different from their own and in preparation for supporting individuals in another country following a mass casualty event. Finally, the developmental stage of the individual may have an impact on grief reactions, how needs for support are expressed, and risk and resilience trajectories (Alvis et al. 2022).

Neurobiology of Grief and Loss

To understand the biological mechanisms that underlie our brain's response to bereavement, we must begin with an appreciation of how our brains encode social relationships. Much of our knowledge about the neurobiology of affiliative behaviors was gained from partner preference studies in monogamous prairie voles as compared with non-monogamous vole species. From this model, we have learned multiple genetic and epigenetic mechanisms that regulate social attachment behaviors, including the importance of vasopressin 1a receptor distribution in mediating partner preference and paternal care (Sadino and Donaldson 2018). Behavioral effects after use of intranasal vasopressin suggest the potential for therapeutic modulation of these systems in human disorders of social functioning (Guastella et al. 2010; Thompson et al. 2006), but such studies are relatively small, and clinical translation is ongoing. Oxytocin similarly plays an important role in maternal nurturing, bonding, and social recognition (Froemke and Young 2021). Intranasal oxytocin shows promise as a prosocial intervention, with administration of a single dose sufficient to induce an increase of attachment security in insecurely attached adults (Buchheim et al. 2009).

In addition to the affiliative social learning inherent in partner preference, evidence demonstrates that pair bonding also causes activation of stress circuitry. For example, if a mate is missing, the prairie vole will experience a corticosteroid response that fuels searching for the partner (Bosch et al. 2009). A recent synthesis of animal data and human cognitive theories hypothesizes that in humans, our cognitive trace of bonding includes the notion that one's partner will "always" be one's partner. As we mentioned at the start of this chapter, loss initiates confusion between an encoded notion of forever and new sensory information that a partner is no longer present (O'Connor and Seeley 2022). It is important to note, however, that there are many outstanding questions regarding how the neurobiology of pair bonding seen in animals translates to human experience.

Our understanding of how *self* and *other* are reflected in brain structures and circuits is more limited, but imaging studies have identified the medial prefrontal cortex as a key region for our neural representation of self. Activation in the medial prefrontal cortex increases when thinking about oneself, and similarity in the neural representation between self and other is increased depending on how closely we identify with the other person (e.g., friend vs. acquaintance vs. a celebrity known by name). Of particular interest to understanding prolonged grief, loneliness is associated with reduced similarity between self and others—perhaps a neural trace of how social disconnection feels (Courtney and Meyer 2020).

The most important point to glean from the available neuroscientific data is that social learning is at the core of attachment. How we encode our most important bonds is key to understanding how we may adapt to a change in our external reality when a loved one dies. It follows that bereavement, which forces us to confront a world without our loved one, requires new learning as well. Given evidence that the formation of close attachments affects brain circuitry, it is unsurprising that loss of important relationships does the same. In one study of healthy control subjects who did not report symptoms of psychiatric distress, several kinds of losses, including the death of a close relative or a romantic relationship breakup, were associated with loss of volume in the amygdala and changes in the size of other structures that regulate stress and response to reward (Acosta et al. 2021). Of note, these changes were observed on average 4.5 years after the loss, suggesting that changes in brain structures relevant to emotional processing persist well after a loss experience, even in individuals without threshold psychiatric symptoms.

As with all complex human behaviors, friendship and love cannot be reduced to a single neuropeptide, gene, or brain region. Nor can the normative reaction to bereavement or the potentially maladaptive response that can occur with prolonged grief. In more colloquial terms, we can imagine that the changes initiated by bonding with a loved one, shared memories, and a sense of similarity of this other person to oneself come together to form a representation of *us* across the brain that then must adapt to loss. It is as though the metaphysical reality of someone missing from the world is now out of sync with the neurobiological stamp of that person on our mind. Sharing a conceptual framework like this is a gift to a bereaved person who is struggling to understand why they keep thinking of calling their deceased spouse or thinking that they hear their loved one's voice calling their name. This ongoing neural representation of self-other reflects in part the painful reality of grief: for the living, it feels as if a piece of them is missing, because it is.

General Approaches to Managing Grief

The key task of grief is not *forgetting* or *moving on*; instead, it is making sense of a world without the person. Imagine the grief that follows loss as a bolt of lightning that strikes and damages a tree. It will leave a scar, such that it will be obvious when the event occurred from looking at the tree's rings; however, when someone successfully navigates the grief process, they reengage with life, and many more tree rings are added on top of the scar. The person ultimately reengages with social connections, adds life milestones, and sees the event with perspective—sad, but one of many other positive and negative memories of their lost loved one. However, the scarring—the memory of the lost person—remains.

What do people need following loss to facilitate the process of grieving? Most people do not need psychotherapy, although of course many have found this resource invaluable. They need human connection. They need a safe, structured space to talk about the loss and its impact. A colleague of ours often reminds clinicians responding to disasters that they should show up as a person first, then as a medical or mental health professional. Responders should be aware that following mass casualty events, such as natural disasters or the 9/11 terrorist attacks, it is generally recommended to focus first on fostering physical safety and ensuring access to food, basic life supplies, and shelter. Mental health practitioners providing immediate support are advised to validate and normalize immediate emotional reactions and prioritize being fully present to the bereaved individual instead of focusing on doing something.

We hear so frequently from bereaved individuals that they do not want to talk about the loss and are afraid that if they start crying, they will not be able to stop. However, the meaning-making process is disrupted by avoidance, and individuals should be encouraged, within their comfort level, to *avoid avoiding*. Research seems to indicate that there are more and less effective ways to facilitate these conversations. Critical incident stress debriefing (CISD; later renamed critical incident stress management) was developed to provide a group-based intervention for discussing a trauma and its impact in the short-term aftermath of the event. The goal of CISD is to reduce postincident distress and prevent the development of posttraumatic stress disorder (PTSD). It seeks to do this by providing a venue for emotional catharsis and processing of traumatic memories and includes strategies for educating individuals about common stress reactions and ways to label and accept difficult emotions. Although CISD has been widely employed after mass casualty events (e.g., the 9/11 terrorist attacks, school shootings, natural disasters), a rigorous Cochrane review of single-session individual CISD concluded that it may have either no impact on the prospective development of PTSD or may be harmful, particularly for those who quickly develop prominent mental health symptoms after an event (Rose et al. 2003). The review authors instead recommended a *screen-and-treat* approach, devoting resources to identifying those individuals at greatest risk, screening them with appropriate measures, and providing timely evidence-based treatment. Individual conversations with friends, family, or spiritual advisors on an individual's own timeline may also prove to be more helpful than structured debriefings.

Psychiatric Conditions Following Loss

It is helpful to consider conditions that can emerge following grief, such as depressive disorders, PTSD, and prolonged grief disorder (PGD; generally synonymous with prolonged complex bereavement disorder [PCBD] and complicated grief), as initially normal grief reactions that become chronic, pervasive, severe, and life-impairing as the acute post-loss or disaster period evolves into the longer term. In the acute period, the disaster mental health professional can educate survivors about these possible long complications of normal grief, ideally permitting early identification and mitigation.

Although we describe some differences among these conditions, it is also important to note that there is substantial symptom overlap, and they have been found to co-occur. For example, one 42-month longitudinal study of 172 individuals who lost loved ones in a plane disaster found that chronic PCBD was present in 18.8% and chronic depression and PTSD were present in 6.2% and 10.3%, respectively. These researchers found a nearly complete overlap between class membership in the chronic PCBD and depression groups and that 65% of individuals with chronic PTSD also met criteria for probable chronic PCBD (Lenferink et al. 2017).

Loss has long been understood as a contributing factor to the onset of depression. In earlier DSM nomenclature, there was a "bereavement exclusion," which disallowed the diagnosis of major depressive disorder (MDD) in the 2 months following a loss to avoid overpathologizing normal grief reactions. However, this restriction was lifted in DSM-5 (American Psychiatric Association 2013). Clinicians should be aware that the presence of ongoing functional impairment, feelings of worthlessness as a person, and thoughts of suicide (separate from a wish to reunite with the loved one) are suggestive of MDD over and above "normal" grief reactions.

Interpersonal psychotherapy specifically formulates grief as a key stressor that can lead to depression. This intervention helps the patient rebuild or establish relationships and reconnect to a meaningful life through collaborative problem-solving, extensive affect labeling, and interpersonal skills building (Weissman et al. 2008). Similarly, there is substantial evidence for the efficacy of cognitive-behavioral therapy (CBT) for grief-related depression. CBT focuses on challenging negative automatic thoughts (e.g., excessive self-blame for circumstances of a loss) and behavioral exercises, including encouraging reengagement with activities that could bring a sense of joy and fulfillment.

Under certain circumstances, a diagnosis of PTSD can also be considered following a loss. Indeed, even before the inclusion of PTSD in DSM-III (American Psychiatric Association 1980), symptoms of PTSD were often described as sequelae of grief and loss (Krupnick and Horowitz 1981). Concepts surrounding posttraumatic reactions can be found in literature as far back as Hammurabi's lost warriors and Homer's *Odyssey*. When DSM was revised in subsequent editions, the symptoms associated with PTSD were revised and expanded, as were the inciting events that would qualify as traumatic. In the recently released DSM-5-TR (American Psychiatric Association 2022), losses that occur because of accidents and/or have violent elements may meet the exposure criterion (Criterion A). Of note, this would definitionally preclude the diagnosis of PTSD following loss for many individuals, including the expected and "peaceful" death of a child with terminal cancer. However, it may apply to other situations, such as the loss of family members in a natural disaster or violent conflict. PTSD criteria comprise 20 symptoms distributed across four domains: avoidance of trauma reminders, intrusive symptoms (e.g., upsetting memories of the event), negative thoughts and cognitions (e.g., self-blame, lack of trust in others), and hyperarousal (e.g., exaggerated startle response). Evidence-based treatments for PTSD, including symptoms resulting from traumatic loss, include prolonged exposure therapy and cognitive processing therapy.

Over the past two decades, there was a concerted effort, led by researchers including Kathy Spear and Holly Prigerson, to validate a psychiatric diagnosis specifically related to problematic grief sequelae. It should be noted that at that time, there was robust debate in academic literature regarding the utility and validity of a grief-specific disorder and whether it would pathologize a normative experience. PGD was ultimately included as a psychiatric diagnosis in DSM-5-TR (American Psychiatric Association 2022), released in March 2022, following the inclusion of PCBD as a condition in need of further study in DSM-5 approximately 9 years earlier. Box 15–1 lists the DSM-5-TR criteria for PGD. The diagnosis of PGD includes the following elements: 1) 12 or more months since the loss (a time requirement), 2) the presence of a constellation of symptoms, 3) distress or impairment, and 4) reactions that are longer and more intense than what can be expected on the basis of the individual's particular culture and context. Research has shown that approximately 10% of adults may develop PGD following a loss (American Psychiatric Association 2022).

Box 15–1. Prolonged Grief Disorder

A. The death, at least 12 months ago, of a person who was close to the bereaved individual (for children and adolescents, at least 6 months ago).

B. Since the death, the development of a persistent grief response characterized by one or both of the following symptoms, which have been present most days to a clinically significant degree. In addition, the symptom(s) has occurred nearly every day for at least the last month:

1. Intense yearning/longing for the deceased person.
2. Preoccupation with thoughts or memories of the deceased person (in children and adolescents, preoccupation may focus on the circumstances of the death).

C. Since the death, at least three of the following symptoms have been present most days to a clinically significant degree. In addition, the symptoms have occurred nearly every day for at least the last month:

1. Identity disruption (e.g., feeling as though part of oneself has died) since the death.
2. Marked sense of disbelief about the death.
3. Avoidance of reminders that the person is dead (in children and adolescents, may be characterized by efforts to avoid reminders).
4. Intense emotional pain (e.g., anger, bitterness, sorrow) related to the death.
5. Difficulty reintegrating into one's relationships and activities after the death (e.g., problems engaging with friends, pursuing interests, or planning for the future).
6. Emotional numbness (absence or marked reduction of emotional experience) as a result of the death.
7. Feeling that life is meaningless as a result of the death.
8. Intense loneliness as a result of the death.

D. The disturbance causes clinically significant distress or impairment in social, occupational, or other important areas of functioning.

E. The duration and severity of the bereavement reaction clearly exceed expected social, cultural, or religious norms for the individual's culture and context.

F. The symptoms are not better explained by another mental disorder, such as major depressive disorder or posttraumatic stress disorder, and are not attributable to the physiological effects of a substance (e.g., medication, alcohol) or another medical condition.

PGD is highly treatable with evidence-based psychotherapy. Holly Prigerson and colleagues have developed an approach called prolonged grief disorder therapy (PGDT), which draws in part on CBT (Prigerson et al. 2022). The two aims of PGDT are 1) acceptance of the reality and finality of the loss and 2) restoration of a sense of autonomy and social connection. The PGDT therapist focuses on extensive psychoeducation regarding grief emotions, supporting the patient to set future-oriented goals, facilitating social support by bringing other close people into the session, and addressing avoidance through exposure exercises.

When evaluating this work, it is important to note that the studies in which the criteria for PGD were validated included mostly White and female-identifying individuals in later life, usually studied following the death of a male spouse. The grief experiences of people of color, including individuals identifying as African American, is vastly understudied (Granek and Peleg-Sagy 2017). Without culturally contextualized considerations, one could plausibly overpathologize or underpathologize the grief experiences of individuals with diverse and intersecting identities. Treatment studies for prolonged grief need to be culturally responsive and include diverse populations.

Risk Screening

Ongoing work has focused on the development of a risk screener for adverse mental health outcomes following loss that can be administered prior to an anticipated loss (e.g., to a caretaker when their loved one is under palliative care) and after loss at regular intervals. One example of such a screener is the Bereavement Risk Inventory and Screening Questionnaire, which was developed because of the limited clinical utility of previously developed measures (Roberts et al. 2017). This scale evaluates multiple pre-loss and post-loss risk and protective factors, such as perceived social support, personal history of psychiatric diagnoses, loss of meaning and purpose, traumatic circumstances of death (e.g., perception of the death as painful; witnessing aggressive medical procedures), anxious or avoidant personality traits, difficulties with acceptance and guilt, and having an active caretaking role. The routine use of screening measures such as this one in medical settings would help to triage individuals to bereavement-specific services, which are often quite limited.

Resilience

As we noted above when defining grief and resilience, there is substantial debate regarding the definition of resilience. For example, epidemiological studies have focused on resilience as resistance to illness despite exposure. Here, we define resilience, broadly, as the ability to adapt, recover, and grow following life's challenges, including personal loss. One's ability to manage stress has a strong genetic component, but research shows that many resilience factors can be fostered with practice (Southwick et al. 2023) (Table 15–1).

Although a full review of the literature on resilience is beyond the scope of this chapter, we address a few that are particularly robust with respect to their evidence base (see Table 15–1 for a longer explanation of resilience factors). First, as we saw in Zara's story ("I think I made a friend"), social support is vital for recovery. Studies have shown that across a variety of traumatic events and populations (e.g., 9/11 terrorist attacks, emergency responders or survivors, bereaved spouses, combat veterans, COVID-19 frontline health care workers and their loved ones), greater perceived social support conveys protection against the development of a range of psychiatric conditions. The presence and support of a disaster mental health professional supplements available social support. Second, the funerary and memorial rituals inherent in the world's religions, which often integrate group gatherings, offer comfort to believers by helping them make meaning of the loss. These same rituals were disrupted by the COVID-19 pandemic, which may have contributed to persistent and distressing grief reactions in faith communities (Sneed et al. 2020). Third, having a range of personal coping resources has been shown to have protective effects. Such resources include the ability to reframe the loss and challenge negative automatic thoughts (e.g., guilt, self-blame), acceptance rather than avoidance of difficult emotions, and connecting to sources of joy and happiness amid one's suffering, (Southwick et al. 2023). Psychotherapy, support groups, or self-help resources may assist individuals in building up these factors in anticipation of or following a loss.

With respect to meaning making, it is important to consider the role of posttraumatic growth (PTG), which may be defined as a silver lining or unsought gift in response to trauma. PTG is a positive change that comes because of or following an emotional struggle in the aftermath of a traumatic event; this can include new or dependent relationships, a new sense of personal strengths or capabilities, a reorienting or sharpening of one's priorities in life, and/or changes in spiritual beliefs and practices (Tedeschi and Calhoun 1996). During the first wave of the COVID-19 pandemic in New York City, a survey of frontline health care workers found that 80% of respondents endorsed at least one dimension of PTG (Feingold et al. 2022). With PTG, distress is intrinsic to the experience; it should not and cannot be avoided. Indeed, the aforementioned study of health care workers found that those individuals with probable PTSD on the basis of a

TABLE 15–1. Activities to foster resilience factors

Factor	Enhancement activities
1. Foster realistic optimism and positive emotions	Use cognitive-behavioral therapy tools to identify negative automatic thoughts and challenge them with more realistic and helpful thoughts Use activities such as scheduled worry time to address rumination Use behavioral activation approaches, including scheduling pleasant activities Focus on gratitude through journaling, reminiscing, or conversation with others
2. Face fear directly	Use activities such as fear hierarchies to gradually counter avoidance Face fears with social support Learn skills to master fear (e.g., deep breathing, mindfulness approaches, acceptance-based approaches)
3. Have a personal moral compass	Identify core values Discuss values with a role model Act according to personal values Employ altruism to derive meaning from personal suffering Identify and challenge negative automatic thoughts that may contribute to moral distress
4. Embrace faith and spirituality	Engage in prayer or daily meditation if doing so is in line with personal preference Engage in physical practice (e.g., yoga, martial arts) or creative practice (e.g., poetry, singing) (Re)engage with a trusted faith community
5. Use social support networks	Devote time to social relationships even if there is low motivation to do so Schedule social interaction, including brief phone calls Ask for help

TABLE 15–1. Activities to foster resilience factors *(continued)*

Factor	Enhancement activities
6. Rely on resilient role models	Identify individuals who have faced adversity before and learn from the adaptive ways they have navigated these challenges Observe the skill(s) of this individual, break down the skill into segments, practice, and get feedback Be aware that no role model is perfect and that successful coping may involve learning from different individuals
7. Attend to physical well-being	Develop increasingly ambitious goals for physical exercise after consulting with a health provider (Re)engage with healthy sleep habits, including limiting electronics and time spent awake in bed due to rumination Develop a vocabulary for stress awareness and identify activities that address increasingly intense negative emotions Avoid skipping meals because of poor appetite
8. Devote time to brain fitness	Continue lifelong learning, including through engaging with podcasts, books, or online courses Take on a new hobby or interest or reengage with an old one
9. Employ cognitive and emotional flexibility	Accept limits of personal control, blame, and responsibility Appraise situations with a broadening perspective to open new possibilities Learn from failures Rely on humor at times to reframe situations Employ a broad set of strategies (e.g., dialectical behavior therapy, acceptance and commitment therapy) to regulate emotions
10. Connect to a sense of meaning and purpose	Search for meaning in both the experiences of daily life and moments of suffering to promote posttraumatic growth

Note. For further details of each resilience factor, see Southwick et al. 2023.

screening measure tended to endorse greater PTG. Other work has demonstrated an inverse U-shaped relationship between PTG and PTSD, whereby individuals with moderate PTSD have the highest PTG (Whealin et al. 2020). Plausibly, persons with few or mild symptoms have little impetus to reflect on the impact of the event(s), whereas those with much more severe symptoms may be so affected that they cannot devote cognitive and emotional resources to identifying sources of growth.

DePierro and colleagues (2024) recently developed a 24-item self-report measure of these resilience factors, called the Mount Sinai Resilience Scale, which evaluates how frequently people rely on a given factor and how effective each one is for them. This scale may be helpful in evaluating baseline risk for psychopathology following loss and processes of psychological recovery over time.

Conclusion

Loss is a ubiquitous experience, particularly in the age of simultaneous large-scale global disasters, and disaster mental health professionals should be prepared to help survivors navigate through it. The grief that follows can take many forms. For a subset of individuals, these grief reactions are persistent and impairing and may meet criteria for one or more DSM-5-TR psychiatric disorders, including PGD. Individuals may lean on resilience factors such as social support; sources of meaning and purpose (e.g., meaning derived from participating in the caretaking for a deceased loved one); and cognitive reframing to manage and recover from the acute distress associated with grief, whether or not this distress rises to the level of a psychiatric diagnosis. To help survivors, disaster mental health professionals should include resilience promotion in their toolkit. Further work is needed to examine the cross-cultural applicability of PGD criteria, screening tools, and treatments. At the same time, it is crucial that countries and individual institutions make financial investments in disseminating evidence-based interventions for prolonged grief sequelae so that at-risk individuals do not fall through the cracks.

References

Acosta H, Jansen A, Kircher T: Larger bilateral amygdalar volumes are associated with affective loss experiences. J Neurosci Res 99(7):1763–1779, 2021 33789356

Alvis L, Zhang N, Sandler IN, et al: Developmental manifestations of grief in children and adolescents: caregivers as key grief facilitators. J Child Adolesc Trauma 16(2):447–457, 2022 35106114

American Psychiatric Association: Diagnostic and Statistical Manual of Mental Disorders, 3rd Edition. Washington, DC, American Psychiatric Association, 1980

American Psychiatric Association: Diagnostic and Statistical Manual of Mental Disorders, 5th Edition. Arlington, VA, American Psychiatric Association, 2013

American Psychiatric Association: Diagnostic and Statistical Manual of Mental Disorders, 5th Edition, Text Revision. Washington, DC, American Psychiatric Association, 2022

Bonanno GA, Malgaroli M: Trajectories of grief: comparing symptoms from the DSM-5 and ICD-11 diagnoses. Depress Anxiety 37(1):17–25, 2020 31012187

Bosch OJ, Nair HP, Ahern TH, et al: The CRF system mediates increased passive stress-coping behavior following the loss of a bonded partner in a monogamous rodent. Neuropsychopharmacology 34(6):1406–1415, 2009 18923404

Buchheim A, Heinrichs M, George C, et al: Oxytocin enhances the experience of attachment security. Psychoneuroendocrinology 34(9):1417–1422, 2009 19457618

Courtney AL, Meyer ML: Self-other representation in the social brain reflects social connection. J Neurosci 40(29):5616–5627, 2020 32541067

DePierro JM, Marin DB, Sharma V, et al: Development and initial validation of the Mount Sinai Resilience Scale. Psychol Trauma 16(3):407–415, 2024 37796549

Feingold JH, Hurtado A, Feder A, et al: Posttraumatic growth among health care workers on the frontlines of the COVID-19 pandemic. J Affect Disord 296:35–40, 2022 34587547

Froemke RC, Young LJ: Oxytocin, neural plasticity, and social behavior. Annu Rev Neurosci 44:359–381, 2021 33823654

Granek L, Peleg-Sagy T: The use of pathological grief outcomes in bereavement studies on African Americans. Transcult Psychiatry 54(3):384–399, 2017 28540767

Guastella AJ, Kenyon AR, Alvares GA, et al: Intranasal arginine vasopressin enhances the encoding of happy and angry faces in humans. Biol Psychiatry 67(12):1220–1222, 2010 20447617

Krupnick JL, Horowitz MJ: Stress response syndromes: recurrent themes. Arch Gen Psychiatry 38(4):428–435, 1981 7212973

Lenferink LIM, de Keijser J, Smid GE, et al: Prolonged grief, depression, and posttraumatic stress in disaster-bereaved individuals: latent class analysis. Eur J Psychotraumatol 8(1):1298311, 2017 28451067

O'Connor M-F, Seeley SH: Grieving as a form of learning: insights from neuroscience applied to grief and loss. Curr Opin Psychol 43:317–322, 2022 34520954

Prigerson HG, Shear MK, Reynolds CF 3rd: Prolonged grief disorder diagnostic criteria—helping those with maladaptive grief responses. JAMA Psychiatry 79(4):277–278, 2022 35107569

Roberts K, Holland J, Prigerson HG, et al: Development of the Bereavement Risk Inventory and Screening Questionnaire (BRISQ): item generation and expert panel feedback. Palliat Support Care 15(1):57–66, 2017 27516152

Rose S, Bisson J, Wessely S: A systematic review of single-session psychological interventions ("debriefing") following trauma. Psychother Psychosom 72(4):176–184, 2003 12792122

Sadino JM, Donaldson ZR: Prairie voles as a model for understanding the genetic and epigenetic regulation of attachment behaviors. ACS Chem Neurosci 9(8):1939–1950, 2018 29513516

Saito M: Japan's tsunami survivors call lost loves on the phone of the wind. Reuters, April 7, 2021. Available at: https://widerimage.reuters.com/story/japans-tsunami-survivors-call-lost-loves-on-the-phone-of-the-wind. Accessed April 3, 2024.

Sneed RS, Key K, Bailey S, Johnson-Lawrence V: Social and psychological consequences of the COVID-19 pandemic in African-American communities: lessons from Michigan. Psychol Trauma 12(5):446–448, 2020 32525371

Southwick SM, Charney DS, DePierro JM: Resilience: The Science of Mastering Life's Greatest Challenges, 3rd Edition. New York, Cambridge University Press, 2023

Tedeschi RG, Calhoun LG: The Posttraumatic Growth Inventory: measuring the positive legacy of trauma. J Trauma Stress 9(3):455–471, 1996 8827649

Thompson RR, George K, Walton JC, et al: Sex-specific influences of vasopressin on human social communication. Proc Natl Acad Sci USA 103(20):7889–7894, 2006 16682649

Weissman MM, Markowitz JC, Klerman G: Comprehensive Guide to Interpersonal Psychotherapy. New York, Basic Books, 2008

Whealin JM, Pitts B, Tsai J, et al: Dynamic interplay between PTSD symptoms and posttraumatic growth in older military veterans. J Affect Disord 269:185–191, 2020 32339132

16

Psychological First Aid

Edward M. Kantor, M.D.
David R. Beckert, M.D.

The majority of organized emergency and disaster response agencies in the United States now use or recommend Psychological First Aid (PFA) as a primary support tool for working with individuals exposed to a major disaster or mass casualty event (Hobfoll et al. 2007; National Institute of Mental Health 2002; Ng and Kantor 2010). The core elements of PFA are generally defined as contact and engagement, safety and comfort, stabilization, information gathering, practical assistance, connection with social supports, information on coping, and linkage with collaborative services. PFA has found a role in reducing intergroup variations in the approach to exposed individuals and has evolved into a more standardized approach for both mental health professionals and first responders alike during and after a disaster event.

During the coronavirus disease 2019 (COVID-19) pandemic, PFA was at times employed to support both health care workers and the general public (Shah et al. 2020). In some cases, it was paired with Skills for Psychological Recovery (SPR), which serves as a next-step additional tool for psychological support and a referral mechanism that focuses on resilience building to distressed individuals who may not meet criteria for more focused illness-based treatments (Berkowitz et al. 2010; Williams et al. 2020). PFA is not a treatment for posttraumatic stress disorder (PTSD) or other psychiatric diagnoses. Rather, it is a mechanism to sensitively approach exposed individuals, attempt to understand their situation, offer early available support, and help connect to relevant resources. Once an individual is engaged, next steps are based on their specific needs and circumstances. PFA may also serve as an important triage tool to help identify and differentiate general distress from a more specific or severe psychiatric illness (North 2017).

In this chapter we outline the history and evolution of PFA, describe the goals and basic elements that inform its implementation, review key components, and highlight some resources and caveats when working with varied populations.

History and Evolution

After the 9/11 terrorist attacks in 2001, early mental health interventions for disaster survivors received increased attention in the United States. Federal support for disaster response planning required that states address mental health issues to receive disaster funding. Although sources vary in reporting its origin, PFA, as a basic concept, is not new in the psychological literature. It shares its roots with much of the early crisis and disaster literature that evolved in the first half of the twentieth century. In the military and civilian response communities, various forms of critical incident stress debriefing (CISD) formerly prevailed as the primary intervention for police, fire, and emergency medical services workers (McEvoy 2005). Otherwise, a great variety of approaches were used by unaffiliated mental health responders, who applied their individual or group early treatment of choice to the disaster exposed. As a result of several expert consensus conferences and literature reviews (National Institute of Mental Health 2002), it became clear that components of psychological debriefing, such as that used in CISD (now known as critical incident stress management), could worsen stress symptoms in some individuals and did not lower the rate of PTSD among those who participated as a whole. Note that *psychological* debriefing is distinctly different from *operational* debriefing, which is used to evaluate response and organizational effectiveness and learn about what worked and what might be improved as an important part of quality improvement efforts.

Although the evidence is still evolving, it appears that early interventions that reconnect victims with family, social supports, and known relevant resources may prove to be the most effective way to facilitate recovery (Hobfoll et al. 2007; Orner et al. 2006). At its essence, PFA is an attempt to attune to the specific human needs and emotional style of the individual and in the context of their expressed needs at the moment of intervention. It emphasizes empathic listening coupled with nonjudgmental responses, as well as an attempt to support individual coping styles and connect the individual to helpful social supports.

The roots of PFA can be found in the evolving literature of crisis intervention and traumatic stress. As far back as the 1950s, a special article in the *Journal of the American Medical Association* titled "Psychological First Aid in Community Disasters" (Drayer et al. 1954), written by the American Psychiatric Association Committee on Civil Defense (forerunner of the association's Committee on Psychiatric Dimensions of Disaster), outlined many of the basic premises used in more formal PFA training. Twenty years later, Beverly Raphael (1977) used the term and added some of the basic approaches to bereavement intervention. Much of the recent disaster literature continues to support the interventions and objectives (outlined in Table 16–1) that promote safety, help to return a sense of control, and link individuals to relevant supports in the community or to people or institutions of particular significance to the survivor (Orner et al. 2006).

Developing Standard

In the United States, PFA implies a very specific and more manualized approach initially intended for mental health workers to use in early response that was developed through the National Child Traumatic Stress Network (NCTSN) and the National Center for PTSD (NCPTSD). From what was previously a generic term for these basic interventions, a semistructured field guide has evolved for use by mental health providers and other responders who are at baseline well trained in their usual practice but not necessarily experienced in crisis and disaster work. PFA guidelines emerged more rapidly as evidence accumulated against the routine use of psychological debriefing because of its potential for worsening symptoms and increasing the risk of developing PTSD (see also Chapter 17, "Psychotherapies"). Those findings and the lack of alternative safe practices have cemented PFA concepts into general use. NCCTS and NCPTSD released the first edition of the *Psychological First Aid (PFA) Field Operations Guide* after Hurricane Katrina (Brymer et al. 2006). The guide was revised to accommodate new materials and information, and a second edition was released in 2006 (Brymer et al. 2006). A later version of the field guide, *PFA for Medical Reserve Corps*, resulted from collaboration between NCTSN and the Civilian Volunteer Medical Reserve Corps National Mental Health Work Group (Brymer et al. 2008). The widespread dissemination of the field operations guide and integration of PFA by groups such as the American Red Cross into their own disaster mental health training further advanced acceptance of PFA by academic medi-

TABLE 16–1. Basic objectives of Psychological First Aid

Establish human connection in a nonintrusive, compassionate manner

Enhance immediate and ongoing safety and provide physical and emotional support

Calm and orient emotionally overwhelmed and distraught survivors

Help articulate immediate needs and concerns; gather information as appropriate

Offer practical assistance and information to address needs

Connect survivors with relevant support networks, family, friends, and helping resources

Support positive coping and empower survivors to take an active role in recovery

Provide information to help cope with the psychological impact of disasters

Facilitate continuity and ensure linking to other sources of support after disaster responders have left

Source.   Adapted from Brymer et al. 2006.

cine, public health agencies, the military, and state and local governments (National Child Traumatic Stress Network 2009).

The PFA field operations guide attempts to use evolving research but at the same time "do no harm." In its introduction, the document describes PFA as an "evidence-informed," rather than evidence-based, strategy because much of the material is drawn from the crisis, trauma, and bereavement literature and all recommendations had not yet been scientifically validated in disaster settings (Brymer et al. 2006; Ruzek et al. 2007). The rapidity of response and the inherent chaos and danger, along with limited resources, make it challenging to conduct studies on the effectiveness of interventions during the immediate disaster response. Taking this into account, the authors of the *PFA Field Operations Guide* considered the concerns and warnings in the literature, and there has been a growing consensus of support among trauma and disaster mental health experts for PFA as a useful tool.

Basics of Psychological First Aid

Detailed knowledge of the elements and goals of PFA helps to inform accurate implementation. The basic elements are described in Table 16–2.

Among the key resources in the *PFA Field Operations Guide* is a series of specific techniques and sample scripts meant to serve as examples for responders working with persons exposed to disaster situations. Recommendations for learning PFA include an initial didactic core through read-

TABLE 16–2. Elements and goals of Psychological First Aid

Element	Goals
1. Contact and engagement	• Respond to contacts initiated by survivors or initiate contacts in a nonintrusive, compassionate, and helpful manner
2. Safety and comfort	• Enhance immediate and ongoing safety • Provide physical and emotional comfort
3. Stabilization	• Calm and orient emotionally overwhelmed or disoriented survivors
4. Information gathering	• Identify immediate needs and concerns • Gather additional information • Tailor Psychological First Aid interventions
5. Practical assistance	• Offer practical help to survivors in addressing immediate needs and concerns
6. Connection with social supports	• Help establish brief or ongoing contacts with primary support persons and other sources of support, including family members, friends, and community helping resources
7. Information on coping	• Provide information about stress reactions and coping to reduce distress and promote adaptive functioning
8. Linkage with collaborative services	• Link survivors with available services needed at the time or in the future

Source. Adapted from Brymer et al. 2005.

ings, classroom instruction, or online course material. Additional supervised practical exercise is also recommended.

Special Populations

The PFA field guide format includes specific resources and tools for working with children, older adults, bereaved persons, and other special populations. Several adaptations and translations of the guide have evolved from the original for a variety of users and situations. Although PFA was initially intended for mental health providers, over time it has become a tool for other practitioners and responders. Adaptations of the *PFA Field Operations Guide* were created for community-based religious professionals and school-based responders; adaptations and variations of the guide are available at the NCTSN website (www.nctsn.org/treatments-

and-practices/psychological-first-aid-and-skills-for-psychological-recovery/
nctsn-resources).

Cultural Implications

The needs and responses of individuals from different cultures and backgrounds play a critical part in early disaster response initiatives, including
PFA. More information is coming to light, but very little is known for certain about how generic mental health assumptions and interventions
should be defined or modified for demographic subgroups of people and
for specific disaster types. The World Health Organization (WHO) issued a
directive asking response organizations to discourage mental health professionals from responding to disaster areas where they are not familiar with
the language or the culture (Inter-Agency Standing Committee 2007).

The *PFA Field Operations Guide* has been translated into Spanish,
Japanese, German, Swedish, and Italian, and it continues to evolve with
sensitivity to cross-cultural issues and other languages. However, relevance
and effectiveness studies are yet to be fully completed, and the distribution
effort has not been without some controversy. International providers have
implied that simply translating and exporting the guide may create a
"Westernization" of a crisis and grief response and may not have relevance
in the affected group (Watters 2010). An emerging strategy for more effective intervention may be to pair up international responders with local
mental health professionals familiar with the local culture and social service system or to pair them with native social supports, such as religious,
community service, or educational professionals. Even so, there have been
questions about the relevance and usefulness of materials developed in the
United States for use in non-Western cultures. In an effort to address these
concerns, the *PFA Field Operations Guide* includes nonspecific *culture
alerts* interspersed throughout that highlight potentially sensitive areas of
understanding and intervention as they relate to other cultures.

These culture alerts are useful for clues on how to initially approach
and interact with survivors, but they do not speak in depth to specific cultural norms. As pointed out by WHO's Inter-Agency Standing Committee
(2007) in its guidance for mental health professionals thinking of responding to disasters in other countries, there is no substitute for having a
solid understanding of the regional culture and language, prior disaster
experience, and knowledge of the legal environment at the disaster scene.
One example is the update issued by the American Psychological Association, based on the Inter-Agency Standing Committee guideline, for mental health professionals considering participation in the 2010 Haiti
earthquake relief effort. They recommended that unaffiliated volunteers

be discouraged from traveling to affected regions without meeting specific culture-based criteria or sponsorship by established relief organizations (IASC Reference Group for Mental Health and Psychosocial Support in Emergency Settings 2010).

Children and Adolescents

The *PFA Field Operations Guide* integrates several strategies designed to facilitate work with children and their parents (see Chapter 19, "Child and Adolescent Psychiatric Interventions"). It also offers child-specific tip sheets for parents and other caregivers to use with children in their charge. Variations focus on how parents can help their own children and how school personnel can use the techniques at times of disaster or school crises. Over the past 10 years, many situation- and population-specific variations of PFA have been produced.

Conclusion

This chapter is not a substitute for PFA training, although the goals and basic elements are presented in a way that can hopefully influence a responder's approach to early intervention in disaster. Key issues related to PFA are presented in Table 16–3.

Some components of PFA are knowledge based and can be obtained through additional readings or a short online training course. Developing the skills and attitudes that translate these concepts and interventions into practice may require a bit more training. This can be accomplished through live scenarios and through practical skill sessions mentored by seasoned instructors. Many agencies and courses use the PFA concepts, including the American Red Cross, the Medical Reserve Corps, the American Psychiatric Association, and other disaster response organizations.

Efforts are underway to further evaluate and standardize PFA, particularly in the response community. In 2014, McCabe et al. (2014, p. 621) proposed a competency-based training model for PFA, suggesting that the various sources offering training and resources "have not systematically addressed pedagogical elements necessary for optimal learning or teaching." Their article addressed the need for a more consistent curriculum, as well as the use of public health core competencies. Core competency frameworks have been established by both the public health community and organized medicine. Unfortunately, each group structures their competencies differently. The need for collaboration was identified and attempted in the early 2000s with the establishment of the Civilian Medical Reserve Corps, and although the disconnect was recognized, the systems remain quite separate

TABLE 16–3. Teaching points

Disaster mental health professionals and responders should make an effort to do the following:

- Understand the origins and evolution of Psychological First Aid (PFA) in disaster response
- Be aware of the strengths and limitations of PFA as an evidence-informed approach
- Become familiar with the basic goals and principles of PFA
- Recognize that any mental health intervention, including PFA, may have cultural implications
- Obtain information about major PFA training resources and consider completing a competency-based course involving practical exercises

---

(Kantor et al. 2005). Even so, there is merit in the concept, and there would likely be value in bringing public health, academic medicine, and related allied practitioner groups together to develop shared competencies and identify reciprocal language in disaster response overall.

Despite the difficulty of conducting disaster outcomes research in a timely and ethical way, the widespread adoption of PFA allows for continuing review as more data become available. As physicians, psychiatrists must approach disaster settings with an awareness of their own skills and limitations, as well as the full range of potential medical and psychiatric issues that may require care beyond the basic elements of PFA. Although PFA attends to urgent immediate needs, the use of PFA by psychiatrists in acute disaster settings will hopefully lead to earlier specific assessment, diagnosis, and therapeutic opportunities, with effective triage and referral criteria as psychiatric illness is uncovered.

Additional Resources

National Child Traumatic Stress Network: Psychological First Aid for Youth Experiencing Homelessness. Los Angeles, CA, National Child Traumatic Stress Network, 2009. Available at: www.nctsn.org/sites/default/files/resources/pfa_youth_experiencing_homelessness.pdf. Accessed April 15, 2023.
National Child Traumatic Stress Network: Psychological First Aid (PFA) and Skills for Psychological Recovery (SPR) (includes a 5-hour interactive course that puts the participant in the role of a provider in a postdisaster scene). Los Angeles, CA, National Child Traumatic Stress Network, 2023. Available at: https://learn.nctsn.org/course/index.php?categoryid=11. Accessed April 15, 2023.
Watson, PJ. Early interventions for trauma-related problems, in Textbook of Disaster Psychiatry, 2nd Edition. Edited by Ursano R, Fullerton C, Weisaeth L, Raphael B. Cambridge, UK, Cambridge University Press, 2017, pp 87–100

References

Brymer M, Layne C, Pynoos R, et al: Psychological First Aid: Field Operations Guide, 2nd Edition. Los Angeles, CA, National Child Traumatic Stress Network/National Center for PTSD, September 2006. Available at: www.nctsn.org/sites/default/files/resources//pfa_field_operations_guide.pdf. Accessed April 15, 2023.

Berkowitz S, Bryant R, Brymer M, et al: Skills for Psychological Recovery Field Operations Guide. Los Angeles, CA, National Child Traumatic Stress Network/National Center for PTSD, 2010. Available at: www.nctsn.org/sites/default/files/resources/special-resource/spr_complete_english.pdf. Accessed on April 15, 2023.

Brymer M, Jacobs A, Layne C, et al: Psychological First Aid for Medical Reserve Corps Field Operations Guide. Los Angeles, CA, National Child Traumatic Stress Network/National Center for PTSD, March 2008. Available at: www.nctsn.org/sites/default/files/assets/pdfs/MRC_PFA_04_02_08.pdf. Accessed April 15, 2023.

Drayer CS, Cameron DC, Woodward WD, et al: Psychological first aid in community disasters: prepared by the American Psychiatric Association Committee on Civil Defense. JAMA 156:36–41, 1954

Hobfoll SE, Watson P, Bell CC, et al: Five essential elements of immediate and mid-term mass trauma intervention: empirical evidence. Psychiatry 70(4):283–315, discussion 316–369, 2007 18181708

IASC Reference Group for Mental Health and Psychosocial Support in Emergency Settings: Mental Health and Psychosocial Support in Humanitarian Emergencies: What Should Humanitarian Health Actors Know? Geneva, Switzerland, 2010. Available at: https://interagencystandingcommittee.org/sites/default/files/migrated/2018-10/MHPSS%20Protection%20Actors.pdf. Accessed July 10, 2024.

Inter-Agency Standing Committee: IASC Guidelines on Mental Health and Psychosocial Support in Emergency Settings. Geneva, Switzerland, Inter-Agency Standing Committee, 2007. Available at: https://interagencystandingcommittee.org/iasc-task-force-mental-health-and-psychosocial-support-emergency-settings/iasc-guidelines-mental-health-and-psychosocial-support-emergency-settings-2007. Accessed April 15, 2023.

Kantor EM, Beckert DR, Dowdell KJ, et al: Training physicians and health professionals in disaster and bioterrorism: gearing up for the core competency movement in medical education. Oral presentation, National MRC Conference, San Francisco, CA, April 2005

McCabe OL, Everly GS Jr, Brown LM, et al: Psychological first aid: a consensus-derived, empirically supported, competency-based training model. Am J Public Health 104(4):621–628, 2014 23865656

McEvoy M: Psychological first aid: replacement for critical incident stress debriefing? Rochelle Park, NJ, Fire Engineering, 2005. Available at: www.fireengineering.com/fire-ems/psychological-first-aid-replacement-for-critical-incident-stress-debriefing/#gref. Accessed April 15, 2023.

National Child Traumatic Stress Network: About PFA. Los Angeles, CA, National Child Traumatic Stress Network, November 2009. Available at:

www.nctsn.org/treatments-and-practices/psychological-first-aid-and-skills-for-psychological-recovery/about-pfa. Accessed April 15, 2023

National Institute of Mental Health: Mental Health and Mass Violence: Evidence-Based Early Psychological Intervention for Victims/Survivors of Mass Violence: A Workshop to Reach Consensus on Best Practices (NIH Publ No 02-5138). Washington, DC, U.S. Government Printing Office, 2002

Ng AT, Kantor EM: Psychological first aid, in Hidden Impact: What You Need to Know for the Next Disaster: A Practical Mental Health Guide for Clinicians. Edited by Stoddard FJ, Katz CL, Merlino JP. Sudbury, MA, Jones & Bartlett, 2010, pp 115–122

North CS: Epidemiology of disaster mental health: the foundation for disaster mental health response, in Textbook of Disaster Psychiatry, 2nd Edition. Edited by Ursano RJ, Fullerton CS, Raphael B. New York, Cambridge University Press, 2017, pp 37–38

Orner R, Kent A, Pfefferbaum BJ, et al: The context of providing immediate post event intervention, in Interventions Following Mass Violence and Disasters: Strategies for Mental Health Practice. Edited by Ritchie EC, Watson PJ, Friedman MJ. New York, Guilford, 2006, pp 121–133

Raphael B: Preventive intervention with the recently bereaved. Arch Gen Psychiatry 34(12):1450–1454, 1977 263815

Ruzek JI, Brymer MJ, Jacobs AK, et al: Psychological First Aid. J Ment Health Couns 29:17–49, 2007

Shah K, Bedi S, Onyeaka H, et al: The role of Psychological First Aid to support public mental health in the COVID-19 pandemic. Cureus 12(6):e8821, 2020 32742836

Watters E: The Americanization of mental illness. New York Times Magazine, January 10, 2010. Available at: www.nytimes.com/2010/01/10/magazine/10psyche-t.html. Accessed April 15, 2023.

Williams JL, Rheingold AA, Henschel AV, et al: Novel application of skills for psychological recovery as an early intervention for violent loss: rationale and case examples. Omega (Westport) 81(2):179–196, 2020 29570030

17

Psychotherapies

Individual, Family, and Group

Srini Pillay, M.D.
Kathleen A. Clegg, M.D.
Kristina Jones, M.D.

Psychotherapies can be very helpful in the context of disasters. A recent systematic review of psychological interventions for disasters, pandemics, and trauma found that psychological distress and subclinical symptoms were reduced in 9 of 15 randomized controlled trials, 2 of 3 controlled pre-post studies, and 9 of 9 uncontrolled pre-post studies. A key feature of the psychotherapies was that they were brief and innovative (Lotzin et al. 2023). In another systematic review and meta-analysis of 27 studies, post-disaster psychotherapeutic interventions were found to be effective (Semerci and Uzun 2023).

A scoping review of 45 studies of trauma-informed psychological interventions to treat anxiety, depression, and posttraumatic stress symptoms in youth following natural and biological disasters was conducted by Burkhart et al. (2023). The most implemented interventions were cognitive-behavioral therapy (CBT), trauma-focused CBT (TF-CBT), and eye movement desensitization and reprocessing (EMDR). Although methodologies were varied, overall, there was a significant decrease in posttraumatic stress symptoms, distress, anxiety, and depression regardless of whether the participant received CBT, TF-CBT, or EMDR.

In general, these data are based on population averages, and it is impossible to predict which individuals will respond to a proven treatment. For this reason, in the disaster setting, psychotherapy must be tailored to the needs of the individual. There is no one-size-fits-all approach that can be mechanically applied across the board.

Targets of Psychotherapy

A review of the disaster psychology literature (Norris et al. 2002) defined outcomes of disasters into categories labeled as follows:

1. Specific psychological problems (diagnostic disorders according to the *Diagnostic and Statistical Manual of Mental Disorders*; American Psychiatric Association 2022)
2. Nonspecific distress (troubling symptoms associated with reactions to extreme stress)
3. Health problems and concerns such as somatic complaints and substance abuse
4. Chronic problems in living such as increased daily hassles secondary to the disaster
5. Psychosocial resource loss such as disruption of personal hardiness and social support
6. Problems specific to youth such as separation anxiety, developmental regression, and externalizing behavior problems

Psychotherapy in the disaster setting might target any of these categories of disability.

Planning psychological interventions after disasters includes five key elements: 1) promoting a sense of safety, 2) calming, 3) a sense of self and community, 4) enhancing connectedness such as resuming socializing with friends, and 5) enhancing hope (Stoddard et al. 2009).

Therapist-Patient Relationship

In the disaster setting, a formal therapist-patient relationship is rare. However, even in less formal situations, clinicians should obey the ethical codes of their discipline, the licensing regulations of the relevant state(s), and the laws of the state in which they are practicing at the time. For this reason, it would be prudent to look up any local laws prior to entering the disaster area.

It is common for clinicians to perform many of the nonclinical tasks of social work such as helping people connect to public and private resources. Ideally, the psychotherapy intervention itself should be a short-term, emotionally supportive, and pragmatic intervention, although in certain instances a longer-term relationship may be indicated. This may occur online or through referral to a local therapist.

Early Interventions

Some of the commonly practiced interventions are crisis intervention, psychoeducation, psychological debriefing, and defusing.

Crisis Intervention

Crisis intervention is a technique invented by a psychiatrist, Erich Lindemann, after the Boston Cocoanut Grove fire of 1942 (Lindemann 1944/1994). When a crisis occurs, the people affected by it lose their equilibrium and may display a range of physical, emotional, or cognitive symptoms. Often, there is a form of shell shock, with a sense of helplessness, panic, or fear and an inability to walk, talk, or sleep. Patients are often in a state of autonomic imbalance, trapped in a fight-or-flight state. When this is the case, the primary goal of psychotherapy is to ensure the safety of the patient (e.g., by inquiring into the degree of suicidal or homicidal ideation or by helping them find resources relevant to everyday living) and to help them attain some autonomic recovery. To achieve this, the therapist should focus on establishing a supportive relationship, identifying gaps in resources, exploring alternative options for filling these gaps, and obtaining a firm commitment from the patient and ensuring availability of resources to decrease the uncertainty that is already a destabilizing factor in the disaster setting.

A therapist who intervenes in a crisis must balance adopting a firm and directive position with providing support and hope. This will help to limit confusion, shock, helplessness, emotional lability, aggression, or unresolved grief. The therapist and patient should provide inputs for goal setting, planning, and constructive coping. If the patient remains severely distressed or impaired, a referral to a local provider may be necessary. It is important to be realistic and to build on small improvements gradually.

Psychoeducation

The crux of psychoeducation involves consolidating the goal of recovery by reducing the uncertainty and unpredictability of the future as much as possible. In the context of a crisis, it helps to distribute brochures about common symptoms that are experienced, to educate mental health professionals in public forums, to provide contact numbers of relevant resources, and to use electronic media where possible.

The purpose of psychoeducation is to reduce the confusion and feelings of helplessness after a disaster. Giving adequate information to public officials, teachers, parents, first responders, and anyone else who is responsible for the emotional welfare of others will help to equip these helpers to provide better care and to feel more confident in their ability to function effectively under difficult conditions. Often, the spokespersons may be not the therapists themselves but trusted public figures whom therapists can support and inform prior to their communications.

Psychological Debriefing

Psychological debriefing refers to discussions that occur 48–72 hours after an event. In general, these discussions encourage people affected by a disaster to discuss and describe the factual and emotional aspects of their disaster experience. The assumption is that people who can speak about their experiences will be able to cognitively restructure their experiences.

There are various kinds of debriefing, such as critical incident stress debriefing and critical incident stress management. Although debriefing has been successfully used in military combat settings and in relief workers (Knobler et al. 2007), several key reviews have concluded that it may in fact be harmful. For example, one study of 11 trials with single-session interventions involving some form of emotional processing or ventilation by encouraging recollection or reworking of the traumatic event, accompanied by normalization of emotional reaction to the event, found no short-term benefit in reduction of posttraumatic stress disorder (PTSD) symptoms at 3–5 months, and at 1 year there was an increased risk of PTSD symptoms (Rose et al. 2002). Debriefing had no impact on depression, anxiety, or psychiatric morbidity. The subsequently published National Institute of Clinical Health and Care Excellence (NICE) guidelines recommended that psychological debriefing should not be used to prevent PTSD (National Institute for Health and Care Excellence 2018). Another review of 11 studies found that no psychological intervention can be recommended for routine use following traumatic events and that multiple-session interventions, like single-session interventions, may have an adverse effect on some individuals (Roberts et al. 2009).

More recently, many studies included within the review by Roberts and colleagues and the NICE analysis have been criticized on multiple levels, including that they 1) used debriefing in one-to-one settings rather than in a group and 2) used debriefing with individuals exposed to personal physical traumas rather than those exposed in a work capacity

(Tamrakar et al. 2019). These authors concluded that psychological debriefing may be worth reconsidering when it applies to the original population it was intended for: emergency personnel and first responders.

A recent meta-ethnographic systematic review suggested that debriefs were consistently evaluated by trauma-exposed workers as helpful (Richins et al. 2020). Although debriefing does not help to prevent PTSD, it is helpful for workers to integrate their experiences, normalize their reactions, and promote recovery. In keeping with these findings, a recent systematic review and meta-analysis of debriefing in group settings found that although debriefing did not reduce the risk of PTSD symptoms, there was evidence that it was associated with reduced anxiety and alleviated problematic alcohol use (Vignaud et al. 2022). When these debriefings are helpful, they involve catharsis, peer support, and normalization of distress. Team briefing after a traumatic event is now frequently recommended (O'Toole and Eppich 2022).

One way to reconcile these seemingly conflicting reports is that debriefing works when people are properly trained to do it. One such 5-day training program was recently shown to be widely appreciated by the trainees (Johnson et al. 2023).

American Red Cross Debriefing

American Red Cross debriefing (ARCD) involves crisis intervention, defusing, and debriefing. Although this debriefing also involves the patient telling their story and venting, there are significant distinctions from the International Critical Incident Stress Foundation (ICISF). The ARCD method is more about coping with the frustrations after an incident rather than focusing on the critical incident itself. The process is relatively unstructured, using techniques such as empathy, accepting, and active listening, with a focus on coping strategies and active support. ARC's emphasis is on supporting their staff, not just the survivors of a disaster or their communities. Also, for ARC, debriefing is just one of many stress management tools. In contrast, the ICISF focuses on structured debriefing and managing critical incident stress. Their approach is designed to address the specific details of the critical incident, providing a systematic method for helping individuals process their experiences and mitigate stress. This comparison highlights that whereas ARCD prioritizes support and coping mechanisms for staff, the ICISF emphasizes a more formalized process centered on the incident itself.

Defusing metaphorically relates to deactivating a bomb by removing the fuse. This is typically used when frustrations are at their peak, and ventilation can help to facilitate constructive communication. Also, whereas debriefing is usually about a past event, defusing can also be about the present or about preempting a worsening of the situation in the future.

ARC defusing is commonly directed toward rapidly relieving a stressful working situation (e.g., conflict among coworkers), and disaster mental health service workers are often positioned close to first responders so they can detect and respond to problems efficiently. Because emotional hot spots can emerge rapidly and unexpectedly, these defusings must be correspondingly fluid and timely, allowing for ventilation and conflict resolution.

Critical Incident Stress Defusing

Critical incident stress defusing is a method of ventilation most often administered within 12 hours of a critical incident to allow people to ventilate and process their thoughts, emotions, and experiences with the goal of normalization and validation. This is usually a smaller group than the debriefing group and is less structured and formal.

Psychological First Aid

The idea behind Psychological First Aid (PFA; Snider et al. 2011) is that people without extensive medical training can provide immediate help without having to be trained in psychotherapy. The main components are empathy and compassion. The goals are to reduce the risk of harm and psychological distress and to provide practical assistance such as connecting the person with adequate resources. However, crisis intervention goes beyond this by providing diagnostic and lethality assessments, collaborative problem-solving, referrals for mental health follow-up, and follow-up to determine the efficacy of the intervention.

Trauma-Related Therapy

Most people in disasters are quite resilient. Trauma is not an inevitable and definite consequence. In addition, therapists who are used to treating trauma in a clinical setting will be faced with very different priorities, such as acute stress in the disaster setting. Because debriefing techniques are at best questionable for the prevention of PTSD in the disaster setting, the goals of psychotherapy should be geared toward the reduction of emotional distress and the enhancement of resilience.

Cognitive-Behavioral Therapy

CBT has been shown to be effective in the context of disasters. For example, two studies have found that CBT is helpful to adolescents in the context of earthquakes and war (Qouta et al. 2012; Shooshtary et al. 2008). On the morning of December 26, 2003, at 05:28 (local time) a major earthquake measuring 6.5 on the Richter scale struck southeastern Iran. The epicenter of the earthquake, with a depth of 10 km, was near the city of Bam, which was located 180 km southeast of the provincial capital of Kerman and 975 km southeast of Tehran. The Iranian government estimated the deaths from the earthquake at 41,000, with some figures exceeding 50,000. More than 10,000 survivors were injured. Children and adolescents who were close to the epicenter were vulnerable to deficits in cognition and attention, social skills, personality style, self-concept and self-esteem, and impulse control. This had impacts on the formation of stable attachments, acquisition of affect regulation, development and integration of self-concepts, and socialization. In this context, CBT proved to be very helpful.

CBT may involve various components, including psychological debriefing, managing intrusions (e.g., with thought stopping), addressing avoidance, reducing hyperarousal, and cognitive interventions. The debriefing addresses the purpose of the meeting and involves listening to the concrete experience of the patient, reviewing early thoughts and sensory experiences, examining reactions, and normalization. When addressing intrusions, it is helpful to normalize this phenomenon to the group. After making a list of traumatic events and reminders so they can be brought to conscious awareness, it is helpful to help the patient find a safe place in imagination. Imagery techniques include 1) imagining the image as if it were on a television, 2) imagining the image as if it were on the therapist's or patient's hand, 2) putting a frame around the image and replacing the image with a positive image within that same frame, 3) looking away from the image, and 4) having imaginary helpers.

Touch and movement can also contribute to therapeutic effects. In addition, a step derived from EMDR can be added. This involves deliberately recalling the traumatic image with the eyes open while simultaneously tracking with the eyes the side-to-side rhythmical movement of the therapist's hand. Dream restructuring and rehearsal relief and homework can also help address intrusions.

To address avoidance, homework review and the discussion of good and bad avoidance can be helpful. Imaginal exposure, drawing, writing, and talking can all be used in a graded manner to face the situations that are being avoided. For hyperarousal, making a distinction between being scared and simply experiencing bodily sensations can be helpful. In addition, muscle relaxation, breath control, positive self-statements, and sleep hygiene can all help. For the cognitive components, normalizing traumatic events and reactions, psychoeducation, and becoming aware of traumatic reminders can all facilitate recovery.

With CBT, patients are encouraged to express themselves, to interact with peers and families, and to seek support from their families whenever they are distressed. One study found that coping skills treatment such as systematic desensitization and implosive therapy, an exposure-based treatment, was similarly effective in reducing the frequency and intensity of intrusions and avoidance.

Trauma-Focused CBT

TF-CBT has been shown to be effective in disasters (O'Callaghan et al. 2013) and typically includes both behavioral techniques, such as exposure, and cognitive techniques, such as cognitive restructuring or reappraisal. CBT that includes exposure to the traumatic memory uses imagery, written narratives about the trauma, or reading the traumatic memory out loud. CBT that includes exposure to trauma-related stimuli typically uses in vivo exposure (directly facing a feared object or situation) or teaching patients to identify triggers of reexperiencing and distinguishing between the past and present. Cognitive restructuring focuses on teaching patients to identify dysfunctional thoughts and thinking errors; elicit rational alternative thoughts; and reappraise beliefs about themselves, the trauma, and the world. The steps in this therapy are defined by the mnemonic PRACTICE: Psychoeducation/parenting, Relaxation, Affective expression and modulation, Cognitive coping, Trauma narration and processing, In vivo mastery, Conjoint sessions, and Enhancing future safety and development.

Although these earlier studies were promising, the treatment efficacy of CBT has come into question over the years. For example, a recent review (Gimigliano et al. 2022) concluded that there is uncertainty about whether behavioral interventions are effective in reducing PTSD symptoms and improving functioning and quality of life when the disorder is triggered by a physical or medical trauma rather than a psychological trauma. Therefore, in the context of a disaster, the specific type of trauma might sway one toward or away from CBT.

Therapist misconceptions include the following erroneous beliefs (Murray et al. 2022):

1. TF-CBT does not work for complex trauma.
2. Stabilization is always needed before memory work.
3. Talking about trauma memories is retraumatizing.
4. Some traumas should not be relived.
5. TF-CBT is a talking therapy (in fact, it involves a lot of doing).
6. PTSD cannot be treated remotely.
7. Dissociation makes working on trauma memories impossible.

8. PTSD is about fear (in fact, it is about the full range of negative emotions that can occur during and after traumatic events, including guilt, shame, anger, humiliation, betrayal, disgust, helplessness, hopelessness, and horror).
9. Exposure always needs to be graded.
10. Cognitive therapy for PTSD must be strictly manualized.

However, other evidence suggests that some of these apparent misconceptions may in fact be true. For example, retraumatization has been linked to hypersensitivity to threats to safety, exposure to triggers, posttraumatic stress reactions, and avoidant coping. As with many instances in psychotherapy, there is a delicate balance that must be considered when one is weighing having someone being triggered by talking about a trauma versus not promoting avoidant coping. It is also important to note that there is no evidence that single-session individual psychological debriefing is a useful treatment for the prevention of PTSD after traumatic incidents.

Eye Movement Desensitization and Reprocessing

A review article evaluating EMDR as a group protocol indicated positive effects on 236 children with PTSD following an Italian plane crash (Fernandez et al. 2004). Two other studies served to further the scientific community's understanding of the effects of EMDR among survivors of natural disasters. The first review article (Jarero et al. 2014) showed the positive effects of EMDR as a group protocol among children following a Mexican flood, and the second highlighted the efficacy of EMDR as an individual treatment among 1,500 adult earthquake survivors in Turkey (Konuk et al. 2006).

During a traumatic memory, EMDR uses bilateral stimulation that can occur in a variety of forms, including left-right eye movements, tapping on the knees, headphones, or handheld buzzers known as tappers. It also engages a person in imaginal exposure to trauma while simultaneously performing this stimulation such that patients are required to divide their attention between bilateral stimulation and the retrieval of traumatic memories. The eight steps of EMDR are 1) patient history, 2) preparation, 3) assessment, 4) desensitization, 5) installation, 6) body scan, 7) debriefing and enclosure, and 8) reevaluation.

Family Therapy

The trauma experienced by any given individual also reverberates throughout the family. For family therapies, the existing evidence base suffers from methodological limitations such as small sample sizes and heterogeneous populations. Nevertheless, there is preliminary evidence that family interventions that focus on parenting, multifamily groups, and school-based approaches can be helpful in the disaster setting. The fundamental challenges that families face usually revolve around family relations, interactions, boundaries, and rules.

For example, in the context of a disaster where one parent is lost, a child may be expected to fulfill the roles of the lost parent. Highlighting the nuances around this expectation would be helpful. The responses to a traumatic event may be different among family members, with one person experiencing PTSD and another posttraumatic growth. Highlighting these differences and the implications for relationships may help all individuals in the family cope with their distress, guilt, and interpersonal conflicts. In addition, processing grief together can assist a family in the postdisaster healing process.

Group Therapy

Psychotherapy for PTSD, as well as psychosocial support for stressed and traumatized health care workers and responders, can also be delivered in a group format, either in person, in a videoconferencing format, or via telephone. Crisis intervention psychotherapy is an underutilized form of therapy that may be especially useful during the age of coronavirus disease 2019 (COVID-19). It is a problem-solving, solution-focused, trauma-informed treatment using an individual or systemic/family-centered approach and is delivered as a companion or follow-up to PFA.

From a theoretical point of view, the conceptualization of PTSD as a special case of "unfinished business" posits Gestalt therapy as a treatment of choice for this syndrome. Gestalt therapy offers unique mechanisms for surfacing trauma-related conflicts from the past and solving them in the present through attending to the here and now, body movements and nonverbal behavior, and retelling the traumatic event as if it were happening in the present. It uses fantasy and visualization, the creative enhancement of body language, two-chair and empty chair work, graded experiments, and psychodrama and enactments. However, despite the assets of Gestalt therapy, not much exists in the literature on the utility of this therapy for treating PTSD (Cohen 2003).

Group interventions help reach a larger number of people with a limited number of mental health professionals and can offer additional healing elements that individual approaches do not, including sharing experiences in a peer setting, consensual validation, support and learning from peers, and building a sense of solidarity and camaraderie with fellow group members. The University Hospital of Brooklyn Psychiatry Department developed peer support groups for physicians, resident physicians, and nursing staff via videoconferencing and telephone focusing on issues and emotions related to their frontline clinical work with COVID-19 patients in a medical center that was designated as a COVID-only hospital by the state. Support groups were offered even though group intervention in this area had not been described in detail in the literature at the time of the study (Viswanathan et al. 2020).

In this study, participants said that four to seven weekly groups was the number that seemed to be most helpful. The researchers reported that groups work best if one member of the clinical service takes responsibility for organizing the weekly video conference or teleconference and serves as the group's liaison with the group facilitators. Other important factors include allowing participants to attend with audio only or to listen without verbal participation and offering groups at different periods of the day and evening to accommodate varying work schedules. It is important that employers give employees time to participate in groups such as these.

The 9/11 terrorist attacks in 2001 affected first responders and law enforcement profoundly; many members of the New York City Police Department, Fire Department of New York, Port Authority Police Department, and emergency medical services found themselves experiencing multiple bereavements simultaneously, and a substantial proportion were acutely traumatized. The adjustment from body recovery to a desk job was very difficult for those sidelined because of injury. Others refused to acknowledge PTSD and kept working or volunteering. The culture of law enforcement does not encourage emotional expression, but group therapy was offered on a voluntary basis for anyone who felt like attending. Groups were open, and bereavement support was acceptable to many, sometimes with involvement of clergy for pastoral counseling. The offerings in psychosocial and mental health support also included group debrief support.

Groups were also facilitated to focus on others, discussing how to speak to children whose parents had died, organizing group recreational events for children of all ages, and offering practical and emotional support for widows and their children. At these events, the subject of how to help children's grief and distress and the communal shared shock allowed 9/11 first responders to acknowledge, express, and find words for their own feelings while allowing them to actively help others. Psychotherapy contact cards with referrals inside the department or with trusted providers known to the departments were always on offer, and patients referred themselves. Group supervision for therapists was essential. Alcoholics Anonymous meetings were also added for responders; these meetings were closed to the public because the gruesome details of body recovery were too much for civilian groups. When the 9/11 substance abuse and mental illness program was started, many responders self-referred to individual therapists who were themselves supported by group therapy and supervision.

Pandemic-Related Therapies

Computerized CBT (Liu et al. 2021) is an online self-help intervention delivered over 1 week. The primary goal is to reduce acute psychological distress and symptoms of depression, anxiety, and insomnia in adults. Three modules cover cognitive training, cognitive consolidation, and behavioral interventions. The intervention was tested in a randomized controlled trial during the COVID-19 pandemic in China with 252 adults with COVID-19. Participants were given psychological assessments, psychological support, and consultations about well-being and COVID-19. A significant decrease in depressive and anxiety symptoms was found at 1-month follow-up in the computerized CBT plus treatment as usual (TAU) group compared with a TAU-only group.

The Individualized Short-Term Training Program (Zhou et al. 2020) is a self-help program combined with psychological support to reduce depression and anxiety symptoms in emergency nurses during the COVID-19 pandemic. The intervention covers education and mindfulness-based stress reduction. Psychologists provide online and practical face-to-face training and psychological support to nursing staff. The self-help online training is delivered asynchronously through videos, graphics, and texts so that the support does not rely entirely on the availability of nurses. In an uncontrolled study, the authors of the intervention evaluated the impact of the program on 71 female Chinese nurses working in an emergency isolation department during the COVID-19 pandemic. Significant posttraining reduction was found in anxiety but not in depression.

Online Psychotherapy Tool (OPTT) is a 9-week program that was designed to reduce mental health problems in adults during the COVID-19 pandemic. OPTT includes a self-help module and psychotherapeutic support, with the main focus on self-help. The intervention combines CBT, mindfulness therapy, and problem-based therapy. No study results have been reported yet.

My Health Too (Bureau et al. 2021) is a seven-session CBT-based online self-help program with an option for psychotherapeutic support (i.e., the possibility of calling a CBT-trained psychologist). The program was designed for health care workers to reduce psychological distress during the COVID-19 pandemic and to prevent long-term consequences from the pandemic. It involves a total of seven 20-minute asynchronous video sessions covering psychoeducation on stressors, adaptive behavioral and cognitive coping strategies, mindfulness and acceptance of stressors, promoting action toward values, addressing barriers and motivation, and self-compassion. No results have been published to date.

Climate Change

Anxiety about climate change, sometimes part of eco-anxiety, is defined broadly as negative cognitive, emotional, and behavioral responses associated with concerns about climate change. It can be associated with generalized anxiety disorder and major depressive disorder. One review of treatments for eco-anxiety identified five major themes: practitioners' inner work and education, fostering patients' inner resilience, encouraging patients to act, helping patients find social connection and emotional support by joining groups, and connecting patients with nature.

Conclusion

In the context of disasters, psychotherapies are often supportive, brief, and focused on resilience and reintegration into the community. There are a variety of evidence-based approaches from which to choose but no one-size-fits-all approach.

References

American Psychiatric Association: Diagnostic and Statistical Manual of Mental Disorders, 5th Edition, Text Revision. Washington, DC, American Psychiatric Association, 2022

Bureau R, Bemmouna D, Faria CGF, et al: My Health Too: investigating the feasibility and the acceptability of an internet-based cognitive-behavioral therapy program developed for healthcare workers. Front Psychol 12:760678, 2021 34925163

Burkhart K, Agarwal N, Kim S, et al: A scoping review of trauma-informed pediatric interventions in response to natural and biologic disasters. Children (Basel) 10(6):1017, 2023 37371249

Cohen A: Gestalt therapy and post-traumatic stress disorder: the irony and the challenge. Gestalt Review 7(1):42, 2003

Fernandez I, Gallinari E, Lorenzetti A: A school-based EMDR intervention for children who witnessed the Pirelli Building airplane crash in Milan, Italy. J Brief Ther 2(2):129–136, 2004

Gimigliano F, Young VM, Arienti C, et al: The effectiveness of behavioral interventions in adults with post-traumatic stress disorder during clinical rehabilitation: a rapid review. Int J Environ Res Public Health 19(12):7514, 2022 35742762

Jarero I, Artigas L, Uribe S, Miranda A: EMDR therapy humanitarian trauma recovery interventions in Latin America and the Caribbean. J. EMDR Pract Res 8(4):260–268, 2014

Johnson J, Pointon L, Keyworth C, et al: Evaluation of a training programme for critical incident debrief facilitators. Occup Med (Lond) 73(2):103–108, 2023 36516291

Knobler HY, Nachshoni T, Jaffe E, et al: Psychological guidelines for a medical team debriefing after a stressful event. Mil Med 172(6):581–585, 2007 17615836

Konuk E, Knipe J, Eke I, et al: The effects of eye movement desensitization and reprocessing (EMDR) therapy on posttraumatic stress disorder in survivors of the 1999 Marmara, Turkey, earthquake Int J Stress Manag 13(3):291–308, 2006

Lindemann E: Symptomatology and management of acute grief. 1944. Am J Psychiatry 151(6 Suppl):155–190, 1994 8192191

Liu Z, Qiao D, Xu Y, et al: The efficacy of computerized cognitive behavioral therapy for depressive and anxiety symptoms in patients with COVID-19: randomized controlled trial. J Med Internet Res 23(5):e26883, 2021 33900931

Lotzin A, Franc de Pommereau A, Laskowsky I: Promoting recovery from disasters, pandemics, and trauma: a systematic review of brief psychological interventions to reduce distress in adults, children, and adolescents. Int J Environ Res Public Health 20(7):5339, 2023 37047954

Murray H, Grey N, Warnock-Parkes E, et al: Ten misconceptions about trauma-focused CBT for PTSD. Cogn Behav Therap 15:s1754470x22000307, 2022 36247408

National Institute for Health and Care Excellence: Post-traumatic stress disorder. National Institute for Health and Care Excellence, 2018. Available at: www.nice.org.uk/guidance/ng116/resources/posttraumatic-stress-disorder-pdf-66141601777861. Accessed July 4, 2024.

Norris FH, Friedman MJ, Watson PJ, et al: 60,000 disaster victims speak part I: an empirical review of the empirical literature, 1981–2001. Psychiatry 65(3):207–239, 2002 12405079

O'Callaghan P, McMullen J, Shannon C, et al: A randomized controlled trial of trauma-focused cognitive behavioral therapy for sexually exploited, war-affected Congolese girls. J Am Acad Child Adolesc Psychiatry 52(4):359–369, 2013 23582867

O'Toole M, Eppich W: In support of appropriate psychological debriefing. Med Educ 56(2):229, 2022 34541708

Qouta SR, Palosaari E, Diab M, et al: Intervention effectiveness among war-affected children: a cluster randomized controlled trial on improving mental health. J Trauma Stress 25(3):288–298, 2012 22648703

Richins MT, Gauntlett L, Tehrani N, et al: Early post-trauma interventions in organizations: a scoping review. Front Psychol 11:1176, 2020 32670143

Roberts NP, Kitchiner NJ, Kenardy J, et al: Multiple session early psychological interventions for the prevention of post-traumatic stress disorder. Cochrane Database Syst Rev 3(3):CD006869, 2009 19588408

Rose S, Bisson J, Churchill R, et al: Psychological debriefing for preventing post traumatic stress disorder (PTSD). Cochrane Database Syst Rev 2(2):CD000560, 2002 12076399

Semerci M, Uzun S: The effectiveness of post-disaster psychotherapeutic interventions: a systematic review and meta-analysis study. Asian J Psychiatr 85:103615, 2023 37201380

Shooshtary MH, Panaghi L, Moghadam JA: Outcome of cognitive behavioral therapy in adolescents after natural disaster. J Adolesc Health 42(5):466–472, 2008 18407041

Snider L, Schafer A, Ommeren M: Psychological First Aid: Guide for Field Workers. Geneva, Switzerland, World Health Organization, 2011

Stoddard FJ, Katz CK, Merlino JP: Hidden Impact: What You Need To Know For The Next Disaster: A Practical Mental Health Guide For Clinicians. Group for the Advancement of Psychiatry. Sudbury, MA, Jones & Bartlett, 2009

Tamrakar T, Murphy J, Elklit A: Was psychological debriefing dismissed too quickly? Crisis, stress, and human resilience. Int J 1(3):146–155, 2019

Vignaud P, Lavallé L, Brunelin J, et al: Are psychological debriefing groups after a potential traumatic event suitable to prevent the symptoms of PTSD? Psychiatry Res 311:114503, 2022 35287042

Viswanathan R, Myers MF, Fanus AH: Support groups and individual mental health care via video conferencing for frontline clinicians during the COVID-19 pandemic. Psychosomatics 61:538–543, 2020 32660876

Zhou M, Yuan F, Zhao X, et al: Research on the individualized short-term training model of nurses in emergency isolation wards during the outbreak of COVID-19. Nurs Open 7(6):1902–1908, 2020 33346408

18

Psychopharmacology

Considerations in the Acute and Postacute Disaster Settings

Kristina Jones, M.D.
Kathleen A. Clegg, M.D.

In this chapter, we address acute and postacute psychopharmacological interventions in the hours and days after a disaster. Psychological interventions are first line. A limited number of patients will need treatment for anxiety and insomnia. A still smaller group will require intervention for agitation, irritability, alcohol withdrawal, or delirium. Frontline nursing, medical, and other responders can be supported by psychiatry in both triage and acute treatment. Acute anxiety, insomnia, and agitation are not diagnoses in themselves, but individuals with these symptoms need safe treatments. Acute stress disorder, which is sometimes but not always a predictor of posttraumatic stress disorder (PTSD), has clear expert guidelines; we summarize them near the end of the chapter.

In acute disaster care, psychopharmacological treatment is targeted at specific symptoms rather than efforts to diagnose and treat a disorder. Symptom control rather than identification of syndromes is the goal. Insomnia and anxiety are the most common presentations, followed by panic attack, behavioral dyscontrol, and substance intoxication or withdrawal. Irritability and agitation, as well as hyperactive or hypoactive delirium in the setting of disaster-related medical problems, are less frequent but are behavioral emergencies in which the psychiatrist adds real value to the care of patients presenting in the first hours, days, and weeks after a disaster event.

Similarities Between Disaster Psychiatry and Emergency Psychiatry

The psychiatrist in the acute disaster setting is challenged by a scarcity of evidence for many psychopharmacological interventions from randomized controlled trials. Because the evidence base for psychopharmacological interventions in the acute disaster setting is limited, medications are usually prescribed only on a short-term basis. Disaster psychiatry most resembles emergency psychiatry, with some modifications. Despite the lack of medications specifically approved by the FDA for acute stress disorder, most psychiatric medications used are familiar from emergency psychiatry practice. Medication choices are not the same as those that might be used on an inpatient psychiatric unit. Nurse practitioners, physician assistants, and primary care physicians are familiar with this small list of medications, and most disaster psychiatric interventions are provided by frontline professionals in those roles.

Exacerbation of Psychiatric Illness

Patients with preexisting psychiatric illness often decompensate during disasters. The psychiatrist plays an important role in recognizing and treating recurrence or intensification of major depressive disorders in patients who present with suicidal ideation or attempts or nonsuicidal self-injury. Psychiatry brings the expertise necessary for treating exacerbations of schizophrenia and bipolar disorder and for intervening in relapse of substance use disorders in the context of the extreme stressors that are the hallmark of disaster events.

Psychiatric Triage in the Emergency Department

The psychiatrist is also of great value in assisting the medical teams with immediate postdisaster arrivals to the emergency department (ED). These patients may be in shock, numb, or detached, or they may be distressed or agitated to the point where they may be reluctant to accept an initial medical evaluation. Psychiatrists in the disaster setting can further be called on for capacity evaluations when acute psychiatric symptoms cause patients to refuse medically necessary care.

Symptoms and Safety

The overall goal is to assess for safety and address the immediate symptoms that emerge in the hours and days after the disaster event and to focus treatment on just those symptoms that are impairing patient functioning. For example, a patient whose anxiety is so overwhelming that they cannot secure basic needs such as food, access emergency aid from social services, or contact their workplace will benefit from brief treatment with medication so that they can begin the behavioral tasks involved in stabilization and early recovery from disaster events.

Assisted Evaluations and Triage

An observant psychiatrist can distinguish emotional distress from thought disorganization and distinguish an emotionally shocked patient from one having periods of dissociation. Patients with recent concussion and brief loss of consciousness can just seem "very upset." The psychiatrist can perform an evaluation for disorientation to person, place, and time and for the fluctuating levels of awareness that are the hallmark of early delirium or concussion and will warrant keeping the patient for observation overnight.

Emergency staff who are used to taking detailed histories need to know that it is not necessarily a requirement to take the whole trauma history that traumatized patients usually want to give just hours after the event. Although it is important for the patient to give their full personal narrative later with a therapist, the ED is not the optimal setting or timing. The kind, polite, yet skillful interruption of the patient's narrative is an art we can show our medical colleagues. For example, saying to the patient, "You have a lot more to this story that is important, but I'm going to switch topics now and make sure you are safe. For right now we need to know: Are you suicidal? Do you usually take a medicine you don't have access to? Are you able to drink water? Can we help you reach your family members? Can you problem-solve for what you will do to get help in the next few hours or days?"

To Treat or Not to Treat

During the first few hours and days after a traumatic event, the primary clinical goal is to reduce the patient's terror and decrease neuronal imprinting of horrific events. The aim is to reduce symptom burden and increase functioning. Psychopharmacology should not be applied indiscriminately or without other interventions. Psychopharmacology is less effective than psychological treatments for acute stress disorder. The expert guidelines detailed below recommend psychopharmacology as secondary to psychological interventions. Psychopharmacology should never be used as first-line treatment except when psychological interventions are unavailable or when symptoms are so severe that psychological treatments cannot be tolerated.

What to Prescribe Depends on When

Prior to September 11, 2001, there was prejudice against use of psychotropic medication at the time of an acute trauma because of concern that it might adversely affect a person's psychological processing of the event. This view has been replaced by a call for more research and by international expert guidelines developed for safe use of rapid psychopharmacological intervention in the disaster setting. There is an absence of evidence of harm(s) regarding psychopharmacology in the acute setting. Ethically, it would not be acceptable to randomly assign patients presenting with psychiatric symptoms in a disaster to placebo, so it has been difficult to obtain the type of evidence that exists for other psychiatric disorders. The evidence is often moderate or of poor quality, has small sample sizes, and describes how much a given medication reduces Clinician-Administered PTSD Scale (CAPS) scores or scores on other PTSD rating instruments. An important caveat here: medication should be deployed only if necessary, and only *after* the psychological armamentarium of interventions that are the more effective and appropriate response.

Pharmacological Interventions in Trauma- and Stressor-Related Disorders

The major clinical situations the disaster psychiatrist confronts are acute stress reactions, acute stress disorder, PTSD, symptoms not otherwise specified, and high-risk medical situations.

Acute Stress Reactions

An *acute stress reaction* is defined as a transient normal reaction to traumatic stress within minutes, hours, or the first few days after the trauma. This is not a DSM-5-TR (American Psychiatric Association 2022) diagnosis, although symptoms may be temporarily debilitating. In most cases, medication is not required; symptoms resolve rapidly by ensuring safety and offering Psychological First Aid.

Acute Stress Disorder

Acute stress disorder is a diagnosis defined by DSM-5-TR that may occur after directly experiencing a disaster situation. To meet criteria (Table 18–1), symptoms must last for at least 3 days and persist for 4 weeks after exposure to the traumatic event. It is important to note that patients do not have to meet full criteria to benefit from treatment; treating the core symptoms of fear, extreme anxiety, and insomnia is a key part of disaster psychiatry.

Psychopharmacological Interventions for Anxiety and Insomnia

Anxiety, including panic symptoms, can be effectively reduced with low-dose benzodiazepines. "Z" medications, including Zolpidem and Zaleplon, are not recommended because studies show they are not effective. Intervention for anxiety should include a prescription of 1week's supply or less to avoid tolerance and dependence and to minimize risk of overdose. Medication should be coprescribed with psychological treatments. Psychopharmacological interventions for anxiety and insomnia are presented in Table 18–2.

Side Effects, Risks, and Medication Interactions

Sedation and dizziness are the most common side effects of benzodiazepines. Significant medication interactions occur with other CNS-sedating agents, most importantly narcotics; never prescribe benzodiazepines in patients taking narcotics or receiving opioid addiction treatments such as methadone or buprenorphine (see Chapter 12, "Adult Psychiatric Evaluation"). In a few individuals, including those with traumatic brain injury, disinhibited behavior can occur. Caution must be used in older adults, who may experience increased CNS effects; in patients with substance abuse (especially alcohol); and in patients with a history of dementia.

Clinical evidence suggests that after 21 days, patients can become dependent and withdrawal may occur, with rebound insomnia and anxiety. Patients should use medication first for a few nights, then taper if anxiety improves for use only on an as-needed basis. Patient reports after 2–3 weeks that benzodiazepines have "stopped working" and requests for higher doses should trigger a referral for full psychiatric evaluation for a selective serotonin reuptake inhibitor or other pharmacotherapy.

TABLE 18–1. Summary of DSM-5-TR criteria for acute stress disorder

Criterion A: Being exposed to a traumatic event (either physically, sexually, or mentally) plus

Criterion B: Having more than eight of the following symptoms (clustered in five categories)

Intrusion symptoms

- Recurrent distressing memories of the traumatic event (children may have repetitive game plays in themes mimicking the main event)
- Repetitive dreams related to the traumatic event (in children, may be in the form of night terrors)
- Enactment of the traumatic event recurrence (i.e., flashbacks)
- Intense or prolonged mental or psychological distress in response to the events or themes reminding the patient of the actual traumatic event

Negative mood (numbing)

- Inability to be happy, feel successful, or feel love

Dissociative symptoms

- Having a sense of being detached from self and emotions
- Dissociative amnesia that is not related to intoxication or traumatic brain injury (TBI)

Avoidance symptoms

- Avoidance of thoughts, memories, and feelings about the traumatic event
- Avoidance of external reminders of the traumatic event

Arousal symptoms

- Sleep problems (e.g., difficulty initiating and maintaining quality sleep)
- Irritability and rage attacks with minimum to no provocation
- Highly and abnormally alert to surroundings
- Distractibility
- Unusually strong reflexive reaction to a sudden event in the environment

Criteria C, D, and E: Duration of the symptoms should be between 3 days and 4 weeks and cause significant functional impairment. They should not be related to substance use or other medical conditions (such as TBI).

Source. Adapted from American Psychiatric Association: *Diagnostic and Statistical Manual of Mental Disorders*, 5th Edition, Text Revision. Washington, DC, American Psychiatric Association, 2022. Copyright © 2022 American Psychiatric Association. Used with permission.

TABLE 18–2. Psychopharmacological interventions for anxiety and insomnia in the acute disaster setting

Medication	Dosage	Cautions
Benzodiazepines		
Lorazepam[a]	0.5 mg PO qhs; can also be used two or three times daily, to a maximum of 0.5–2.0 mg/day for patients who are benzodiazepine naive	Never prescribe more than a patient could take all at once without harm (e.g., 5–10 days); never prescribe 30 days' supply
Clonazepam[a]	0.5 mg PO qhs or bid for 7–14 days only; can also be used two or three times daily to a maximum of 2–4 mg/day	
Alternatives to benzodiazepines		
Diphenhydramine[a]	25–50 mg qhs or bid	
Hydroxyzine[a]	10–50 mg qhs	
Trazodone[a]	25–50 mg	Priapism, hypotension at higher doses[b], long half-life
Mirtazapine[a]	7.5–15 mg	May lower blood pressure, sedation
Melatonin[a,c]	2–5 mg	Generally more effective for jet lag or circadian rhythm disruptions, with period of days or weeks to take effect

[a]Use of this medication for anxiety or insomnia has not been evaluated by the FDA.
[b]Trazodone is an antidepressant only in the 400-mg range, where hypotension is common.
[c]New studies suggest that melatonin is highly effective for use in coronavirus disease 2019 (COVID-19) delirium in preference to benzodiazepines.

Posttraumatic Stress Disorder

Posttraumatic stress disorder is similar to acute stress disorder but persists at least 1 month after the exposure to the traumatic event. An important aspect of disaster psychiatry presentations of PTSD is to address negative alterations in mood and behavior. This may include more "fight" than "flight" as well as exacerbation of coexisting psychiatric disorders, most commonly comorbid major depressive disorder and alcohol use disorder.

Symptoms Not Otherwise Specified

Symptoms not otherwise specified are symptoms that do not meet diagnostic criteria but are serious enough to warrant intervention, most commonly insomnia and extreme anxiety. Other important but less common symptoms are agitation, behavioral dysregulation, worsening of preexisting psychotic disorders, exacerbations of mood disorders (including suicidal ideation), and emergent hypomania.

Medical Workup

Although less common than other symptoms, agitation can be seen in the acute phase of disaster. Agitated patients warrant a psychiatric referral for evaluation because they may have an underlying mental illness, substance use disorder, or other disorder. Agitation may be a harbinger of PTSD. For any patient presenting with agitation, a history must be obtained regarding recent alcohol or substance abuse, and appropriate urine or blood drug screens (blood alcohol level, urine screen for drug toxicology) should be performed. A CT or MRI scan is indicated in any patient with a history of head injury, loss of consciousness, or skull trauma or with complex underlying medical problems, such as cancer.

Psychopharmacological Interventions for Agitation

Agitation is managed in the same way as any acute ED presentation if the survivor is dangerous, extremely agitated, or psychotic. Psychopharmacological interventions for agitation are presented in Table 18–3.

Side Effects, Risks, and Medication Interactions

Sedation and dizziness are the most common side effects of medications for agitation. Haloperidol can cause dystonic reactions in vulnerable patients. Young male patients, patients who are neuroleptic naive, patients with mood disorder histories, and older adults require close monitoring for dystonic reactions. Giving 50 mg diphenhydramine in combination with haloperidol and lorazepam is a precautionary measure against dystonic reactions. For a longer duration of antiparkinsonian action, 2 mg benztropine mesylate may be prescribed instead.

Caution must be used in older adults, who should receive the lowest doses less frequently. Benzodiazepines must be given with great caution in older adults because of the risk of falls and hip fractures and hypotension.

TABLE 18–3. Psychopharmacological interventions for agitation in the acute disaster setting

Medications for use in the emergency department	Dose ranges per 24 hours
Haloperidol	0.5–2.0 mg PO or IM q 4 hours with an antiparkinsonian agent
Lorazepam	1–2 mg PO or IM q 4 hours; never use if patient is intoxicated
Diphenhydramine	50 mg PO or IM q 4 hours if there is concern for dystonic reactions
Quetiapine[a]	25–100 mg

[a]Use of this medication for agitation has not been evaluated by the FDA.

Close monitoring and observation by nursing or emergency department staff is important.

Medication interactions of concern include any medication with CNS sedation as a risk, including benzodiazepines, narcotics, mood stabilizers, antiseizure medications, and other antipsychotics. In patients for whom a benzodiazepine is contraindicated, very-low-dose atypical antipsychotics can be used to control agitation or extreme anxiety. All antipsychotic medications include a black box warning not to use them with patients who have dementia because of the risk of cardiovascular accident. In at-risk patients, an electrocardiogram (ECG) is advised if possible. Antipsychotic and other medications may cause QTc prolongation and cardiac complications (Funk et al. 2020). If QTc is >450 msec, avoid antipsychotic agents. Additionally, documentation should be provided clarifying why conventional approaches to agitation (including benzodiazepines or diphenhydramine) are not indicated or that they have been tried but found ineffective.

Quetiapine may be an appropriate agent to consider for off-label use instead of a benzodiazepine when the patient is anxious or agitated or has insomnia and when a benzodiazepine has been ineffective or is not appropriate. For example, quetiapine is useful in patients with substance use disorder; during cocaine or amphetamine intoxication; in patients who are taking methadone, where a benzodiazepine risks respiratory depression; or in patients with prior brain injury. An ECG is recommended for patients with preexisting cardiac disease or known conduction disorders. Do not give quetiapine if QTc is >450 msec.

Earlier small observational studies suggested that low-dose risperidone was effective for hyperarousal in the setting of traumatic stress in burn unit patients (Stoddard et al. 2017). This recommendation has been replaced by use of quetiapine, a relatively recent inclusion in expert guidelines (Crapanzano et al. 2023). Off-label use of this medication for insomnia and anxiety is not supported by data but is very common in clinical settings.

High-Risk Medical Situations

High-risk medical situations are those such as serious medical trauma, including burns, traumatic amputation, fractures, crush injuries, and *all* patients whose symptoms meet the DSM-5-TR criteria for delirium during emergency medical intervention and stabilization. Research shows that physical injury is a huge risk factor for acute stress disorder and PTSD. Intervention may not prevent PTSD from developing, but overlooking the medically injured who are at increased risk for all the above symptoms and disorders is a serious oversight. Delirium itself is a risk factor for PTSD (Breitbart et al. 1996). It is important to work with consultation-liaison colleagues and collaborate with internal medicine and emergency physicians and teams to give psychiatric recommendations when requested and to assure that patients with preexisting psychiatric illness receive appropriate medications. Clinicians should also be on alert for alcohol withdrawal.

Brief Guide to the Guidelines

The American Psychiatric Association's (APA) Guidelines for PTSD revised in 2009 are legacy guidelines and are no longer current (Benedek et al. 2009). Neuroimaging, neurobiology, novel psychopharmacological agents, and disaster psychiatry intervention and outcome research are published in APA journals. At the APA Annual Meetings, disaster psychiatry response successes and disappointments are discussed, and the proceedings are published, with subjects including current disaster psychiatry responses to mass shootings; the coronavirus disease 2019 (COVID-19) pandemic mental health crisis; and climate disasters, particularly the devastating 2021 wildfires in the southwestern United States. Federal agencies such as the military, state resources such as the National Guard, and other state and city response agency personnel actively involved in recent disasters are often at APA meetings to review lessons learned from responses to, for example, mass shootings, environmental disasters, and terror attacks.

Summary of Evidence-Based Guidelines

The most well-researched and updated PTSD treatment guideline is the U.S. Department of Veterans Affairs and U.S. Department of Defense (VA/DoD) clinical practice guidelines, last revised in 2023 (U.S. Department of

Veterans Affairs and U.S. Department of Defense 2023). These guidelines were developed largely for combat and noncombat PTSD and include recommendations for complex PTSD. Additionally, the International Society for Traumatic Stress Studies (2021) has published guidelines that cover psychiatry and psychology. In the United Kingdom, the National Institute for Health and Care Excellence (2018), which independently advises the National Health Service, has published evidence-based streamlined guidelines for primary care physicians and psychiatrists (Forbes et al. 2020). Because these guidelines did not address monitoring and follow-up, another U.K. country, Wales, developed the Cardiff Protocol (Dekker et al. 2019) to help primary care, psychiatry, and disaster response agencies employ guidelines with more safety. Additionally, the American Psychological Association guidelines cover psychological therapies at length and endorse selective serotonin reuptake inhibitors (SSRIs), although only as second line to brief trauma-focused psychotherapy. The recommendations from these national and international expert bodies and professional organizations are summarized in Table 18–4. They are used by the American Red Cross, the World Health Organization, and many humanitarian aid agencies deployed in disaster settings (Bajor et al. 2022).

Guidelines Through the Health Inequity Lens

Guidelines by professional bodies represent expert opinion and best practices. However, populations that can enroll in studies are generally not the ones who are most at risk for psychiatric injury and morbidity after disasters. Importantly, recent critiques and meta-analyses of the guideline development process note that most of the existing guidelines fail to consider intersectionality. Specifically, the problem is that study design favors therapy and ignores issues of inequities in access (Bryant-Davis 2019). Loss of shelter, food insecurity, and poverty disproportionally affect vulnerable people. There is a call for more applicability to real-world patients, more stakeholder involvement, and more rigorous methodology to address this inequity (Martin et al. 2021).

Strategic Summary

Strategic prescribing involves calculating the time from the patient's exposure to the disaster event to the time the patient presents for care. Psychotherapy should be the first-line treatment. Benzodiazepines should be limited to the first month. Trazodone, mirtazapine, melatonin, and diphenhydramine can be used for insomnia. Acute use of antipsychotics after the event should be avoided. If the patient is not functioning after the first month, consider an SSRI or mirtazapine. Do not prescribe a sero-

TABLE 18–4. Summary of psychopharmacology from guidelines for acute stress disorder and PTSD

Medication	Notes and recommendations	Guideline
Medications for acute stress disorder		
Benzodiazepines[a]	No FDA-approved psychopharmacological agents	
	Very brief (7-day) prescription reasonable for sleep	
Trazodone[a]	Reasonable for sleep	
Diphenhydramine[a]	Reasonable for sleep	
Medications not supported by current expert guidelines		
Propranolol	Used off-label for anxiety but has not been shown to prevent PTSD	
Hydrocortisone	No effect outside the medically ill	
Morphine	No longer considered protective after Iraq *New England Journal of Medicine* finding not replicated	
Medications for PTSD		
Paroxetine	FDA approved	
Sertraline	FDA approved	
Fluoxetine[a]	Expert guideline evidence available	
SSRIs	*Not* appropriate for adolescents or young adults because of the small but serious risk of developing new-onset suicidal ideation	

TABLE 18–4. Summary of psychopharmacology from guidelines for acute stress disorder and PTSD *(continued)*

Medication	Notes and recommendations	Guideline
New recommendations		
Venlafaxine[a]	Slight advantage over selective serotonin reuptake inhibitors (Shiner et al. 2020)	VA/DoD
	Cautions: discontinuation syndrome (mild shock-like "brain zaps" sensation, dizziness, headache, vertigo); serotonin-norepinephrine reuptake inhibitors associated with hyponatremia in older adults	Cardiff
PTSD augmentation: expert guidelines (augmenting SSRI/SNRI)		
Quetiapine[a]	Sole recommended agent in ISTSS guideline; not recommended in VA/DoD	ISTSS
Risperidone[a]		NICE
Mirtazapine[a]		ISTSS, NICE, Cardiff
Not supported by current expert guidelines		
Benzodiazepines		
Citalopram, amitriptyline		
Lamotrigine, topiramate, divalproex		

TABLE 18–4. Summary of psychopharmacology from guidelines for acute stress disorder and PTSD (continued)

Medication	Notes and recommendations	Guideline
Tiagabine, guanfacine, ketamine, hydrocortisone, D-cycloserine		
Prazosin	Only for nightmares; no global PTSD symptom reduction by Clinician-Administered PTSD Scale scores	
Olanzapine	Insufficient evidence	
Cannabis and cannabis derivatives	No evidence acutely; weak evidence for chronic PTSD Cannabis may cause harm in the acutely traumatized by intensifying emotions	

[a]Use of this medication has not been evaluated by the FDA for the given indication.

Note. SNRI=serotonin-norepinephrine reuptake inhibitor; SSRI= selective serotonin reuptake inhibitor.

Guidelines. Cardiff=Cardiff Post-traumatic Stress Disorder Prescribing Algorithm; ISTSS=International Society for Traumatic Stress Studies Effective treatments for PTSD; NICE=International Society for Traumatic Stress Studies Effective treatments for PTSD; VA/DoD=Management of Posttraumatic Stress Disorder and Acute Stress Disorder.

Source. American Psychological Association 2017; Dekker et al. 2019; Forbes et al. 2020; Holbrook et al. 2010; National Institute for Health and Care Excellence 2018; U.S. Department of Veterans Affairs and U.S. Department of Defense 2023.

tonin-norepinephrine reuptake inhibitor without follow-up. Be aware that most disaster research indicates that most people are undertreated and receive inadequate doses of recommended medication (Dekker et al. 2019). Use antipsychotic medication only for extreme arousal symptoms such as agitation and behavioral dyscontrol.

Context-Specific Considerations

Acute Stress Disorder

Acute stress disorder should be treated with caution, but it should be treated. DSM-5 expanded the PTSD arousal category to include irritability and rage attacks with minimum to no provocation. These symptoms should be addressed, with guidance from either acute stress disorder or agitation guidelines for prescribing. Benzodiazepine administration can be considered safe, effective, and useful in the immediate postdisaster setting for acute symptoms of extreme arousal, insomnia, and uncontrollable anxiety, all of which may be considered greater risk factors for developing PTSD than the administration of a benzodiazepine per se.

PTSD

Do not treat PTSD with benzodiazepines, even as an augmentation strategy. There is evidence that long-term treatment with benzodiazepines for patients with PTSD are not only ineffective but may do harm (U.S. Department of Veterans Affairs and U.S. Department of Defense 2023). The potential harm outweighs the benefit because benzodiazepines in PTSD may interfere with fear extinction learning and reduce the effectiveness of exposure therapy. Benzodiazepines will not modify the underlying neurobiological disorder; however, many patients say that nothing else relieves their symptoms. All benzodiazepines have a high risk of abuse and dependence, are dangerous in overdose (especially with alcohol), and are highly associated with falls in older patients.

Medicolegal Issues

If prescribing, document that the patient has been made aware of risks and benefits, informed of side effects, and cautioned strongly about tolerance, dependence, and potential for addiction.

Symptoms That Warrant Early Intervention

The presence of irritability, anger, and self-destructive or injurious behavior in the disaster setting should alert the disaster psychiatrist to undertake a full PTSD screening and to provide medication to ensure patient, staff, and community safety.

Assessing for Risky Behaviors

Although it is easy to see disaster as a terrifying, scary, and anxiety-provoking event from which people would seek *flight*, there is also diagnostic utility in exploring symptoms associated with *fight*. These symptoms include anger, irritability, and self-destructiveness. This is so important that research has developed a scale to measure the symptoms to guide clinical intervention, the Posttrauma Risky Behaviors Scale (International Society for Traumatic Stress Studies 2021). This tool has been shown to have psychometric diagnostic utility (Contractor et al. 2021).

Medication Versus Therapy

As suggested by guideline recommendations, the magnitude of benefit of pharmacological interventions has been found to be inferior to that of trauma-focused psychological interventions. Small mean effect sizes of less than 0.4 have been found for the most effective medications, whereas large mean effect sizes of more than 1.2 have been found for CBT-TF and eye movement desensitization and processing (Bisson et al. 2020). It is, however, notoriously difficult to directly compare the results of randomized controlled trials of psychological and pharmacological approaches.

Benefits of Antidepressants

Antidepressants, especially SSRIs, have benefits, particularly in the medically ill and, importantly, in burn patients (Benedek and Wynn 2018; Stoddard et al. 2017). In a rare randomized but not placebo-controlled study completed 4 months after the 1999 earthquake in Turkey that killed more than 15,000 people, 103 patients were randomly assigned to fluoxetine, the reversible monoamine oxidase inhibitor (MAOI) moclobemide, or the atypical antidepressant tianeptine. All patients completing the study had a greater than 50% decrease in PTSD symptoms as assessed with validated standardized scales. The authors concluded that all three medications were equally effective (Onder et al. 2006).

Existing Psychiatric Medication

The disaster psychiatrist is a valuable member of the response team in assisting medical members of the team in dosing, indication, and side effect profiles of off-label use of antipsychotics. Patients already taking neuroleptic medications for schizophrenia, bipolar disorder, or personality pathology may have better outcome by increasing existing doses within safe limits rather than adding an additional agent such as a benzodiazepine, SSRI, or anticonvulsant.

Cautions With Psychopharmacology in the Disaster Setting

Absence of Robust Data

In disaster settings, physicians are compelled to grasp for something to do to treat the overwhelming suffering and distress of patients presenting acutely. This may lead to the use of medications with very limited clinical evidence or study data. The optimism associated with use of a particular medication may not stand the test of time. Without large sample sizes and with only small nonrandomized observational studies, it can be difficult to discern what is effective.

Substances Without Research or FDA Support

In the absence of information, it is tempting to borrow from known treatment of other disorders that have nothing to do with acute psychological and psychiatric trauma. Both great enthusiasm and great confusion abound in disaster psychiatry. Disinformation is prevalent, with wild claims based on impressive results from non-FDA-approved, nonresearched compounds such as cannabis; 3,4-methylenedioxy-methamphetamine (MDMA); ketamine; and psychedelics such as ashwagandha, Ayahuasca, dimethyltryptamine (DMT), and lysergic acid diethylamide (LSD). The recent surge in interest in psychedelic compounds means that the disaster psychiatrist will be asked about them. Therefore, it is important to keep abreast of studies and stay in the lane of approved recommendations rather than generalizing.

Acute consumption of cannabis can be expected to intensify feelings. The VA does not recommend it for chronic PTSD; however, in New York State, veterans groups obtained approval for dispensary cannabis as a medication for chronic PTSD and pain. Under federal law, cannabis has not been classified as a treatment, but in 2024, the U.S. Justice Department moved to reclassify marijuana from a Schedule I substance (meaning no current accepted medical use and with high potential for abuse) to a Schedule III substance (with low to moderate risk of abuse).

Ketamine is approved only for treatment of refractory depression and is being studied in patients with cancer receiving palliative care. Mushrooms available for purchase on the internet and microdosing and nanodosing of ketamine are *not* regulated. Such use has not been studied at all and may be dangerous. As for ashwagandha, Ayahuasca, and other compounds such as DMT and LSD, the psychedelic research era has begun, but it is simply too early for disaster psychiatrists to have an informed, let alone evidence-based, opinion. Ayahuasca may have an MAOI mechanism that confers a risk of serotonin syndrome. Psychedelics are not indicated and likely are dangerous in the treatment of acute stress disorder.

Newer Agents

Riluzole, which is approved as a treatment for amyotrophic lateral sclerosis, modulates glutamatergic transmission. Because glutamate is the most ubiquitous excitatory neurotransmitter in the brain, it seems reasonable that reduction of excitatory signaling in the amygdala might reduce the subsequent brainstem reactivation thought to be responsible for hyperarousal in PTSD. One small study showed modest differences, with significantly greater improvement on hyperarousal symptoms in the riluzole group as measured by the PTSD Checklist-Specific-Subscale D (Spangler et al. 2020). This may suggest why non-SSRI agents such as trazodone (which has α_1-adrenergic blocker action) and, to a lesser degree, risperidone (with serotonin type 2A receptor activity) work for sleep disturbance in PTSD.

Questions Regarding Psychopharmacology, PTSD, and Acute Stress Disorder

Can Medication Prevent PTSD?

Medical, nursing, and social services colleagues and many patients in the disaster setting pose the following question to the psychiatrist: What medication will prevent one from developing PTSD? The feeling in disaster response and recovery is that everybody is shocked and traumatized, so, logically, won't everyone get PTSD? Without minimizing distress or offering false reassurance, the disaster psychiatrist can educate and inform patients about the natural history of stress reactions, the scope of normal reactions, acute stress disorder, and the symptoms of PTSD. The crucial symptom to address is sleep. Whereas most research has considered how PTSD affects sleep, a recent review examining daily studies of sleep and PTSD symptomatology indicated that shorter sleep and poorer sleep quality predict next-day PTSD symptoms, suggesting that the relationship between PTSD symptoms and sleep may be bidirectional (Slavish et al. 2022).

Does Acute Stress Disorder Always Develop Into PTSD?

Importantly, acute stress disorder does not always develop into PTSD. Unlike other areas of medicine, presentation of disaster psychopathology is not linear or additive. Symptoms of an acute stress disorder may resolve with treatment, resolve with time without treatment, or continue and become PTSD. Many patients present with PTSD who have not previously presented for care or been symptomatic. This puts the psychopharmacologist in a data vacuum, without an obvious algorithm for medication treatment.

Limited outcome research suggests that intersectionality is an important way to understand risk of developing PTSD. Factors that should be considered include loss of employment, financial constraints, and relationship difficulties. In a study conducted 5 years after bushfires in Australia, life stressors—many of which were related to ongoing social and economic disruption caused by the fires—contributed the most to delayed onset or lingering PTSD, depression, and distress (U.S. Department of Veterans Affairs and U.S. Department of Defense 2023). Risk factors following mass shootings include pretrauma vulnerability, exposure to the event, resource loss, and maladaptive coping (Ursano et al. 2017). This underscores the need for psychological and social interventions as the primary treatment for disaster-related mental health symptoms.

Do Specific Acute Stress Disorder Symptoms or Situations Predict Progression to PTSD?

Symptoms of acute stress disorder do not predict onset of PTSD, but situations do. The severity of the postdisaster situation is a greater predictor than a specific symptom. Medical injury, bereavement, loss of housing, substance use disorders and prior mental health conditions are stronger predictors of developing PTSD than are physical or psychological symptoms present in the first hours or days. In reviewing the literature of the past decade in preparation for this edition of this book, predictive PTSD symptom phenomena that seemed to make clinical, intuitive, and biological sense have not stood up to more rigorous, larger, and repeated observational studies (Esterwood and Saeed 2020). Increased heart rate and blood pressure in the presence of hyperarousal (insomnia, easy startle response, hypervigilance) was thought to be predictive of later PTSD, but this did not prove to be the case in larger studies. Similarly, DSM-5-TR changes from prior editions reflect new knowledge that dissociation (as well as detachment, numbing) are not predictive of PTSD (Shalev et al. 1998).

Addressing Vulnerable Communities

A disaster psychiatry approach to community includes ensuring that supplies of depot antipsychotic injection are available to seriously and persistently mentally ill patients. Substance use disorder treatment such as methadone clinics, suboxone prescriptions, and acute detoxification for alcohol use disorders must be available during periods of social disruption because of the demonstrated dramatic increases in substance use disorders during disaster events.

Conclusion

Psychopharmacology interventions in disaster psychiatry are always secondary to psychotherapy and other interventions described in this book. The very specific, sparing, and careful administration of psychiatric medication can be of great benefit if given to the patients most likely to benefit. This includes those with significant psychiatric symptoms. Most people who will recover from disaster events with other interventions do so within 3 days to 3 weeks. Those who have disabling anxiety or severe insomnia or who present with agitation or delirium are priorities for psychiatric assistance.

Medically ill patients are not just "bodies"; they are minds and people going through an overwhelming experience. Disaster psychiatry recognizes this humanity and vulnerability and brings to bear psychiatric expertise to help medical colleagues manage this situation. It is increasingly recognized that material resources of housing, jobs, and health care access are critical for surviving a disaster. The intersectionality of risk factors affects people strongly, if not more heavily, than do psychiatric or psychological factors. Psychiatrists are valuable advocates for the mentally ill in disaster settings and can mitigate intense psychological suffering and psychiatric symptoms with thoughtful interventions.

References

American Psychological Association: Clinical Practice Guideline for the Treatment of PTSD. Washington, DC, American Psychological Association, 2017

American Psychiatric Association: Diagnostic and Statistical Manual of Mental Disorders, 5th Edition, Text Revision. Washington, DC, American Psychiatric Association, 2022

Bajor LA, Balsara C, Osser DN: An evidence-based approach to psychopharmacology for posttraumatic stress disorder (PTSD): 2022 update. Psychiatry Res 317:114840, 2022 36162349

Benedek DM, Friedman MJ, Zatzick D, et al: Guideline Watch (March 2009): Practice Guideline for the Treatment of Patients With Acute Stress Disorder and Posttraumatic Stress Disorder. Washington, DC, American Psychiatric Publishing, 2009

Benedek DM, Wynn GH: Pharmacologic treatment of adults with trauma- and stressor-related disorders. in Trauma- and Stressor-Related Disorders. Edited by Stoddard FJ, Benedek DM, Milad MR, et al. New York, Oxford University Press, 2018, p 278

Bisson JI, Baker A, Dekker W, et al: Evidence-based prescribing for post-traumatic stress disorder. Br J Psychiatry 216(3):125–126, 2020 32345407

Breitbart W, Marotta R, Platt MM, et al: A double-blind trial of haloperidol, chlorpromazine, and lorazepam in the treatment of delirium in hospitalized AIDS patients. Am J Psychiatry 153(2):231–237, 1996 8561204

Bryant-Davis T: The cultural context of trauma recovery: considering the posttraumatic stress disorder practice guideline and intersectionality. Psychotherapy (Chic) 56(3):400–408, 2019 31282715

Contractor AA, Jin L, Weiss NH, et al: A psychometric investigation on the diagnostic utility of the posttrauma risky behaviors questionnaire. Psychiatry Res 296:113667, 2021 33360968

Crapanzano C, Damiani S, Casolaro I, Amendola C: Quetiapine treatment for post-traumatic stress disorder: a systematic review of the literature. Clin Psychopharmacol Neurosci 21(1):49–56, 2023 36700311

Dekker W, Baker A, Hoskins M, et al: Cardiff Post-traumatic Stress Disorder Prescribing Algorithm. Cardiff, Wales, Traumatic Stress Wales, 2019

Esterwood E, Saeed SA: Past epidemics, natural disasters, COVID19, and mental health: learning from history as we deal with the present and prepare for the future. Psychiatr Q 91(4):1121–1133, 2020 32803472

Forbes D, Bisson JI, Monson CM, et al (eds): Effective Treatments for PTSD, 3rd Edition. New York, Guilford, 2020

Funk MC, Beach SR, Bostwick JR, et al: QTc prolongation and psychotropic medications. Am J Psychiatry 177(3):273–274, 2020 32114782

Holbrook TL, Galarneau MR, Dye JL, et al: Morphine use after combat injury in Iraq and post-traumatic stress disorder. N Engl J Med 362(2):110–117, 2010 20071700

International Society for Traumatic Stress Studies: Posttrauma Risky Behaviors Questionnaire. Chicago, IL, International Society for Traumatic Stress Studies, 2021. Available at: https://istss.org/wp-content/uploads/2024/08/Posttrauma-Risky-Behaviors-Questionnaire.pdf. Accessed August 7, 2024.

Martin A, Naunton M, Kosari S, et al: Treatment guidelines for PTSD: a systematic review. J Clin Med 10(18):4175, 2021 34575284

National Institute for Health and Care Excellence: Post-Traumatic Stress Disorder (NICE Guideline NG116). London, National Institute for Health and Care Excellence, December 5, 2018. Available from: www.nice.org.uk/guidance/ng116. Accessed April 4, 2024.

Onder E, Tural U, Aker T: A comparative study of fluoxetine, moclobemide, and tianeptine in the treatment of posttraumatic stress disorder following an earthquake. Eur Psychiatry 21(3):174–179, 2006 15964747

Shalev AY, Sahar T, Freedman S, et al: A prospective study of heart rate response following trauma and the subsequent development of posttraumatic stress disorder. Arch Gen Psychiatry 55(6):553–559, 1998 9633675

Shiner B, Leonard CE, Gui J, et al: Comparing medications for DSM-5 PTSD in routine VA practice. J Clin Psychiatry 81(6):20m13244, 2020 33049805

Slavish DC, Briggs M, Fentem A, et al: Bidirectional associations between daily PTSD symptoms and sleep disturbances: a systematic review. Sleep Med Rev 63:101623, 2022 35367721

Spangler PT, West JC, Dempsey CL, et al: Randomized controlled trial of riluzole augmentation for posttraumatic stress disorder: efficacy of a glutamatergic modulator for antidepressant-resistant symptoms. J Clin Psychiatry 81(6):20m13233, 2020 33113596

Stoddard FJJr, Sorrentino E, Drake JE, et al: Posttraumatic stress disorder diagnosis in young children with burns. J Burn Care Res 38(1):e343–e351, 2017 27359192

Ursano R, Fullerton C, Weisaeth L, et al (eds): Textbook of Disaster Psychiatry, 2nd Edition. New York, Cambridge University Press, 2017

U.S. Department of Veterans Affairs, U.S. Department of Defense: Management of Posttraumatic Stress Disorder and Acute Stress Disorder. Washington, DC, U.S. Department of Veterans Affairs, 2023

19

Child and Adolescent Psychiatric Interventions

Kunmi Sobowale, M.D.
Linda Chokroverty, M.D.

Disasters uniquely affect the mental health of infants, children, and adolescents because of demographic and developmental factors (Masten and Osofsky 2010; Peek 2008). Demographically, children live in areas of the world that are more prone to disasters, such as wars, droughts and famines, or flooding. Developmentally, children's understanding of disasters and perception of risk may be limited (Shibley and Stoddard 2011). They may regress in their behaviors or blame themselves. Because of their size and less developed coordination, children are at greater risk than adults of suffering injuries or death. The loss of social connections in the wake of a disaster, especially educational disruption, adversely affects child socioemotional development.

Children crucially rely on others for their care. Caregivers (parents and other adults providing daily care) are central in this role, but children's experiences of disaster and their ability to buffer related stress also depend on communal and societal factors. Therefore, a broader socioecological perspective that includes the child, the family or caregiver, and the community is needed to support children's mental health (UNICEF

2018a). Furthermore, when it comes to intervention, all phases of the disaster cycle, from predisaster to recovery, should be considered.

In this chapter, we take a tiered approach to prevention and intervention, including universal, targeted, and indicated levels (Figure 19–1) as we go through each disaster cycle phase. Universal interventions are designed to reach and impact an entire population or population group regardless of their risk or protective factors. Targeted interventions focus on the specific needs of subgroups of the population that have risk factors or barriers to accessing support or services. Indicated interventions address the needs of individuals with signs or symptoms of a specific mental health condition. Most children have the resources to face adversity and recover with universal interventions alone. However, some severely impacted children and those with elevated baseline vulnerabilities will need more support. Mental health professionals can play a role at all of these levels of prevention and intervention; however, depending on the setting, professionals may not be able or willing to be involved in universal or targeted efforts.

Two important caveats should be noted. First, we consider individuals younger than age 18 years to be children (United Nations 1989) and those ages 18–22 years to be transitional youth, although we recognize that developmentally, there is much variance in children's mental and physical capacities. Second, the literature on child mental health interventions in the context of disasters is limited, so many interventions are evidence informed or based on research from the trauma literature.

Predisaster Phase

The role of the mental health professional is traditionally at the indicated intervention level in the postdisaster phase, treating children with moderate to severe mental health difficulties several weeks to months after a disaster. For several reasons, we advocate for an increased role for mental health professionals in the predisaster phase using universal and targeted interventions (see Chapter 2, "Disaster Prevention and Climate Change," Chapter 3, "Needs Assessment," and Chapter 7, "Engaging in Disaster Response"). First, 100 million children annually experience a disaster worldwide (Save the Children 2007), and 14% of children in the United States experience a disaster by age 18 (Becker-Blease et al. 2010). As a result, mental health professionals will encounter children who will be exposed to a future disaster or who are already survivors.

Furthermore, children with existing mental health difficulties are at higher risk of developing mental health issues in the postdisaster phase

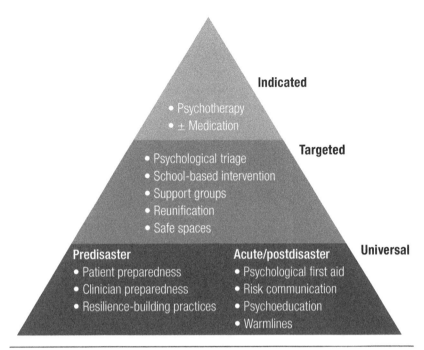

Indicated
- Psychotherapy
- ± Medication

Targeted
- Psychological triage
- School-based intervention
- Support groups
- Reunification
- Safe spaces

Universal

Predisaster
- Patient preparedness
- Clinician preparedness
- Resilience-building practices

Acute/postdisaster
- Psychological first aid
- Risk communication
- Psychoeducation
- Warmlines

FIGURE 19–1. Levels of disaster mental health interventions.

(Bonanno et al. 2010; Guo et al. 2020). Preparedness can reduce the need for later indicated interventions, which are crucial yet often inaccessible for children with significant mental health difficulties. Specifically, preparedness reduces the risk of physical injury and increases a child's sense of control. Increased control decreases the traumatic features of events (Epel et al. 2018)—perceived helplessness, novelty, and, to some extent, the unpredictability of events—through advance planning and disaster simulation. Indeed, predisaster stress, often related to last-minute preparations or evacuation, is associated with worsened postdisaster maternal mental health (La Greca et al. 2022). Clinician-emphasized preparedness could decrease last-minute evacuation, which may bolster maternal mental health and thereby protect child mental health.

Thus, in a world with increasing disasters, it is incumbent on mental health professionals to increase preparedness efforts. Clinicians working with marginalized populations and people residing in disaster-prone areas are strongly encouraged to discuss or share information on disaster preparedness (see Chapter 13, "Specific Needs of Submarginalized Populations"). In addition to direct care, mental health professionals can consult with primary care providers and educators. Given the seasonality of certain disasters (e.g., wildfires), preparation efforts may be more successful when disasters are top of mind.

Practically, for clinicians in the predisaster phase, this means using universal interventions such as encouraging disaster preparedness and promoting factors that support resilience. Indicated interventions are limited in this phase, although treating existing mental health issues, including adverse childhood experiences that increase risk and decrease preparedness behaviors (Eisenman et al. 2009; Guo et al. 2020), will likely be protective. Although hospitals often have disaster planning in place for mass casualties or other patient surges, the community itself, where most disasters happen, is often underprepared. More could be done to keep people safe and promote resilience.

For children and caregivers, resilience-promoting activities include positive childhood experiences (PCEs), emergency planning, and basic stress management skills. PCEs are "favorable experiences between birth to age 18 characterized by internal and external perceived safety, security, and support; and positive and predictable qualities of life" (Narayan et al. 2018, p. 20) (Table 19–1). PCEs are about safe and nurturing relationships and enriching environments. For example, household routines can emotionally regulate children and their caregivers by providing predictability. During the coronavirus disease 2019 (COVID-19) pandemic, children in families with routines were less likely to develop mental health issues (Bates et al. 2021; Glynn et al. 2021). Clinicians can help foster healthy routines by encouraging families to eat together and dedicate time to talk and play with their children daily. Professionals should reinforce and praise the health-promoting actions that caregivers are already doing to support their children.

Emergency planning for families reduces the risk of harm in disaster situations. If one is prepared for certain possibilities, it is easier to make rational decisions in highly stressful situations such as disasters. Clinicians should inquire whether families have a "go bag," a collection of essential supplies that can be taken quickly in an emergency. Families can be referred to the website Ready.gov (www.ready.gov), which lists items to stock in an emergency kit. If space allows, families will also benefit from preparing kits with nonelectronic materials for entertainment (e.g., playing cards, drawing supplies, books) and soothing items (e.g., fidget toys, squeeze balls, preferred stuffed animals). A family disaster plan detailing family communication and evacuation routes is crucial. The plan should include instructions and a portable item to facilitate reunification, such as a paper listing phone numbers, a home address, and a meeting place. Children separated from their caregivers are more likely to experience abuse (Seddighi et al. 2021), leading to a higher risk of mental health problems.

TABLE 19–1. Examples of positive childhood experiences

A positive self-image

A predictable home routine

Beliefs that give comfort

A sense of belonging or enjoyment in school

Beliefs that give comfort

A sense of belonging or enjoyment in school

At least one good friend who is supportive

A caring noncaregiver adult

An adult in the home who makes a child feel safe and protected

Opportunities to have a good time

Opportunities to participate in community traditions

Clinicians who plan to be involved in disaster relief efforts can prepare by creating a therapeutic supply kit with art materials, hand puppets, building blocks, toy emergency vehicles, doctor's kits, and dolls of varying races/ethnicities. Further, they can consider training in interventions used in the acute and postdisaster phases discussed later in this chapter.

Sharing age-appropriate ways for caregivers to support children during disasters is essential. For example, children can learn "drop, cover, and hold on" to decrease injury during an earthquake. Fortunately, many resources, including television programs (e.g., *Sesame Street*), have information on family disaster preparedness and talking to children about disasters (Table 19–2). Clinicians can also share mobile apps such as the Federal Emergency Management Agency and Substance Abuse and Mental Health Services Administration behavior health apps, which have preparedness tips covering a wide range of disaster scenarios.

Before a disaster, clinicians should work with communities to support emergency planning. To do this, a clinician needs familiarity with existing assets at local schools, community-based organizations, and social services where children and their families eat, work, learn, and play. Knowledge of schools' preparedness practices (e.g., reunification plans) is important because some activities, such as active shooter drills, do not use best practices and may traumatize children (Schildkraut and Nickerson 2022). Knowing best practices allows mental health professionals to intervene as consultants by offering expertise on whether and how to conduct such drills. Being abreast of school-based mental health services and socioemotional learning programs that support child well-being is important. These services can be protective and are crucial in the aftermath of a disaster. For

TABLE 19–2. Resources on disaster preparedness for families and clinicians

Organization	Resources	Description
American Academy of Child and Adolescent Psychiatry	Disaster and Trauma Resource Center, www.aacap.org/AACAP/Families_and_Youth/Resource_Centers/Disaster_Resource_Center/Resources_for_Parents_Disaster.aspx	Psychoeducational materials for families on child mental health in a variety of disasters
American Academy of Pediatrics	Disaster Preparedness Resources for Families, www.aap.org/en/patient-care/disasters-and-children/resources-for-families	Family readiness kit and other planning materials
	Clinical Professional Resources for Disaster Preparedness, www.aap.org/en/patient-care/disasters-and-children/professional-resources-for-disaster-preparedness	Materials for pediatric clinician preparedness
American Red Cross	Prepare With Pedro Hazard Storybooks, www.ready.gov/kids/prepare-pedro; www.redcross.org/get-help/how-to-prepare-for-emergencies/teaching-kids-about-emergency-preparedness/prepare-with-pedro.html	Free books on disaster preparedness for different types of disasters developed through a partnership with FEMA and American Red Cross
		Activity sheets for children on preparedness in different scenarios
Federal Emergency Management Agency	FEMA mobile products, www.fema.gov/about/news-multimedia/mobile-products	Information on disaster preparedness and shelter and recovery center locations in the United States
National Child Traumatic Stress Network	Disaster resources, www.nctsn.org/what-is-child-trauma/trauma-types/disasters	Information on family preparedness and coping for a variety of disasters

TABLE 19–2. Resources on disaster preparedness for families and clinicians (*continued*)

Organization	Resources	Description
	Help Kids Cope app, www.nctsn.org/resources/help-kids-cope	Mobile application to help parents talk to their children about various disasters during predisaster, acute disaster, and postdisaster phases
Ready.gov	Ready Kids activities, www.ready.gov/kids	Preparedness activities for kids, teens, families, and communities
Sesame Workshop	Emergency videos, https://sesameworkshop.org/topics/emergencies	Information on disaster preparedness

children in a marginalized group, peers and adults at a community-based organization can provide safe and nurturing relationships.

Organizations with emergency plans to reach children and offer alternative ways for them to socialize post disaster can provide a sense of normalcy and foster recovery. Mental health professionals can support organizations that lack contingencies to develop emergency plans. The Urban Institute (Fedorowicz et al. 2020) and the Ready.gov website have resources on this topic. Children are more likely than adults to live in poverty, which is a risk factor for postdisaster mental illness. Social services such as diaper banks, free tax return preparation, and the Supplemental Nutrition Assistance Program (SNAP) can all boost resilience by lessening financial constraints. Clinicians should share these resources with families in need (i.e., provide a targeted intervention) when appropriate.

Forming relationships with the media to ensure that public health announcements benefit schools and parents is vital. Collaboration with media representatives is necessary to plan helpful announcements and to provide warnings to families about forthcoming graphic images and guidance for parents needing professional help for their children (Shibley and Stoddard 2011). These efforts can be a lot of work for an individual clinician. Local psychiatric, pediatric/family medicine, social work, psychological, and teachers' associations are all part of disaster response networks where multidisciplinary collaboration can occur. These networks can also facilitate clinical interventions via telepsychiatry for children, adolescents, and families (see Chapter 4, "Technology").

Acute Phase

In the immediate aftermath of a disaster, safety and basic needs take priority over all else. Major disruptions in routine activities such as school, childcare, recreation, and parental employment are likely to occur. Caregivers' ability to look after their children may become impaired because of various distractions and stressors, such as extreme losses incurred by a disaster. Additionally, separations and delays in reunification among children or youth and family members are to be expected. Children and youth are at far greater risk for harm, such as abuse, neglect, and crime victimization, when separated from their families or in cases of compromised parenting. These secondary circumstances of separation and disruption may add another layer of stress on stresses created directly by the disaster event itself.

Mental health professionals have a role to play in assisting affected children or youth and families in reestablishing controls and connections through the principles of Psychological First Aid (PFA), a universal intervention (see also Chapter 16 for details), the goal of which is "to reduce distress, assist with current needs and promote adaptive functioning" (Brymer et al. 2005). The core actions include the following: "listen, protect, connect, model calm and optimistic behavior, teach." These actions are approached from a family, child or youth, and parent or caregiver standpoint rather than an individual standpoint, and developmental adjustments according to the age of the child or youth must be made. Several online courses and mobile phone apps on PFA are available for reference (Table 19–3).

PFA can be modified for children and youth. These modifications are summarized briefly in following subsections.

Listen to Concerns and Pay Attention to Behaviors

Allow children and teens to express their concerns. If factual inaccuracies exist in their understanding of the event, validate their feelings but correct misperceptions, which might contribute to their distress. Younger children or those with or special needs may express themselves nonverbally, such as through play and restless or disruptive behaviors. Observe nonverbal communication and pay attention to behaviors and body language and, as appropriate, play or interact with the child to see and hear more of what they are experiencing. Fears, worries, and recurring themes of destruction and loss might be conveyed in play. Older children and teens might also be nonverbal or inhibited about expressing themselves, and that is permitted. No one of any age should be forced to speak about things they do not want to at that moment. Engaging older youth might be possible through interactive games and expressive arts such as drawing or modeling clay figures, which often have a calming effect and can lower psychological defenses that might prevent the expression of difficult feelings. Listening to parents' concerns about their children's well-being and questions that might arise around stress reactions is an effective way of providing validation and support to parents who likely feel overwhelmed and unable to provide the usual parental oversight and reassurance children need. Paying attention to factors that raise the risk for future psychopathology in children is an important triage process (see Chapter 11, "Infant, Child, and Adolescent Psychiatric Evaluation") because referral for clinical care may be needed. Such risks include high trauma exposure, disrupted social supports (including maladaptive parenting), and a prior history of mental health disorders (Pine and Cohen 2002).

During the first few days following a disaster, safety, reunification, and adjustment to predictable and familiar routines are prioritized. Formal and structured interventions are neither possible nor advised. Practi-

TABLE 19–3. Training resources for clinicians on acute disaster and postdisaster interventions

Intervention	Resources	Description
Psychological First Aid	Psychological First Aid (PFA) Field Operations Guide, 2nd Edition, www.nctsn.org/resources/psychological-first-aid-pfa-field-operations-guide-2nd-edition	NCTSN manual
	Psychological First Aid (PFA) Online, www.nctsn.org/resources/psychological-first-aid-pfa-online	NCTSN online course and materials
	PFA Mobile, www.nctsn.org/resources/pfa-mobile	Mobile application
	Psychological First Aid, www.coursera.org/learn/psychological-first-aid	Online course from Coursera
Skills for Psychological Recovery	Skills for Psychological Recovery (SPR) Field Operations Guide, www.nctsn.org/resources/skills-for-psychological-recovery	NCTSN manual
	Skills for Psychological Recovery (SPR) Online, www.nctsn.org/resources/skills-psychological-recovery-spr-online	Online course and materials
Cognitive Behavioral Intervention for Trauma in Schools (CBITS)	https://app.traumaawareschools.org/interventions	Online course and materials from the Center for Safe & Resilient Schools and Workplaces

Note. NCTSN=National Child Traumatic Stress Network.

tioners should approach the situation not with intentions to provide psychotherapies or medications but rather with flexibility. Clinicians should facilitate a return to normal functioning and help healthy child development to occur despite the adversities at hand. The creation of a safe transitional space in the emergency setting, outfitted with toys and materials (for information regarding kits for clinicians and families, see the "Predisaster Phase" section) and guided by caring adults, allows children and youth to play and engage in age-appropriate and normalizing activities such as games and expressive arts. Play is universal and a right, as named by the United Nations Convention on the Rights of the Child (United Nations 1989). Further, play itself has healing and therapeutic powers because it facilitates communication, fosters emotional wellness, enhances social relationships, and increases personal strengths (Schaefer and Drewes 2014). Telepsychiatric interventions (Meersand and Gilmore 2017), including play and video games, are increasing access to child psychiatric consultation for disaster response, including for the many remote disasters.

The conceptualization of use of the transitional space for play and recreation in emergency settings has been popularized. Examples include the Kids' Corner, implemented by child psychiatrists and other child professionals at the Family Assistance Center in New York City after the 9/11 terrorist attacks in 2001 and in Sri Lanka after the 2004 tsunami (Chokroverty and Sriskandarajah 2007) and Child Friendly Spaces, assembled by larger nongovernmental organizations responding to disasters (Inter-agency Network for Education in Emergencies 2011; UNICEF 2018b). These spaces are well suited for carrying out PFA in all forms with children, youth, and parents or caregivers. They may be overseen by paid and/or volunteer child professionals, paraprofessionals, and informed adult community members. The unique perspectives provided by mental health professionals may offer additional guidance and education to caregivers on developmentally expected reactions and health-promoting practices. For example, ways to provide guidance and education on what to expect and how to help include 1) not "correcting" children's aggressive toy play but allowing it, while explaining how the feelings and ideas are being expressed, and 2) removing television and electronic devices that enable unwelcome news media exposures or distract from physical play (Chokroverty and Sriskandarajah 2007).

Protect Children and Youth

Children, especially very young ones, and youth must be reunited with parents or caregivers as soon as possible because separation causes more distress and the act of reuniting itself alleviates that distress and provides reassurance that they are safe and cared for and that their loved ones are also safe. Preserving the parent-child bond in emergencies is possibly the most protective way to intervene at all stages of disaster. Indeed, recent findings from a large-scale longitudinal study of children in the United States showed that parent monitoring and communication were protective factors for children's mental health during the COVID-19 pandemic (Hamatani et al. 2022).

Children and youth who have lost a parent in a disaster need another adult to step in immediately and provide consistent and reliable caregiving and much support. They may need additional counseling to help them through if they have traumatic grief, a situation in which normal bereavement is interfered with and complicated by the recent traumatic event (Cohen et al. 2017). Helping all children and families resume as many routines as possible around meals, sleep, and self-care is protective and provides grounding and normalization during acutely chaotic and difficult external conditions. Sleep hygiene and sleep routines (e.g., maintaining consistent bedtimes, sleeping in a dark room) help people of all ages settle into more restful sleep and are highly protective during difficult times. Additionally, paying attention for violent or suicidal behaviors exhibited by children, youth, or adults is paramount (Becker and Correll 2020), and the involvement of mobile crisis teams and possibly law enforcement may be necessary.

Connect Families With Each Other and to Services

As noted, reuniting families is essential. In the early stages of an emergency, helping parents or caregivers identify and find resources (e.g., for bereavement, health care, food) they might need for their families or themselves is helpful. Adults and youth who have a substance use disorder will need guidance and connection to resources supporting harm reduction, emergency services, and detoxification and rehabilitative services (Du et al. 2020; Gray and Squeglia 2018). During crisis situations, connection to these services and to peer support systems for people with a substance use disorder is of utmost importance to decrease negative impacts on the family.

Model Calm and Optimistic Behavior

Children turn to their parents' or caregivers' reactions to inform their own responses to situations. Therefore, having a calm demeanor and—even if distressed—being honest and sincere with children and youth about uncertainties is important. Parents who are highly anxious or agitated may have a negative impact on their children. These parents need further support from mental health clinicians to learn and use coping techniques. If unable to do so, parents should identify alternative caregivers who can provide calm reassurance to children while seeking their own mental health support. Mental health clinicians will also need to manage their own stress reactions and engage in self-care (see Chapter 6, "Rescuing Ourselves") in order to be able to model for and reassure adults, children, and youth who have been directly impacted by disasters.

Provide Psychoeducation

Children, youth, and parents or caregivers benefit from psychoeducation in the form of both written materials and live discussions. This information includes descriptions of normal stress reactions, coping techniques, activities that are calming, healthy lifestyle habits, parenting techniques, and when to seek further help for more serious mental health concerns.

Psychological debriefing (PD) is a controversial one-time intervention used in the period immediately following a traumatic event. It is a single group discussion in the first 72 hours of an event, comprising a narrative review of the event, ventilation of feelings, and normalization of reactions, with the goal of preventing more serious future conditions such as posttraumatic stress disorder (PTSD). A critical systematic review of studies on PD in adults, however, showed neither benefit nor negative results (Rose et al. 2003), raising concerns about its use and whether the natural course of recovery is preferred over PD (Pfefferbaum et al. 2015; Raphael and Wooding 2004). The few pediatric studies on PD are largely empirical and have had methodological problems. These studies have shown mixed results regarding mental health outcomes. Thus, a strong evidence base is lacking for PD in this population. Experts also worry that early reexposures following a major trauma could be stressful or traumatic for some children and youth. As a result, PD is not recommended for the younger population in the earliest stages of a disaster. Instead, PFA, although also lacking controlled studies but drawing from evidence-informed practices, remains the first-line acute intervention recommended by professional groups such as the American Academy of Child and Adolescent Psychiatry (AACAP) (Pfefferbaum et al. 2013).

Prescribe Medications With Extreme Caution

Medications in the acute phase of disaster have little or no role in children and youth (Table 19–4). However, if medications were previously prescribed for physical, developmental, or mental health disorders (e.g., selective serotonin reuptake inhibitors for depression or anxiety or insulin for diabetes), efforts to maintain continuity of treatment would be ur-

---

TABLE 19–4. Prescribing for children after disasters

- The use of psychotropic medications is discouraged in socially disorganized disaster settings because the recommended follow-up monitoring may be impossible. For antidepressants, the FDA recommends *weekly* check-ins for the first month after a new prescription or dosage change, then follow-up visits *every 2 weeks* for the next month, with *monthly* meetings thereafter. For monitoring treatment, it is also helpful to have the patient complete a symptom inventory for the condition being treated before each meeting.

- Although prescription of psychotropic medications acutely in a hospital setting may be indicated, it is usually not indicated to prescribe during a disaster in a community setting, where specialized follow-up may be inaccessible. These tables are appropriate for use primarily in the hospital.

- After disasters, medications such as analgesics, benzodiazepines, and stimulants are sometimes diverted for illegal purposes.

- Prescribing psychotropic medications when no child psychotherapy is available is discouraged. Optimally, antidepressants should be prescribed in conjunction with therapy and closely monitored, but psychotherapy is often not available in rural or postdisaster settings.

- Antipsychotic medications may be prescribed by physicians in hospital settings where follow-up is possible. However, children should not be given antipsychotic medications without baseline blood tests or without close monitoring of blood tests and Abnormal Involuntary Movement Scale examinations by physicians.

---

gently needed to avoid relapse or breakthrough symptoms. Unlike with adults, who may use antianxiety (benzodiazepines) or sleep (hypnotics) medications to help with their acute stress, such medicines can have paradoxical effects on the younger population, resulting in disinhibited or disorganized behaviors. Also, the window of safety with such agents is narrower for younger children. Low-dose diphenhydramine or melatonin (both available over the counter in the United States) are relatively benign and may be used with caution, if at all, because they lack evidence for use under these circumstances. Behavioral methods such as calming techniques or activities, sleep hygiene, and other health-oriented routines are preferred. Parents must be educated about the difference between medication use for adults and children in the acute setting.

Postacute Phase

The postacute phase, defined as weeks to months following a disaster, brings many challenges. Traditional sources of support, such as schools or early education settings, may remain compromised. Existing limited child mental health services will likely be at a lower capacity. Levels of distress will probably be elevated. Despite these challenges, most children recover successfully. Therefore, as in the acute phase, interventions must balance supporting all affected individuals with triaging and referring those most likely to develop worsened or new mental health issues. Universal interventions supporting basic needs, social connections, and routines should continue. For all responders who interact with children, education on how children of different ages respond to and understand stressful and traumatic events is helpful (see Chapter 11). A targeted approach with less intensive, skills-based group interventions should be used for children at risk or with moderate symptoms, whereas those with enduring (several months postdisaster) or severe symptoms need intensive treatment, often delivered by mental health professionals. This may be individual treatment, but group interventions are also efficacious (Davis et al. 2023; Salloum and Overstreet 2008) and may be the only viable option given limited access.

Families

Universal family interventions can help all children. One recommendation is for families to focus on non-disaster-related activities (e.g., reading, singing, walking, drawing). Clinicians can encourage families to resume routines if possible because they are emotionally regulating. Play can promote recovery by allowing children to take an active role by using fantasy, which can help regulate and facilitate the processing of a traumatic experience. Depending on the disaster, caregivers can use nontraditional ways (e.g., videoconferencing, online games) to connect to loved ones and peers socially. Minimizing potentially triggering or traumatizing exposures from the news or social media is warranted, given their adverse effects on child mental health (Ohnuma et al. 2023). Caregivers can encourage children to reduce social media exposure by changing settings (e.g., indicating a preference not to see posts on a particular topic, using topic filters). Although nondisaster activities can promote mental health, supporting older children and adolescents who want to contribute to recovery efforts is one way to increase their agency and sense of control.

Psychoeducation may prevent further distress or harm. For example, caregivers can provide information on earthquake aftershocks to prepare children (see Table 19–2). Psychiatrists can counsel caregivers to share age-appropriate information in a calm manner when possible. They should avoid unrealistic reassurances such as saying, "Nothing bad is going to happen." Children should not be forced to talk, but caregivers should let them know they are available if they want to talk. Relatedly, educating caregivers to normalize their children's emotions rather than dismissing or minimizing them is important. Caregivers can also model coping skills by expressing emotions. For example, a parent could say, "Having to leave home because of the flood is really frustrating."

Schools and Communities

Schools are crucial for disaster recovery for children. Children spend most of their time in school. In addition to providing learning opportunities, schools provide supportive peer and staff relationships. Parents generally trust teachers and school counselors, who have frontline access to their children. Many schools in the United States have mental health services on campus, where many children receive care (Ali et al. 2019), and could be sites for delivery of mental health services. Indeed, a study of three schools after Hurricane Katrina showed that 98% of children accessed trauma-focused psychotherapy in school compared with only 37% in an offsite clinic (Jaycox et al. 2010).

Teachers and other school staff can intervene in multiple ways. Teachers may assist with communicating and educating their students about normal responses to disasters, modeling healthy ways of coping, and instilling self-efficacy and hope. Teachers can also be trained to deliver classroom-based interventions such as art therapy and group therapy (Jaycox et al. 2009). These services can be effective, as demonstrated by a meta-analysis of posttraumatic stress outcomes conducted by Fu and Underwood (2015), which revealed that school-based interventions administered by teachers and paraprofessionals benefited children exposed to natural and human-made disasters. One school intervention clinicians should be familiar with is Cognitive Behavioral Intervention for Trauma in Schools (CBITS; Jaycox et al. 2012). It is an evidence-based manualized group cognitive-behavioral therapy (CBT) program that includes 10 group sessions, 1–3 individual sessions, and parent and teacher education sessions (see Table 19–3). Schools are also a place to monitor students' mental health over time. Clinicians can assist teachers in identifying those children who may benefit from evaluation or treatment (Schreiber et al. 2006).

Clinicians can work with school administrators to implement practices that may be helpful as well as to identify those that may be detrimental to mental health. In the broader community, reopening churches and other houses of worship and community-based after-school programs also creates a sense of structure, routine, and support. Communities can support children through ordinary activities such as sports or cultural events. Communal healing events that bring people together promote social support and meaning-making of disaster. Rite-of-passage events such as graduation ceremonies can help foster a sense of normalcy. Clinicians can deliver Skills for Psychological Recovery, a modular targeted intervention that is effective in the postdisaster phase in community settings. A training course is freely available (see Table 19–3).

Caring for Carers

Support for caregivers and other individuals who interact with children is needed so that they can help children. In this work, clinicians need to use a trauma-informed approach because disasters may bring up past trauma for those supporting children. Clinicians can consider recommending clinically vetted mobile health applications to adults. For example, COVID Coach is a free, publicly available mental health app developed by the U.S. Department of Veterans Affairs that provides psychoeducation and stress management skills. It was widely used during the COVID-19 pandemic (Jaworski et al. 2021). Notably, the app does not collect individual data, which may be appealing to families.

The Individual Child

For the individual child, several interventions are helpful. As emphasized in PFA, it is essential to ensure that children have their basic needs of food, shelter, and clothing met. Clinicians should be aware of social services for children and families in need. Most children recover with family and community support alone. For children needing more help, clinicians should stay abreast of referral resources for clinical mental health care. When possible, children and their families should be given options to decide how they want to receive services (in person, online, or both) in line with trauma-informed practices.

Children with persistent psychopathology, including sustained posttraumatic stress symptoms, usually necessitate indicated interventions with more intensive and structured psychotherapy. Many psychological interventions for children are trauma focused. Trauma-focused CBTs (TF-CBTs) have the most robust evidence in children and adolescents (Dorsey et al. 2017). These therapies usually include psychoeducation about trauma, teaching coping skills (e.g., relaxation, stress management, cognitive restructuring), and exposure through trauma narratives and drawings. Parent involvement is often used to support child participation. Training in TF-CBT for children is available online for practitioners. Narrative exposure therapy, related to but distinct from TF-CBT, has good adult evidence and emerging pediatric evidence for the treatment of multiple traumas (Fazel et al. 2020). Another therapy for trauma considered probably efficacious in children is eye movement desensitization and reprocessing (Dorsey et al. 2017).

Children can be distressed for reasons other than trauma. Adjustment to changing circumstances (e.g., a displaced child living in a new setting) can lead to distress. In such cases, family and community interventions are likely to promote healthy adaptation. Children who develop depression may benefit from CBT or behavioral activation rather than TF-CBT. Substance use–related issues also can cause distress and should be treated (Gray and Squeglia 2018).

Grief is a normative response to loss that usually does not result in mental illness. Practical ways for mental health professionals to help grieving children include identifying safety concerns such as suicidality. Instructing caregivers of young children to use factual information about death is necessary to avoid confusing children who may interpret a euphemism about death literally. Special attention must be paid to children and youth who lose a parent because losing a primary caregiver without adequate support from remaining family and caregivers can have devastating consequences. Clinicians should inform parents or caregivers about children's higher propensity to blame themselves for the loss even when there is no fault. Some resources to share with families are the National Alliance for Children's Grief website (https://nacg.org) and AACAP's Facts for Families series educational tip sheet titled "Grief and Children." For more information on this topic, see Schonfeld et al. (2015).

Medications are rarely indicated in the wake of a disaster, but they may be necessary if a child is chronically overwhelmed or to target a specific, problematic symptom such as insomnia. If medication is needed, it should be used at the minimum dose and duration. Behavioral and psychological alternatives are preferred.

Recommendations Addressing the Long-Term Effects of the COVID-19 Pandemic on Children and Families

Recently, the National Academies of Sciences, Engineering, and Medicine addressed the long-term effects of the COVID-19 pandemic disaster on children from high-risk communities (National Academies of Sciences, Engineering, and Medicine 2023). Authors of the report documented that the pandemic has caused significant disparities in child bereavement, with racial and ethnic minorities accounting for 65% of children who lost a primary caregiver because of COVID-19. The report identified adverse effects on children's education and mental health, including increased school absenteeism, decreased literacy and numeracy, and increased depression and anxiety. There have also been increases in stress levels among parents and in household chaos.

The National Academies report "propose[d] a path to recover and rectify the inequities resulting from and exposed by the pandemic" and future disasters through 10 recommendations. The full report presents the effects of the pandemic and is a road map for implementing new policies and mobilizing congressional, state, or local funding to address the negative effects of pandemics on low-income and racially and ethnically minoritized children and families. It is one of the earliest national evidence-based disaster initiatives designed to benefit children and families.

Conclusion

Disasters have impacts on infants, children, and adolescents; their families; and entire communities. Intervention should include these three tiers of influence. Effective preparation may mitigate the impact of disasters on children and their families. When preparing to meet the postdisaster needs of children, it is important to evaluate and consider their developmental needs, as well as the needs of their parents, families, and schools. Pediatric services, child mental health services, and other child-serving entities should have specific plans and staff disaster training to anticipate and meet the needs of children, families, and staff and should coordinate their planning with other disaster agencies in the community. Acutely and post disaster, children's mental health needs range from universal support using PFA for acute distress to indicated psychotherapeutic treatment for disorders that may persist, such as PTSD or depression. Most children recover with universal interventions. Psychopharmacological treatment is rarely indicated. Evidence to better prepare for and mitigate the impact of disasters on children and adolescents continues to grow.

References

Ali MM, West K, Teich JL, et al: Utilization of mental health services in educational settings by adolescents in the United States. J Sch Health 89(5):393–401, 2019 30883761

Bates CR, Nicholson LM, Rea EM, et al: Life interrupted: family routines buffer stress during the COVID-19 pandemic. J Child Fam Stud 30(11):2641–2651, 2021 34404970

Becker M, Correll CU: Suicidality in childhood and adolescence. Dtsch Arztebl Int 117(15):261–267, 2020 32449889

Becker-Blease KA, Turner HA, et al: Disasters, victimization, and children's mental health. Child Dev 81(4):1040–1052, 2010 20636681

Bonanno GA, Brewin CR, Kaniasty K, et al: Weighing the costs of disaster: consequences, risks, and resilience in individuals, families, and communities. Psychol Sci Public Interest 11(1):1–49, 2010 26168411

Brymer M, Layne C, Pynoos R, et al: Psychological First Aid: Field Operations Guide, 2nd Edition. Los Angeles, CA, National Child Traumatic Stress Network/National Center for PTSD, September 2005. Available at: www.nctsn.org/sites/default/files/resources//pfa_field_operations_guide.pdf. Accessed April 15, 2023.

Chokroverty L, Sriskandarajah N: A model for acute care of children and adolescents exposed to disasters, in Responses to Traumatized Children. Edited by Hosin AA. London, Palgrave Macmillan, 2007, pp 66–90

Cohen J, Mannarino A, Deblinger E: Treating Trauma and Traumatic Grief in Children and Adolescents, 2nd Edition. New York, Guilford, 2017

Davis RS, Meiser-Stedman R, Afzal N, et al: Systematic review and meta-analysis: group-based interventions for treating posttraumatic stress symptoms in children and adolescents. J Am Acad Child Adolesc Psychiatry 62(11):1217–1232, 2023 36948393

Dorsey S, McLaughlin KA, Kerns SEU, et al: Evidence base update for psychosocial treatments for children and adolescents exposed to traumatic events. J Clin Child Adolesc Psychol 46(3):303–330, 2017 27759442

Du J, Fan N, Zhao M, et al: Expert consensus on the prevention and treatment of substance use and addictive behaviour-related disorders during the COVID-19 pandemic. Gen Psychiatr 33(4):e100252, 2020 34192233

Eisenman DP, Zhou Q, Ong M, et al: Variations in disaster preparedness by mental health, perceived general health, and disability status. Disaster Med Public Health Prep 3(1):33–41, 2009 19293742

Epel ES, Crosswell AD, Mayer SE, et al: More than a feeling: a unified view of stress measurement for population science. Front Neuroendocrinol 49:146–169, 2018 29551356

Fedorowicz M, Arena O, Burrowes K: Community Engagement during the COVID-19 Pandemic and Beyond: A Guide for Community-Based Organizations. Washington, DC, Urban Institute, 2020

Fazel M, Stratford HJ, Rowsell E, et al: Five applications of narrative exposure therapy for children and adolescents presenting with post-traumatic stress disorders. Front Psychiatry 11:19, 2020 32140112

Fu C, Underwood C: A meta-review of school-based disaster interventions for child and adolescent survivors. J Child Adolesc Ment Health 27(3):161–171, 2015 26890398

Glynn LM, Davis EP, Luby JL, et al: A predictable home environment may protect child mental health during the COVID-19 pandemic. Neurobiol Stress 14:100291, 2021 33532520

Gray KM, Squeglia LM: Research review: what have we learned about adolescent substance use? J Child Psychol Psychiatry 59(6):618–627, 2018 28714184

Guo J, Fu M, Liu D, et al: Is the psychological impact of exposure to COVID-19 stronger in adolescents with pre-pandemic maltreatment experiences? A survey of rural Chinese adolescents. Child Abuse Negl 110(Pt 2):104667, 2020 32859393

Hamatani S, Hiraoka D, Makita K, et al: Longitudinal impact of COVID-19 pandemic on mental health of children in the ABCD study cohort. Sci Rep 12(1):19601, 2022 36379997

Inter-agency Network for Education in Emergencies: Guidelines for Child Friendly Spaces in Emergencies. New York, Inter-agency Network for Education in Emergencies, 2011. Available at: https://inee.org/resources/guidelines-child-friendly-spaces-emergencies. Accessed April 4, 2024.

Jaworski BK, Taylor K, Ramsey KM, et al: Exploring usage of COVID Coach, a public mental health app designed for the COVID-19 pandemic: evaluation of analytics data. J Med Internet Res 23(3):e26559, 2021 33606656

Jaycox LH, Cohen JA, Mannarino AP, et al: Children's mental health care following Hurricane Katrina: a field trial of trauma-focused psychotherapies. J Trauma Stress 23(2):223–231, 2010 20419730

Jaycox LH, Langley AK, Stein BD, et al: Support for students exposed to trauma: a pilot study. School Ment Health 1(2):49–60, 2009 20811511

Jaycox LH, Kataoka SH, Stein BD, et al: Cognitive behavioral intervention for trauma in schools. J Appl Sch Psychol 28(3):239–255, 2012

La Greca AM, Brodar KE, Tarlow N, et al: Evacuation- and hurricane-related experiences, emotional distress, and their associations with mothers' health risk behaviors. Health Psychol 41(7):443–454, 2022 35727322

Masten AS, Osofsky JD: Disasters and their impact on child development: introduction to the special section. Child Dev 81(4):1029–1039, 2010 20636680

Meersand P, Gilmore KJ: Play Therapy: A Psychodynamic Primer for the Treatment of Young Children. Washington, DC, American Psychiatric Association Publishing, 2017

Narayan AJ, Rivera LM, Bernstein RE, et al: Positive childhood experiences predict less psychopathology and stress in pregnant women with childhood adversity: a pilot study of the benevolent childhood experiences (BCEs) scale. Child Abuse Negl 78:19–30, 2018 28992958

National Academies of Sciences, Engineering, and Medicine: Addressing the Long-Term Effects of the COVID-19 Pandemic on Children and Families. Washington, DC, National Academies Press, 2023

Ohnuma A, Narita Z, Tachimori H, et al: Associations between media exposure and mental health among children and parents after the Great East Japan Earthquake. Eur J Psychotraumatol 14(1):2163127, 2023 37052091

Peek L: Children and disasters: understanding vulnerability, developing capacities, and promoting resilience—an introduction. Child Youth Environ 18(1):1–29, 2008

Pfefferbaum B, Shaw JA; American Academy of Child and Adolescent Psychiatry Committee on Quality Issues: Practice parameter on disaster preparedness. J Am Acad Child Adolesc Psychiatry 52(11):1224–1238, 2013 24157398

Pfefferbaum B, Jacobs AK, Nitiéma P, et al: Child debriefing: a review of the evidence base. Prehosp Disaster Med 30(3):306–315, 2015 25868757

Pine DS, Cohen JA: Trauma in children and adolescents: risk and treatment of psychiatric sequelae. Biol Psychiatry 51(7):519–531, 2002 11950454

Raphael B, Wooding S: Debriefing: its evolution and current status. Psychiatr Clin North Am 27(3):407–423, 2004 15325485

Rose S, Bisson J, Wessely S: A systematic review of single-session psychological interventions ('debriefing') following trauma. Psychother Psychosom 72(4):176–184, 2003 12792122

Salloum A, Overstreet S: Evaluation of individual and group grief and trauma interventions for children post disaster. J Clin Child Adolesc Psychol 37(3):495–507, 2008 18645741

Save the Children: Rewriting the Future for Children: Annual Report 2007. Westport, CT, Save the Children. 2007. Available at: www.savethechildren.org/content/dam/usa/reports/annual-report/annual-report/sc-2007-annualreport.pdf. Accessed April 4, 2024.

Schaefer CE, Drewes AA: The Therapeutic Powers of Play: 20 Core Agents of Change, 2nd Edition. Hoboken, NJ, Wiley, 2014

Schildkraut J, Nickerson AB: Lockdown Drills: Connecting Research and Best Practices for School Administrators, Teachers, and Parents. Cambridge, MA, MIT Press, 2022

Schonfeld DJ, Demaria T, Krug SE, et al: Providing psychosocial support to children and families in the aftermath of disasters and crises. Pediatrics 136(4):e1120–e1130, 2015 26371193

Schreiber M, Gurwitch R, Wong M, et al: Listen, Protect, Connect—Model and Teach: Psychological First Aid (PFA) for Students and Teachers. Washington, DC, U.S. Department of Homeland Security, 2006. Available at: https://files.eric.ed.gov/fulltext/ED496719.pdf. Accessed April 4, 2024.

Seddighi H, Salmani I, Javadi MH, et al: Child abuse in natural disasters and conflicts: a systematic review. Trauma Violence Abuse 22(1):176–185, 2021 30866745

Shibley H, Stoddard F: Child and adolescent psychiatry interventions, in Disaster Psychiatry: Readiness, Evaluation and Treatment. American Psychiatric Publishing, Washington, DC, 2011, pp 287–312

United Nations: Convention on the Rights of the Child, New York, 20 November 1989. United Nations Treaty Series, Vol 1577. New York, United Nations, 1989. Available at: https://treaties.un.org/Pages/ViewDetails.aspx?src=TREATY&mtdsg_no=IV-11&chapter=4&clang=_en. Accessed February 26, 2023.

UNICEF: Community-based mental health and psychosocial support in humanitarian settings. New York, UNICEF, 2018a. Available at: www.unicef.org/media/52171/file. Accessed April 4, 2024.

UNICEF: Displaced families face aftermath of indonesia earthquake and tsunami. New York, UNICEF, 2018b. Available at: www.unicef.org/stories/displaced-families-face-aftermath-indonesia-earthquake-and-tsunami. Accessed April 4, 2024.

20

Geriatric Psychiatry Interventions

Helen Kyomen, M.D.
Robert Roca, M.D.
Kenneth Sakauye, M.D.

Disasters occur when a community is "not appropriately resourced or organized to withstand the impact, and whose population is vulnerable because of poverty, exclusion or socially disadvantaged in some way" (Mizutori 2020). Even if older adults live in communities that are appropriately resourced or organized to respond to disasters, they may have certain personal susceptibilities that make them vulnerable to disasters. Many—but not all—older adults are a vulnerable population because of 1) frailty that substantially limits their reserve capacity and ability to rebound adequately from stressors in a timely fashion, 2) diminished psychosocial networks and supports that significantly exclude them from accessing mainstream community resources, and 3) decreased economic flexibility due to reduced or fixed incomes or even poverty.

Disasters are preventable. Hazards can be prevented from progressing to disasters by helping communities prepare, reduce their risks, and become more resilient (International Federation of Red Cross and Red Crescent Societies 2024). In this chapter, we provide a framework for how communities can help prevent hazards from progressing to disasters in vulnerable older adults and can intervene with vulnerable older adults when disaster does strike.

How Disasters Can Be Different for Vulnerable Older Adults Compared With Younger Adults

Disaster-related actions taken for persons of all ages include preparedness, risk reduction, and interventions. Older adults who have developed and expanded their coping abilities over a lifetime have been found to have improved abilities to adapt and achieve heightened resilience (Foster 1997; McClain et al. 2018; Perez-Rojo et al. 2022; Pietrzak et al. 2013; Rafiey et al. 2016). However, about 80% of older adults have at least one chronic health condition that may make them more vulnerable during a disaster than individuals without any chronic illnesses. Together with aging-related physiological, sensory, cognitive, and functional changes, these chronic conditions may cause increased special needs in frail older adults (Aldrich and Benson 2008). It is especially important to consider the impacts of frailty, diminished psychosocial networks and supports, and decreased economic flexibility on each factor of preparedness, risk reduction, and interventions in such vulnerable older adults (Table 20–1).

Preparedness involves a general evaluation of risk. Although many different types of hazards can progress to disasters, and each poses its own set of unique risks, there is a general perspective for identifying who has the greatest risk for negative outcomes on the basis of a dose-response hypothesis. The Substance Abuse and Mental Health Services Administration (SAMHSA) outlined six broad groups in decreasing order of risk for psychiatric sequelae after a disaster (Table 20–2). This list applies equally to the older adult population.

Having essential descriptive characteristics (e.g., age, gender, family composition, cognitive function, physical function, health status, level of interaction with neighbors, participation in community activities) (Hattori et al. 2021) and needs assessment information about each of the six groups in the hierarchy would provide a basic sense of the potential magnitude of resources and risk reduction that may be needed in disaster situations. However, such data can be lacking for the young-old, middle-old, and very/oldest-old subgroups of older adults because of underreporting about, lack of attention to, and lack of statistics specific to older adults.

Although SAMHSA risk group 5 (government officials, groups that identify with victims, and businesses impacted by the disaster) and group 6 (the community at large) are considered to be at lower risk, older indi-

TABLE 20–1. Factors that influence vulnerability in the older adult population during disasters

Factors that increase vulnerability

    Decreased sensory awareness (e.g., from cognitive impairment)

    Preexisting medical conditions and frailty

    Impaired physical mobility

    Socioeconomic limitations (e.g., low income, low reading skills, language barriers)

    Preexisting psychiatric morbidity

    Social isolation

Factor that serves as a buffer

    Positive social supports

Source. Sakauye 2011.

TABLE 20–2. Dose-response hypothesis of risk

SAMHSA risk group hierarchy (from most to least at risk)

1. Seriously injured victims; bereaved family members

2. Victims with high exposure to trauma; evacuees

3. Bereaved extended family members and friends; rescue and recovery workers; service providers involved with death notifications and bereaved families

4. People who have lost homes, jobs, pets, or valued possessions; mental health providers; clergy and chaplains; emergency health care providers; school personnel involved with survivors or families of victims; media personnel covering the disaster

5. Government officials; groups that identify with target victim group; businesses with financial impacts

6. Community at large

Note. SAMHSA=Substance Abuse and Mental Health Services Administration.
Source. U.S. Department of Health and Human Services 2023.

viduals in these groups may perceive their stress as extreme because of uncertainty about the future; insecurity; loss of a supportive community, infrastructure, or essential services; having no doctors, churches, stores, phone or internet service, transportation, or mail; interruption of treatment; and seeing little or no progress toward recovery. The following case exemplifies a typical older adult's response in the absence of direct exposure to trauma.

Vignette

Mrs. R, an 85-year-old woman, was living in a life care community when Hurricane Katrina hit New Orleans. The residents relocated to Baton Rouge and did not experience any direct trauma. Mrs. R showed no problems until 2 months after returning to her residence, when staff noticed moderate depression with anxiety, as well as cognitive impairment. Her family had not returned, she had lost touch with many of her old friends, there was no telephone service, 90% of the staff members were new, and news reports left her convinced that it would take 10 years just to remove the debris from the city. Mrs. R felt hopeless and was mourning the loss of her city.

Social supports, which are a primary buffer against stress, are often lost after a disaster and compound the impact of loss. The American Association for Geriatric Psychiatry (AAGP) Disaster Preparedness Task Force prepared a position statement about the needs of older adults (Sakauye et al. 2009). An unexpected finding by this group included the fact that older adults typically request less disaster financial aid than do younger groups. This may be related to the perceived stigma about receiving aid, an increased desire for self-reliance, concern about loss of other entitlements, and lower reading skills or language barriers that increase difficulty navigating bureaucratic systems. Whatever the reason, older adults have greater difficulty achieving economic recovery after a disaster. Outreach and direct offers of assistance to older adults are frequently required rather than waiting for a call for help.

Older adults seem to have a higher propensity not to heed governmental warnings to evacuate. In part, their choice may be due to prior successful disaster experiences, which may give them a false sense of security and result in an increased tendency to refuse to leave their home in the face of a pending disaster.

Older adults who are at highest risk for negative outcomes include the following:

- Persons who are of advanced age
- Persons who are frail or have complex medical illness
- Persons who have cognitive impairment (e.g., dementia, major neurocognitive disorder [MNCD] or minor neurocognitive disorder [mNCD])
- Persons with severe mental illness or chronic disability due to mental illness (e.g., schizophrenia, affective disorder, depression)
- Persons with impaired mobility
- Persons with sensory impairment
- Persons who lack close family caregivers or local social supports

Dementia or MNCD is a special issue because older adults with dementia or MNCD lack the capacity to understand or cope with stress, have an inability to communicate needs, and have a much higher risk for developing delirium during illness. Since 2013, DSM-5 (American Psychiatric Association 2013) has included the diagnostic class *neurocognitive disorders* to replace older diagnostic terms such as dementia, delirium, amnestic, and other cognitive disorders. MNCD refers to a subdiagnosis indicating greater severity of mental disorders such as cognitive disorders, various forms of dementia, and head trauma. A pivotal addition is mNCD, which is defined by a noticeable decrement in cognitive functioning that goes beyond normal changes seen in aging. Although dementia or MNCD clearly implies severe dysfunction, mNCD can be expected to limit coping as well because of measurable declines in memory and executive function.

Psychiatric Outcomes of Disasters in Older Adults

The hierarchy of responses first described by Lindemann (1944/1994) after the 1942 Cocoanut Grove nightclub fire is still the most commonly used conceptual framework for estimating the mental health effects of disasters. In response to acute trauma, people may experience a range of reactions. The majority of people cope well, many have immediate minor stress responses, some experience delayed responses of anxiety and depression, and a few develop persistent posttraumatic stress disorder (PTSD). This model can be graphed as illustrated in Figure 20–1, with increasingly fewer people showing persisting problems over time. In general, most people are resilient, including older adults.

Estimates of rates of specific mental illnesses following a disaster differ widely by the type of disaster, extent of the destruction, speed of recovery from the disaster, and individual factors. The Community Advisory Group surveyed 815 adults who lived in the areas hit by Hurricane Katrina and who requested help from the Red Cross (Kessler et al. 2008). Interviews were conducted 5–8 months after the disaster and again 1 year after that. Although an age breakdown was not provided for the sample, 41.8% showed serious mental illness or PTSD 18 months after the hurricane, and 6.4% showed persisting suicidal ideation. In general, in the geriatric population, mood, anxiety, and PTSD symptoms that are seen in younger adults occur less reliably, and acute stress may be expressed in a somatic way. A rise in substance abuse does not appear to be as much of a problem as in younger populations.

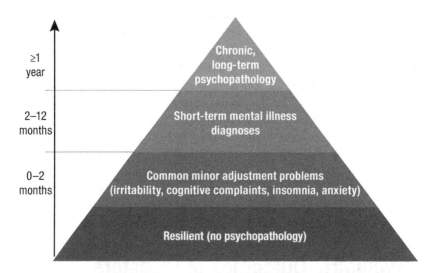

FIGURE 20–1. Hierarchy of responses to trauma.

This schematic illustrates that many people cope well after a trauma, although most will show mild adjustment difficulties early on. Intermediate effects after 2 months demonstrate that many (approximately one-third) will develop a major mental illness diagnosis. Some will experience long-term problems, but the majority of trauma victims will not.

Mild memory impairment following trauma has been an underrecognized problem in the older adult population. After Hurricane Katrina, this was commonly referred to by the locals as "Katrina brain." It has been a general finding that anxiety often leads to a memory disorder. In older persons under extreme stress, one often sees entrenched memories, such as in PTSD, or the converse of amnesia or thought blocking. The neurobiological basis has been speculated to be a disruption of frontocingulate circuits due to hypothalamic-pituitary-adrenal axis and cortisol dysfunction causing disruption of cholinergic and frontal dopamine circuits. Interconnections among the thalamus, amygdala, and hippocampus suggest a reason for the strong association between memory and stress. The main reasons to be aware of the association of stress and memory impairment are to avoid overdiagnosing MNCD in older adult persons after a disaster and to avoid making cognitive impairment worse through use of benzodiazepines and other tranquilizers.

A different array of psychiatric disorders may be associated with disasters such as pandemics that have direct pathophysiological effects on the central nervous system. For example, during the coronavirus disease 2019 (COVID-19) pandemic, delirium was the most common serious psychiatric disorder seen among older adults infected with the virus. At times, it was the predominant presenting symptom, overshadowing the pulmonary signs and symptoms typically associated with the illness. COVID-19 delirium has been speculated to be caused by infection of the central nervous system by the virus, by *cytokine storms* precipitated by the immune response to the virus, and/or the effects of the virus on other organ systems (e.g., hypoxia due to respiratory failure). Some of these mechanisms have been invoked as possible explanations for other psychiatric manifestations of COVID-19, such as the emergence or exacerbation of major mood and psychotic disorders. These mechanisms may also play a role in the emergence of some of the late sequelae of COVID-19, including "brain fog"—a core component of so-called *long COVID*—and PTSD, a condition associated with severe illness requiring care in an intensive care unit.

In 2011, a powerful earthquake and subsequent tsunami resulted in a nuclear accident in Fukushima, Japan—the first complex disaster in history that included both natural and nuclear power disasters. Among patients already diagnosed with dementia who were exposed to these disasters, Miyagawa et al. (2021) noted a difference in the manifestation of the behavioral and psychological symptoms of dementia (BPSD). There was a significant increase in the BPSD of agitation and irritability in the early post–complex disaster phase and a significant increase in the BPSD of hallucinations and delusions in the late post–complex disaster phase.

Disaster Intervention Strategies for Older Adults

Disaster response can be conceptually divided into three phases: immediate response (first week or so), early or acute response (1 week to 2 months), and late or postacute response (2 months and longer). In all phases, care providers must be alert to the risk of negative psychiatric outcomes after a disaster and should know the signs of emotional distress.

In general, for the older adult, at any phase of response, it is important to do the following:

- Triage for patients at risk
- Check for prior psychiatric history
- Avoid interruption of psychotropic medication treatment
- Screen for depression, anxiety, cognitive impairment, and psychosis
- Check for substance use
- Avoid medications on the Beers Criteria for potentially inappropriate medications in older adults (2019 American Geriatrics Society Beers Criteria Update Expert Panel 2019)

Patients with known psychiatric illness or cognitive problems need additional support, as well as continuation of existing medications. Because of compromised health or cognitive impairment, older adults are more likely to need social support to mitigate the effects of stress. In addition, responses to each phase (immediate, acute, and postacute) emphasize different issues.

Immediate Response

Psychological First Aid (PFA) should be provided as an immediate response. PFA involves addressing immediate needs, ensuring immediate physical safety, attending to physical comfort, promoting social engagement, protecting from additional trauma or trauma reminders, attending to grief and spiritual issues, helping with finding family if separated from them, attending to traumatic grief, and stabilizing emotionally overwhelmed survivors (see also Chapter 16, "Psychological First Aid"). Continuation of medical treatment regimens must be assured, and psychotropic medication may be needed for anxiety or sleep if the benefits outweigh the risks of treatment. PFA has been provided in both group and individual venues. Strategically, the goal of psychological first response is aimed at providing a sense of control and mastery over the trauma.

PFA for patients with MNCD is qualitatively different from that for other individuals. One can anticipate agitation after a trauma in most patients with MNCD. Even minor life changes can feel catastrophic to a patient with MNCD and can cause agitation. Having an attachment figure to reassure and protect the individual in times of stress is far more beneficial than taking medication. However, if medications are needed, the main guideline in MNCD care after a disaster is to avoid using medications listed in the Beers Criteria for potentially inappropriate medication use in the older adult (2019 American Geriatrics Society Beers Criteria Update Expert Panel 2019). Medications that are usually inappropriate include sedative psychotropics (e.g., chlorpromazine, doxepin, trazodone), antihistamines (e.g., diphenhydramine), or other medications with high anticholinergic potential. Starting dosages for older adult patients, especially for those who are frail or have MNCD, should be at least 50% less than the usual starting dosages for younger patients.

Acute Response

Screening high-risk patients and doing evaluations on the high-risk group are important in the acute response phase. A triage tool for vulnerable older adults was developed after Hurricane Katrina to identify compromised elders without family help. Developed by Dyer et al. (2008), this simple screening instrument taps three main areas: 1) not having any social support or being separated from social supports; 2) existing health, memory, or activities of daily living (ADL) limitations; and 3) need for case management. In addition, it is essential to avoid interruption of psychiatric and medical treatment to minimize the risk of relapse.

After high-risk or symptomatic individuals are identified, they should be referred for treatment or further evaluation. Appropriate response is impossible to achieve if a large geographic area has been devastated and the social infrastructure has been destroyed. In the absence of hospitals, gas, water, electricity, roads, food distribution, housing, sewage, medical supplies, telephones, and professionals, patients cannot receive help locally. Arrangements must be available for evacuation to intact service areas if needed. If communication systems are intact, or once they are restored, some of this acute support may be provided by means of telepsychiatry, including telephone-only services. Such access was a critical lifeline to needed services during the height of the COVID-19 pandemic.

The most common needs in this phase are primarily social and environmental. Important goals are to reunify families, rebuild the infrastructure to make life livable, provide reliable information, continue medications, evacuate the most severely impaired to a place where hospital care can be provided, and offer social support to the most isolated individuals. The last of these—social support to isolated older adults—was especially critical during the protracted period of quarantining during COVID-19, and an inspiring array of creative approaches to this problem were devised in short order during the pandemic. Such approaches included increased use of telehealth, more depression screening, availability of free home deliveries, communication by email and video chat, and more outreach calls.

MNCD care requires a stable and expectable environment, preferably with familiar people or family. Adding psychotropic medications should be avoided, but if patients need them, they should not be given highly sedating medications, benzodiazepines, or highly anticholinergic medications. Restraints should also be avoided because they often increase agitation. Behavioral management techniques include stimulus control, cognitive-behavioral techniques (e.g., skill elicitation, differential reinforcement), reorientation, structured social activities, and staff training on improving communication techniques.

Postacute Response

In the postacute phase, some patients will need formal psychiatric treatment. Psychotherapy and psychotropic medications may be needed. Patients with MNCD may seem worse after a disaster, although it is unclear whether the apparent deterioration in cognition and ADL functions is permanent or whether the patient can recover. The appearance of psychiatric symptoms, such as psychosis, depression, or agitated behaviors, is assumed to be reversible.

There is no best treatment approach for anxiety disorders, partly because there are many subtypes of anxiety disorders and most studies focus only on generalized anxiety disorder or PTSD. Few outcome studies have specifically addressed older adults. Typically, the psychotherapy choice consists of eclectic models that are matched with the person. According to our review of the literature, the following treatment hierarchy is applied: First, patients are taught palliative or distraction techniques (relaxation exercises, meditation, soothing thoughts). If symptoms persist, cognitive-behavioral therapy is tried. The goal is to help the patient gain control over specific symptoms through problem-solving skills, guided imagery, or psychoeducation. Some patients will need more time-intensive, insight-oriented therapies that focus on developing awareness and understanding of unconscious influences on present behaviors and unconscious resistances. Medication approaches have shifted to use of antidepressants—namely, selective serotonin reuptake inhibitors or serotonin-norepinephrine reuptake inhibitors—as the initial trial. In older adults, treatment of major psychiatric disorders, such as major depression or psychosis, does not differ from traditional approaches.

It is important to recognize that the postacute impact may extend well beyond the immediate aftermath of the disaster. To some observers, it seems paradoxical that most trauma victims do well in the acute phase, which is sometimes referred to as the "honeymoon period." However, calling it a honeymoon period is a misnomer. There is nothing pleasant or vacation-like about this period. Disillusionment, anniversary reactions, grief, anxiety, or depression begin to emerge in susceptible individuals in the postacute period. The explanation for this pattern was first predicted by Maslow's hierarchy of needs (Maslow 1943). When one is in survival mode the motivation is physiological. One is driven to secure food, money, housing, medical care, and basic survival. It is not until one's life is beginning to settle down that one becomes aware of higher-order needs such as psychological distress and worries about one's future. For some, the course of recovery is lengthy and uncertain.

Preparation

Because of the nearly global lack of attention to older adult issues in the literature to date, it is imperative to designate older adults as a special population within state disaster plans. The AAGP Disaster Preparedness Task Force (Sakauye et al. 2009) recommended the following:

- Modify state disaster plans to include special plans for frail older adults and patients with MNCD that address communication needs to ensure that older adults are warned of impending disasters when possible.
- Take special precautions for the frail older adult, such as ensuring access to safe houses, and train care providers on unique population needs (e.g., management of MNCD).
- To avoid interruption of treatment, MedicAlert jewelry or microchip implants can be helpful, as can electronic medical records that can be accessed from distant sites.
- Train first responders how to deal with frail older adults.
- Establish services for frail older adults or persons with MNCD and contingency plans in the event the primary plan falls short.
- Develop plans to prevent separation from family and pets.
- Identify programs that deal with older adults and make prior arrangements with the state or federal agencies in charge to involve these programs in recovery efforts.

Toner et al. (2010) expanded on many of the issues listed above in their book *Geriatric Mental Health Disaster and Emergency Preparedness*. They provided several examples of model disaster response programs, including the collaborative Geriatric Emergency Preparedness and Response initiative and the Canadian model (Emergency Management Policy and Outreach Directorate 2017). They emphasized the importance of team management and training. One model involved special training using character role-play cards to teach how to deliver care to special populations. The dissemination of similar training through the American Red Cross might be an important first step in improving geriatric disaster care.

The Centers for Medicare and Medicaid Services (CMS) Survey and Certification Group developed a website (www.cms.gov/Medicare/Provider-Enrollment-and-Certification/SurveyCertEmergPrep) to provide useful information to CMS central and regional offices; state survey agencies; state, tribal, regional, and local emergency management partners; and health care providers for the development of effective and vital emergency plans and responses. This website uses an all-hazards approach to provide information and tools for dealing with natural, human-made, and technological disruptive events, including pandemic flu, hurricanes, tornadoes, fires, earthquakes, power outages, chemical spills, and nuclear or biological terrorist attacks. Both mandated and voluntary emergency preparedness information and tools are available at the website. The website is updated regularly to include helpful guidance concerning 1) clarification of the roles, responsibilities, and actions of CMS central and regional survey and certification offices; 2) clarification of the roles, responsibilities, and actions of state survey agencies; and 3) effective emergency planning across all health care provider types to ensure the well-being of vulnerable populations—whether in long-term care, acute care, or community-based venues—during a disruptive event.

A final rule regarding emergency preparedness requirements for Medicare and Medicaid participating providers and suppliers was published in the *Federal Register* by the CMS and the U.S. Department of Health and Human Services on September 16, 2016. This regulation became effective November 16, 2016. Health care providers and suppliers affected by this rule were to be adherent and apply all regulations 1 year after the effective date, on November 15, 2017. On September 30, 2019, CMS published in the *Federal Register* "The Medicare and Medicaid Programs; Regulatory Provisions To Promote Program Efficiency, Transparency, and Burden Reduction; Fire Safety Requirements for Certain Dialysis Facilities; Hospital and Critical Access Hospital (CAH) Changes To Promote Innovation, Flexibility, and Improvement in Patient Care Final Rule," which revised some of the original emergency preparedness requirements for providers and suppliers (Centers for Medicare and Medicaid Services 2019, 2023).

Conclusion

It is important to recognize that many older adults are survivors who may be underrecognized sources of resilience, adaptive coping, and response in times of crises, yet they are still at risk for psychiatric problems after a trauma, especially if they are frail or have a cognitive or health disability. ADL limitations and cognition should be assessed in all vulnerable older adults, and family support should be assessed for limitations. It is crucial to continue existing treatment to prevent potential relapse of any preexisting illness. It is also important to avoid benzodiazepines, sedative antihistamines, anticholinergic medications, and polypharmacy because of known risks for falls and confusion.

References

American Psychiatric Association: Diagnostic and Statistical Manual of Mental Disorders, 5th Edition. Arlington, VA, American Psychiatric Association, 2013
2019 American Geriatrics Society Beers Criteria Update Expert Panel: American Geriatrics Society 2019 updated AGS Beers Criteria for potentially inappro-

priate medication use in older adults. J Am Geriatr Soc 67(4):674–694, 2019 30693946

Aldrich N, Benson WF: Disaster preparedness and the chronic disease needs of vulnerable older adults. Prev Chronic Dis 5(1):A27, 2008 18082016

Centers for Medicare and Medicaid Services: The Medicare and Medicaid Programs; Regulatory Provisions To Promote Program Efficiency, Transparency, and Burden Reduction; Fire Safety Requirements for Certain Dialysis Facilities; Hospital and Critical Access Hospital (CAH) Changes To Promote Innovation, Flexibility, and Improvement in Patient Care Final Rule. Federal Register, September 30, 2019. Available at: www.federalregister.gov/documents/2019/09/30/2019-20736/medicare-and-medicaid-programs-regulatory-provisions-to-promote-program-efficiency-transparency-and. Accessed February 26, 2023.

Centers for Medicare and Medicaid Services: Quality, safety and oversight group—emergency preparedness: emergency preparedness for every emergency. Baltimore, MD, U.S. Centers for Medicare and Medicaid Services, September 6, 2023. www.cms.gov/Medicare/Provider-Enrollment-and-Certification/SurveyCertEmergPrep. Accessed February 26, 2023.

Dyer CB, Regev M, Burnett J, et al: SWiFT: a rapid triage tool for vulnerable older adults in disaster situations. Disaster Med Public Health Prep 2(Suppl 1):S45–S50, 2008 18769267

Emergency Management Policy and Outreach Directorate: An Emergency Management Framework for Canada, Third Edition. Ottawa, Public Safety Canada, 2017. Available at: www.publicsafety.gc.ca/cnt/rsrcs/pblctns/2017-mrgnc-mngmnt-frmwrk/index-en.aspx. Accessed July 5, 2024.

Foster JR: Successful coping, adaptation and resilience in the elderly: an interpretation of epidemiologic data. Psychiatr Q 68(3):189–219, 1997 9237317

Hattori Y, Isowa T, Hiramatsu M, et al: Disaster preparedness of persons requiring special care ages 75 years and older living in areas at high risk of earthquake disasters: a cross-sectional study from the Pacific coast region of western Japan. Disaster Med Public Health Prep 15(4):469–477, 2021 32425149

International Federation of Red Cross and Red Crescent Societies: What is a disaster? Geneva, Switzerland, International Federation of Red Cross and Red Crescent Societies, 2024. Available at: www.ifrc.org/our-work/disasters-climate-and-crises/what-disaster. Accessed April 5, 2024.

Kessler RC, Galea S, Gruber MJ, et al: Trends in mental illness and suicidality after Hurricane Katrina. Mol Psychiatry 13:374–384, 2008 18180768

Lindemann E: Symptomatology and management of acute grief. 1944. Am J Psychiatry 151(6 Suppl):155–190, 1994 8192191

Maslow AH: A Theory of Human Motivation. Psychol Rev 50:370-396, 1943

McClain J, Gullatt K, Lee C: Resilience and Protective Factors in Older Adults. Culminating Capstone project, Dominican University of California, San Rafael, California, May 2018. Available at: https://scholar.dominican.edu/cgi/viewcontent.cgi?article=1305&context=masters-theses. Accessed April 5, 2024.

Miyagawa A, Kunii Y, Gotoh D, et al: Effects of the Great East Japan Earthquake and the Fukushima Daiichi Nuclear Power Plant accident on behavioural and psychological symptoms of dementia among patients. Psychogeriatrics 21(5):709–715, 2021 34089277

Mizutori M: Time to say goodbye to "natural" disasters. Geneva, Switzerland, United Nations Office for Disaster Risk Reduction, 2020. Available at:

www.preventionweb.net/drr-community-voices/time-say-goodbye-natural-disasters. Accessed July 10, 2024.

Perez-Rojo G, López J, Noriega C, et al: A multidimensional approach to the resilience in older adults despite COVID-19. BMC Geriatr 22(1):793, 2022 36221056

Pietrzak RH, Van Ness PH, Fried TR, et al: Trajectories of posttraumatic stress symptomatology in older persons affected by a large-magnitude disaster. J Psychiatr Res 47(4):520–526, 2013 23290559

Rafiey H, Momtaz YA, Alipour F, et al: Are older people more vulnerable to long-term impacts of disasters? Clin Interv Aging 11:1791–1795, 2016 27994445

Sakauye K: Geriatric psychiatry interventions, in Disaster Psychiatry: Readiness, Evaluation, and Treatment. Edited by Stoddard FJ, Pandya A, Katz CL. Washington, DC, American Psychiatric Publishing, 2011, pp 313–326

Sakauye KM, Streim JE, Kennedy GJ, et al: AAGP position statement: disaster preparedness for older Americans: critical issues for the preservation of mental health. Am J Geriatr Psychiatry 17(11):916–924, 2009 20104050

Toner JA, Meirswa TM, Howe JL (eds): Geriatric Mental Health Disaster and Emergency Preparedness. New York, Springer, 2010

U.S. Department of Health and Human Services: Mental Health All-Hazards Disaster Planning Guidance (DHHS Publ No SMA 3829). Rockville, MD, Center for Mental Health Services, Substance Abuse and Mental Health Services Administration, 2003. Available at https://store.samhsa.gov/product/SMA03-3829. Accessed July 5, 2024.

21

Humanitarian Mental Health

Psychosocial Response in the Context of Conflict, Climate Change, and Refugee Crisis

Giuseppe Raviola, M.D., M.P.H.
Vinh-Son Nguyen, M.D.
Sander Koyfman, M.D., M.B.A.

Rapidly Shifting Postpandemic Global Context

In 2021, the annual threat assessment of the U.S. intelligence community (Office of the Director of National Intelligence 2021) reported that the United States and its allies would face a diverse array of threats, which are now playing out amid the global disruption resulting from the coronavirus disease 2019 (COVID-19) pandemic. This is occurring against the backdrop of great power competition, the disruptive effects of ecological degradation and a changing climate, an increasing number of empowered nonstate actors, and rapidly evolving technology. The complexity of the threats, their intersections, and the potential for cascading events in an increasingly interconnected and mobile world create new challenges for the international community.

Escalating tensions in the world, including the 2022 Russian invasion of Ukraine, the 2023 Israel-Gaza crisis, global economic issues spurred by both energy and food insecurity, and rapidly emerging and evolving technologies, continue to be disruptive to traditional business and society, creating unprecedented vulnerabilities. Over the past several decades it has become increasingly challenging to predict the impact of such challenges on the global landscape (Office of the Director of National Intelligence 2023). Over the past several years we have increasingly operated in a new state of *polycrisis*, defined by a cross-cutting, cascading set of global challenges that spans pandemic, climate (e.g., droughts, floods, megastorms, wildfires, extreme heat and cold), and conflict (Lawrence et al. 2022). These overlapping and varied scenarios are accompanied by resulting food and water shortages, lack of safety, and—by extension—human migration and growing refugee emergencies, new conflicts over resources, and unstable political and national actors. COVID-19; structural racism; health inequities; climate change; and other concurrent health, economic, and social crises intersect and have had adverse impacts on the mental health of both individuals and providers of care. The postpandemic global context is therefore increasingly defined by growing complexity and uncertainty.

All of these global concerns should inspire an urgency to synthesize current knowledge in disaster readiness. Organizations must attend to these crises holistically, prioritizing mental health across sectors (an in-all-policies public health approach to mental health) without losing sight of the care of people living with preexisting mental health conditions (Kienzler 2019). Doing so would enshrine what has been common knowledge for generations but finally is being acknowledged, often through the lens of self-care, in a growing array of settings. Synthesis of current knowledge should include best practices in disaster psychiatry as well as draw from the fields of global health, mental health and psychosocial support (MHPSS), and global mental health delivery.

Global health delivery describes the practice of implementing interventions to improve health care delivery in low-resource settings, with attention to epidemiology, pathophysiology, culture, economics, politics, and social determinants, as well as clinical care (Farmer et al. 2013; Harvard Medical School 2023). The field of global health can inform practices that restructure the work force, build mental health knowledge and capacity outside the health sector, and use *task sharing*, the engagement of community members and nonclinicians to scale community preparedness on the basis of core psychosocial principles. Global health delivery begins with the question of how health systems can efficiently provide health services to all who need them in equitable ways. Attention must be given to the complex social and structural forces that inform ill health, including poverty, inequality, and environmental degradation, which requires a broad-based agenda of social change (Farmer et al. 2013). With climate change and COVID-19 has come a growing emphasis on responses to humanitarian crises in the context of conflict and displacement. The field of global health has integrated the concepts of MHPSS, which refers to any type of local or outside support that seeks to protect or promote psychosocial well-being and to prevent or treat mental disorders, particularly in the context of emergency responses (United Nations High Commission for Refugees 2023b).

Refugees, migrants, internally displaced people, and asylum seekers are living on the frontline of the climate emergency and inform our current understanding of the practice of disaster psychiatry, humanitarian crisis response, and global mental health delivery (United Nations High Commission for Refugees 2023a) (Table 21–1). In 2022, 89.3 million people were living forcibly displaced lives worldwide, with 83% hosted in low- and middle-income countries and 72% hosted in neighboring countries (United Nations High Commission for Refugees 2021). Human trafficking is an additional global health crisis, with war and conflict offering hunting grounds for traffickers (Nazer and Greenbaum 2020; United Nations Office on Drugs and Crime 2022).

Beyond the clinical sphere, as we attempt to resettle newly displaced refugees, further consideration should be given to social and structural considerations such as employment and volunteer opportunities for survivors forced into refugee and evacuation settings to gain and apply mutual support skills, with interpreters when needed. Current systems may hinder such engagement of skills and good will, often with the best of intentions. Refugees may be treated as "guests," unable to do paid work. Response planners should anticipate ways to enhance the agency and self-sufficiency of the populations they serve as a psychological imperative for those who have suffered loss of home, job, and meaning. For example, Afghan evacuees in reception centers in the United States demanded to be given resources to teach children to decrease children's distress and idle time, as well as to feel useful themselves. Altruistic activities enhance resilience as children recover from displacement and disasters, and these activities become paths for whole-family engagement.

Even when resettled, refugees may continue to be particularly vulnerable to wage theft, making entry into the mainstream economy that much harder. This requires specialized engagement and protections, with children becoming underequipped spokespersons because they often are

TABLE 21–1. United Nations High Commission for Refugees (UNHCR) selected definitions

Term	Definition
Refugee	A person outside their country of origin who is in need of international protection because of feared persecution or a serious threat to their life, physical integrity, or freedom in their country of origin as a result of persecution, armed conflict, violence, or serious public disorder
Migrant	UNHCR recommends that the word *migrant* not be used as a catchall term to refer to refugees or to people who are likely to be in need of international protection, such as asylum seekers. To do so risks undermining access to the specific legal protections that countries are obliged to provide to refugees.
Internally displaced person	A person who has been forced or obliged to flee from their home or place of habitual residence, in particular as a result of or in order to avoid the effects of armed conflicts, situations of generalized violence, violations of human rights, or natural or human-made disasters and who has not crossed an internationally recognized state border.
Asylum seeker	A general term for any person who is seeking international protection. In some countries, it is used as a legal term referring to a person who has applied for refugee status or a complementary international protection status and has not yet received a final decision on their claim. It can also refer to a person who has not yet submitted an application but may intend to do so or who may be in need of international protection. Not every asylum seeker will ultimately be recognized as a refugee, but every refugee is initially an asylum seeker. However, an asylum seeker may not be sent back to their country of origin until their asylum claim has been examined in a fair procedure, and they are entitled to certain minimum standards of treatment pending determination of their status.

Source. United Nations High Commission for Refugees 2023c.

faster to pick up the language of their new adopted home, through either school or fearlessness. Complex dynamics such as these can and should be considered in resettlement practices. A practical example of an intervention that seeks to address legal inequities that threaten survival of immigrants is Reclamo!, a digital legal tool to help immigrant workers reclaim stolen wages in New York (Nonko 2023).

In addition to addressing social and cultural aspects of vulnerable populations in response to complex crises, expanding collaborative, shared, and even remote-learning platforms is also essential to supporting future expansion of services and research in disaster mental health response to violence and war, climate change, refugee crisis, and other humanitarian crises and disasters. Organizations will increasingly need to attend to the mental health and well-being of essential health care workers and staff as a greater priority. Use of frameworks, care pathways, and associated tools and practices for integrated care takes on greater importance as they move to digital formats. One useful resource for access to such tools is the Mental Health and Psychosocial Support Network (www.mhpss.net), which makes available a variety of open-source tools and resources.

Basic Principles and Practices of Humanitarian Mental Health and Psychosocial Response

The MHPSS framework initially developed in 2007 by the Inter-Agency Standing Committee (IASC) (see Figure 5–1 in Chapter 5, "Communication and Relationships") provides the foundation for effective response across global settings (Inter-Agency Standing Committee 2007). Used in the field of humanitarian response to "emphasize the close connection between psychological aspects of experience and wider social aspects of experience, inclusive of human capacity, social ecology, and culture and values," *psychosocial* interventions are designed to address the psychological effects of conflict, including the effects on behavior, emotion, thoughts, memory and functioning, and social effects, including changes in relationships, social support, and economic status (Meyer 2013). They reflect the World Health Organization (WHO) definition of mental health, "a state of well-being in which an individual realizes his or her own abilities, can cope with the normal stresses of life, can work productively and is able to make a contribution to his or her community. In this positive sense, mental health is the foundation for individual well-being and the effective functioning of a community" (World Health Organization 2022).

Systems

The IASC framework reflects a growing emphasis on needs in the contexts of national and international conflict and displacement, including vulnerable groups and the needs of people with preexisting conditions. Humanitarian emergencies may cause social issues such as family separation; destruction of community structures and social networks; and psychological issues, including depression, grief, anxiety, and stress-related conditions associated with exposure to trauma and displacement (Jones et al. 2009). The MHPSS approach places an emphasis on *functioning*: the ability of an individual to complete daily tasks, including self-care; fulfill relevant social roles as a member of a household, family, and community; and take part in activities such as attending religious events and providing support for community members. It also emphasizes overlap across sectors, including protection concerns, such as sexual or gender-based violence and child abuse (Jones et al. 2009).

Key clinical and care competencies related to the MHPSS approach include the following:

1. A trauma-informed approach grounded in the expectation that most people are resilient and will recover
2. Consideration of how to support existing primary health care workers in providing clinical support
3. Evidence-based approaches to support community members in strengthening community resources
4. Applying principles from the IASC guidelines, balancing clinical services and community-based supports

Awareness and understanding of human rights–related concerns (e.g., accessing resources through the Mental Health and Human Rights Info database at www.hhri.org) is also highly relevant. Of note, in a crisis, the role of the psychiatrist is to be a humanitarian, a colleague, and an advocate while maintaining all the key clinical and training qualifications in taking care of persons with prior and emerging psychiatric needs.

In humanitarian crises, psychiatric clinicians can play a critical role in supporting the training of primary health care workers to care for people in severe distress during a response, as well as serving as leaders by setting an example in sharing care delivery tasks across service provider roles (*task sharing*) (Raviola et al. 2019). Essential elements of task sharing include collaborative care; comprehensive care; establishment of referral pathways, including back referrals; training that is adequate and relevant; support and supervision; incentives and remuneration for providers who are not specialists; and, eventually, career pathways for nonspecialist providers, as a foundation for sustained strengthening of community-based supports.

Parallel key organizational competencies and skills include the following:

1. *Assessment skills to analyze contexts via thorough needs assessments* and coordinating with partners, with attention to avoiding duplication of efforts
2. *Strong managerial skills to oversee and build on existing programs and services,* both during and after humanitarian crises
3. *Ability to elaborate sustained clinical training and supervision models* that are locally acceptable, feasible, and useful in context as well as offering language-appropriate support materials
4. *System design skills for the development of functional data collection systems,* with monitoring and evaluation of data used to improve systems and services
5. *Expertise to facilitate appropriate, well-chosen academic work* such as qualitative or quantitative research methods to evaluate and document completed work

There is need for *longer-term partnerships* between researchers and frontline practitioners to bring research into practice and practice into research (e.g., to ensure humanitarian decision-making based on generated evidence and the implementation of evidence-informed interventions in humanitarian practice) (Tol et al. 2020).

Often, humanitarian MHPSS response requires working within public health systems and in collaboration with government and local leadership. Principles of *building back better* have also been clearly articulated by WHO as crises over the past several decades provided fertile ground for learning how to take every crisis as an opportunity to build better formal mental health services (Epping-Jordan et al. 2015).

The postdisaster time frame serves as a key opportunity to promote medical behavioral integration, adaptation of community resources, and identification of effective system extenders such as teachers or community elders who know the community well (Raviola et al. 2019; see also Friendship Bench at www.friendshipbenchzimbabwe.org). Internationally endorsed tools that can be first consulted in considering humanitarian response include the IASC guidelines (Inter-Agency Standing Committee 2007), the WHO PFA guide (World Health Organization 2011), the

WHO Mental Health Gap Action Programme (mhGAP) intervention guide (World Health Organization 2016), the WHO mhGAP Humanitarian Intervention Guide (World Health Organization 2015a), *UNICEF Operational Guidelines on Community-Based Mental Health and Psychosocial Support in Humanitarian Settings* (UNICEF 2018), and the International Medical Corps Toolkit for the Integration of Mental Health into General Healthcare in Humanitarian Settings (International Medical Corps 2023).

Task Sharing

Task sharing of psychosocial interventions to communities benefits from the strengthening of primary care–delivered mental health services. Psychiatrists can work as part of local teams to elaborate comprehensive, community-based models and systems of care delivery, adapting available international guidance to the crisis. Psychosocial interventions that are delivered outside of health systems require some knowledge of how psychological interventions and psychotherapies (see Chapter 17, "Psychotherapies") have been adapted for use without the presence of specialist providers.

Many psychosocial interventions used in the context of crises in low-resource settings globally have been derived from manualized psychological treatments, such as interpersonal therapy and cognitive-behavioral therapy. Today, there is strong evidence for the effectiveness of components of evidence-based psychological interventions that have been integrated within task-shared models of support using common elements of those interventions to address the precursors of common mental disorders and stress-related disorders (Singla et al. 2017). For example, Problem Management Plus, a scalable, five-session psychological intervention for adults impaired by distress in communities exposed to adversity, integrates elements of managing anxiety and stress, managing problems, behavioral activation, and strengthening social supports (World Health Organization 2015b). Other packages of brief intervention derived from the psychotherapeutic and psychological evidence base include Self-Help Plus, a group-based stress management course (www.who.int/publications/i/item/9789240035119); the Common Elements Treatment Approach, a single treatment approach to address multiple global health problems (CETA Global and Johns Hopkins University, Bloomberg School of Public Health 2014; www.cetaglobal.org); and three-session interpersonal counseling (IPC-3; Global Mental Health Lab 2023; Weissman et al. 2014).

In 2022, WHO and UNICEF introduced the Ensuring Quality in Psychological Support (EQUIP) program to increase the quality of psychological support by improving the competence of helpers and the consistency and quality of training and service delivery (World Health Organization 2021a). The EQUIP platform makes freely available competency assessment tools and e-learning courses to support governments, training institutions, and nongovernmental organizations, both in humanitarian and development settings, to train and supervise the workforce to deliver effective psychological support (World Health Organization 2021a).

The implementation of an MHPSS response to a humanitarian crisis can be envisioned in the context of docking into and strengthening existing formal systems of care, which may be limited depending on the context. In the absence of existing formal mental health systems, accounting for certain key elements of a response in resource-limited settings can engage existing community resources and offer a foundation for the building of services for the longer term. One can consider the essential elements of a task-shared model to build out of disasters collaborative, comprehensive, community-based approaches to care that can also address the complexity of mental health conditions, both common and severe (Figure 21–1).

It is within these emerging collaborative care models that bridge clinical and nonclinical community-based supports that we can expand the reach of mental health support for particularly vulnerable populations. Although each context is different, the skill sets of providers and their interrelationships in an optimal continuum of care can be viewed as a road map for guiding frontline teams in implementing services. Principles underlying the development of collaborative, comprehensive, and community-based care in lower-resource settings include the following (Bolton et al. 2023):

1. Evidence-based practice
2. A collaborative, stepped-care approach at all stages of mental health
3. A family-based approach across the life cycle
4. Integration of MHPSS into community-based services
5. The central role of primary health care providers
6. Dedicated local mental health workers treating multiple and comorbid conditions
7. Support of people living with illness and their families in clinical decision-making
8. Engaging persons with lived experience as providers
9. Workforce care, maintenance, and development

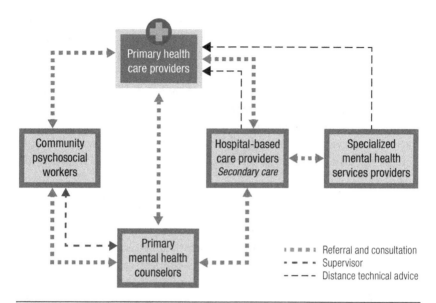

FIGURE 21–1. Complementary roles of five categories of workers delivering components of mental health care in a comprehensive, collaborative, community-based system.

Source. Bolton et al. 2023.

10. Addressing severe mental health conditions
11. Supporting persons with intellectual disabilities and developmental disorders

Practical Applications

In 2010, in response to a devastating earthquake in Haiti, the nongovernmental organization Partners In Health—without a preexisting mental health program at the time—made use of the guidance described here to mount an initial emergency response. The response started with the development of a response coordination team, employing PFA adapted to the context, undertaking initial assessments of pressing local needs, implementing initial management of neuropsychiatric disorders (including psychopharmacological interventions), and establishing appropriate lines of referral (Belkin et al. 2011; Raviola et al. 2012). This initial response included the mapping of existing community-based resources onto a skills package pyramid that anticipated the development of training and programs based on the WHO mhGAP curriculum, as well as the articulation of clinical care pathways, emphasizing task sharing and optimizing the embedding of previously nonexistent mental health skills within cadres of providers and staff (Figure 21–2) (Raviola et al. 2012).

Following the training and implementation of PFA (see Chapter 16), the five essential skills packages for a system pyramid for the initial emergency include 1) case finding, engagement follow-up, and psycho-education (community health workers, teachers, and traditional healers); 2) targeted psychosocial and psychological interventions (social workers, psychologists, and mental health nurses); 3) medication management (generalist physicians); 4) supervision and consultation (clinical supervisors); and 5) quality oversight and quality improvement (a monitoring, evaluation, and quality team) (Belkin et al. 2011). Starting with the initial MHPSS emergency response in Haiti, the system was built and expanded to serve ongoing mental health needs in the context of an ongoing and deteriorating environmental, political, and social crisis in the country, with the iterative elaboration of clinical care pathways to address ongoing mental health service needs, as well as articulation of what were felt by the local teams to be essential system components across broad areas of focus in mental health care delivery (Figure 21–3).

In the year and a half following the earthquake in Haiti, Partners In Health provided 20,000 documented individual and group appointments for mental health and psychosocial needs (Raviola et al. 2012). Increasing numbers of people received care over the subsequent years, including more than 28,000 patient visits between 2016 and 2019 (Raviola et al. 2020). The development of community-based care processes out of the initial earthquake emergency in Haiti were instrumental models in supporting organizational infrastructure and capacity to address new disasters and crises across 10 global sites (United States, Mexico, Peru, Haiti, Sierra Leone, Liberia, Rwanda, Malawi, Lesotho, and Kazakhstan). These included multiple major hurricanes, mudslides, political violence, explosions, the 2014–2016 West Africa Ebola crisis, and the 2020–2023 COVID-19 crisis (Mass.gov, www.mass.gov/info-details/covid-19-community-tracing-collaborative-ctc), as well as leading the Commonwealth of Massachusetts Community Tracing Collaborative (www.pih.org/ma-response). With effective disaster response to unremitting crises as the foundation for developing new programs, and knowing that the frequency of crises may increase, Partners In Health built the capacity to provide more than a quarter-million mental health care visits over 5 years.

Refugees often face stressors and traumas at different phases of displacement: *premigration* (e.g., war, famine, torture, job and property loss,

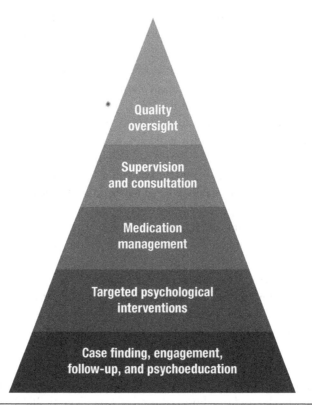

FIGURE 21–2. Skills package pyramid.

In post-earthquake Haiti, the nongovernmental organization Partners In Health mapped existing community-based resources and health care worker cadres onto a pyramid that anticipated the development of training and programs based on the World Health Organization's Mental Health Gap Action Programme curriculum. *Source.* Raviola et al. 2012.

rape), *during transit or migration* (e.g., family separation, physical and sexual assault, extortion, lack of access to services for basic needs), and *postmigration* (e.g., discrimination, acculturation shock, separation from family, detention, poor living conditions, barriers to accessing care). The stressors as categories for assessment can also be organized in terms of *traumatic experiences*, *acculturation*, *resettlement*, and *isolation* (Table 21–2) (Boston Children's Hospital Trauma and Community Resilience Center 2023). These experiences are informed by individual factors, social considerations, and political as well as racial contexts. As a result, a socioecological approach to understanding each individual is needed in both transit and host countries.

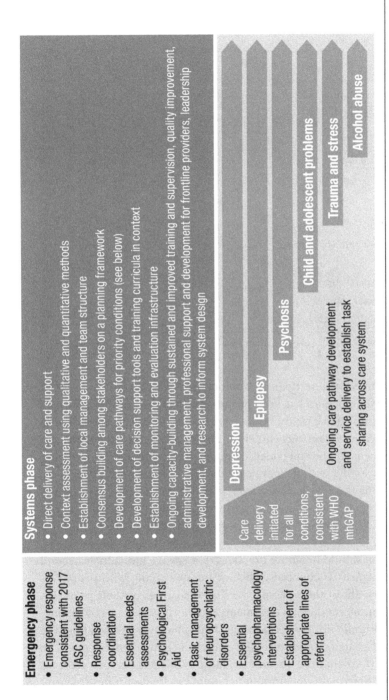

Emergency phase

- Emergency response consistent with 2017 IASC guidelines
- Response coordination
- Essential needs assessments
- Psychological First Aid
- Basic management of neuropsychiatric disorders
- Essential psychopharmacology interventions
- Establishment of appropriate lines of referral

Systems phase

- Direct delivery of care and support
- Context assessment using qualitative and quantitative methods
- Establishment of local management and team structure
- Consensus building among stakeholders on a planning framework
- Development of care pathways for priority conditions (see below)
- Development of decision support tools and training curricula in context
- Establishment of monitoring and evaluation infrastructure
- Ongoing capacity-building through sustained and improved training and supervision, quality improvement, administrative management, professional support and development for frontline providers, leadership development, and research to inform system design

Care delivery initiated for all conditions, consistent with WHO mhGAP

Depression

Epilepsy

Psychosis

Child and adolescent problems

Trauma and stress

Alcohol abuse

Ongoing care pathway development and service delivery to establish task sharing across care system

FIGURE 21–3. Partners In Health mental health response in Haiti, 2010–2023.

The illustration includes the initial emergency response and the long-term systems-building initiative to enhance the health system and community resilience in the face of ongoing, unremitting crisis. ESL=English as a second language; IASC=Inter-Agency Standing Committee; mhGAP=Mental Health Gap Programme; WHO=World Health Organization.

Source. Adapted from Raviola et al. 2020.

TABLE 21–2. Core stressor categories for refugees

Trauma
- Environment
- Social support
- Emotion regulation

Acculturative stress
- Acculturation
- Parenting capacity
- Language

Resettlement
- Basic needs
- Legal status
- Health care and access to services

Isolation
- Informal social support
- Formal social support
- Discrimination, stigma, and bias

Source.   Boston Children's Hospital Trauma and Community Resilience Center 2023.

In the context of resettlement, a multi-tier MHPSS model consistent with the IASC guidelines has been proposed to support trauma-informed and culture-informed care that includes community-based and community-partnered interventions (Im et al. 2021). More specialized mental health treatment can be embedded within an integrated, interdisciplinary primary care setting with primary care doctors, mental health providers, nurses, case managers, social workers, peer navigators, interpreters, and cultural brokers who can develop treatment plans that integrate refugees' cultural narratives, moral frameworks, and intersectional identities (Im et al. 2021).

Evaluation should integrate practices that engage individuals around cultural and spiritual concerns. This includes engaging with people directly to learn about their perspectives on the causes of their problems (their explanatory model); on treatment; and on various forms of healing, including culturally informed traditions. It also includes asking about the role that faith, religion, and spirituality play in helping them to cope. The ETHNIC(S) (Explanation, Treatment, Healers, Negotiate, Intervention, Collaborate, Spirituality/Seniors) mnemonic can be useful in providing culturally responsive care and treatment (Kobylarz et al. 2002).

Consistent with a multimodal approach to the various ways in which refugee populations may experience the hardships they have endured, the Adaptation and Development After Persecution and Trauma (ADAPT) model organizes the psychosocial disruptions caused by mass conflict and displacement into five core pillars: 1) attention to safety and security, 2) attachments, 4) justice, 4) role and identity disruptions, and 5) existential meaning (Silove 2013; Tay et al. 2019) and suggests several cross-cutting, integrative treatment strategies. Programs such as the U.S. government Welcome Corps (https://welcomecorps.org) enable all citizens, including providers, to engage in supporting resettlement for refugees. Participating in this essential work through organized systems such as Welcome Corps is an important way to guard against individual burnout that comes with this work. A team approach allows for a measure of safety to know that the care refugees need and deserve will continue flowing even if an individual volunteer may need to take time off for their own care.

Climate Change, Conflict, Forced Migration, and Refugee MHPSS

Climate change poses a threat to mental health and emotional well-being, spanning direct and indirect effects, including driving forced migrations of populations. Direct effects arise from firsthand experiences of climate change, whereas indirect effects stem from awareness of or bearing witness to changes caused by the climate crisis (Lawrance et al. 2021). Taken together, mental health impacts include driving new cases of mental illness, increased symptoms of illness, increased susceptibility to physical ill health or death for those with diagnosable mental illness, worsened population mental health, and widespread mental and emotional distress. (Lawrance et al. 2021).

It is important to note that healthy psychological processing of crisis, trauma, uncertainty, change, and loss can be part of resilient responses to both direct and indirect experiences, and with support may not create or exacerbate mental illness (Lawrance et al. 2021). At the same time, the absence of psychological distress or mental illness does not mean full health and mental wellness. Efforts to destigmatize accessing mental health resources is a priority for the healthiest and most effective communities (or those that are most rigidly "defended," such as first responders and the military). Heatwaves and extreme high temperatures, extreme weather events, social and economic disruption caused by climate change, food and water insecurity, and increased risk of infectious diseases all relate to climate change and inform the disruption and forced movement of populations (Lawrance et al. 2021). Humanitarian emergencies, including those caused by climate change, may cause additional social issues such as family separation, destruction of community structures and social networks, and psychological issues (Lawrance et al. 2021).

Beyond the MHPSS response for refugee populations in emergency settings, informed by best practices from the IASC and the United Nations High Commission for Refugees, longer-term interventions can address bereavement and healing from trauma. Although various clinical concerns should be addressed, including those related to autonomic hyperarousal and sleep disturbances, displaced persons are confronted with diverse, overlapping symptom constellations as well as existential concerns related to adaptation and longer-term erosion of supportive psychosocial systems and institutions for psychological well-being and mental health (Jou and Pace-Schott 2022; Tay et al. 2019). Embodied trauma is a key consideration in caring for refugees in all phases of response. *Embodied trauma* has been described by O'Brien and Charura (2022) as

> the whole body's response to a significant traumatic event, where mental distress is experienced within the body as a physiological, psychological, biological, cultural, or relational reaction to trauma. Embodied trauma may include psychosomatic symptoms alongside the inability to self-regulate the autonomic nervous system and emotions, resulting in states of dissociation, numbing, relational disconnection, changed perceptions, or nonverbal internal experiences which affect every-day functioning. (p. 6)

Conclusion

In conclusion, a number of robust frameworks have been developed to help pave the way to addressing general and specialized needs of refugees and other vulnerable populations in the current context of climate change, humanitarian crisis response, and global health delivery. However, beyond the organizational and funding challenges for mental health professionals to mount a disaster response to prevent and treat mental distress or illness, it is the work of finding common humanity and proximity to those who are suffering that enables displaced communities to recreate and define their unique place in their adopted homes. This process sometimes can and does take generations, and slower adoption may result in strife and loss of opportunity for all involved. Mental health providers are uniquely trained and positioned to suspend judgment and innovate with newly formed communities and can and should be empowered to do so—even more so as newly trained clinic and hospital employees, mental health workers, primary care clinicians, social workers, psychiatric nurses, psychologists, psychiatrists, and mental health administrators. We all would be better for it.

References

Belkin GS, Unützer J, Kessler RC, et al: Scaling up for the "bottom billion": "5 × 5" implementation of community mental health care in low-income regions. Psychiatr Serv 62(12):1494–1502, 2011 22193798

Bolton P, West J, Whitney C, et al: Expanding mental health services in low- and middle-income countries: a task-shifting framework for delivery of comprehensive, collaborative, and community-based care. Glob Ment Health (Camb) 10(e16):e16, 2023 37854402

Boston Children's Hospital Trauma and Community Resilience Center: Refugee and Immigrant Core Stressors Toolkit. Boston, MA, Trauma and Community Resilience Center, 2023. Available at: www.childrenshospital.org/programs/trauma-and-community-resilience-center. Accessed April 17, 2023.

CETA Global; Johns Hopkins University, Bloomberg School of Public Health: Common Elements Treatment Approach (CETA): a single treatment approach to address multiple global health problems. Houston, TX, CETA Global, 2014. Available at: www.cetaglobal.org; www.jhsph.edu/research/centers-and-institutes/global-mental-health/talk-therapies/common-elements-treatment-approach. Accessed April 17, 2023.

Epping-Jordan JE, van Ommeren M, Ashour HN, et al: Beyond the crisis: building back better mental health care in 10 emergency-affected areas using a longer-term perspective. Int J Ment Health Syst 9:15, 2015 25904981

Farmer P, Kim JY, Kleinman A, et al: Introduction: a biosocial approach to global health, in Reimagining Global Health: An Introduction. Oakland, University of California Press, 2013, p. 12

Global Mental Health Lab: Teachers College, Columbia University. New York, Teachers College, 2023. Three Session Interpersonal Counseling (IPC-3). Available at: www.tc.columbia.edu/gmhlab/projects. Accessed April 17, 2023.

Harvard Medical School: Introduction to Global Health Care Delivery. Boston, MA, Harvard Medical School, 2023. Available at: http://ghsm.hms.harvard.edu/education/courses/global-health-delivery. Accessed on April 17, 2023.

Im H, Rodriquez C, Grumbine JM: A multitier model of refugee mental health and psychosocial support in resettlement: toward trauma-informed and culture-informed systems of care. Psychol Serv 18(3):345–364, 2021 31971439

Inter-Agency Standing Committee: IASC Guidelines on Mental Health and Psychosocial Support in Emergency Settings. Geneva, Switzerland, Inter-Agency Standing Committee, 2007. Available at: https://interagencystandingcommittee.org/iasc-task-force-mental-health-and-psychosocial-support-emergency-settings/iasc-guidelines-mental-health-and-psychosocial-support-emergency-settings-2007. Accessed April 17, 2023.

International Medical Corps: Toolkit for the Integration of Mental Health into General Healthcare in Humanitarian Settings. London, Mental Health Innovation Network, 2023. Available at: www.mhinnovation.net/collaborations/toolkit-integration-mental-health-general-healthcare-humanitarian-settings. Accessed April 17, 2023.

Jones L, Asare JB, El Masri M, et al: Severe mental disorders in complex emergencies. Lancet 374(9690):654–661, 2009 19700007

Jou YC, Pace-Schott EF: Call to action: addressing sleep disturbances, a hallmark symptom of PTSD, for refugees, asylum seekers, and internally displaced persons. Sleep Health 8(6):593–600, 2022 36511279

Kienzler H: Mental health in all policies in contexts of war and conflict. Lancet Public Health 4(11):e547–e548, 2019 31677773

Kobylarz FA, Heath JM, Like RC: The ETHNIC(S) mnemonic: a clinical tool for ethnogeriatric education. J Am Geriatr Soc 50(9):1582–1589, 2002 12383159

Lawrance E, Thompson R, Fontana G, et al: The Impact of Climate Change on Mental Health and Emotional Wellbeing: Current Evidence and Implications for Policy and Practice. Grantham Institute Briefing Paper No 36. London, Institute for Global Health Innovation, Imperial College London, May 2021. Available at: https://spiral.imperial.ac.uk/bitstream/10044/1/88568/9/3343%20Climate%20change%20and%20mental%20health%20BP36_v6.pdf?_gl=1*ab8ehe*_ga*MTU5MDU0Mzk0NS4xNzEyMzMyMzMz*_ga_LME5ZDDFS0*MTcxMjMzMjMzMi4xLjAuMTcxMjMzM-jMzNC42MC4wLjA. Accessed April 17, 2023.

Lawrence M, Janzwood S, Homer-Dixon T: What Is a Global Polycrisis? And How Is It Different From a Systemic Risk? Cascade Institute Discussion Paper No 2022-4. Victoria, BC, Canada, Cascade Institute, September 2022. Available at: https://cascadeinstitute.org/technical-paper/what-is-a-global-polycrisis. Accessed April 17, 2023.

Nonko E: A new digital legal tool helps immigrant workers reclaim their stolen wages. Brooklyn, Make the Road New York, May 26, 2023. Available at: https://maketheroadny.org/a-new-digital-legal-tool-helps-immigrant-workers-reclaim-their-stolen-wages. Accessed August 8, 2023.

Meyer S: UNHCR'S Mental Health and Psychosocial Support for Persons of Concern: Global Review 2013. Geneva, Switzerland, United Nations High Commissioner for Refugees, 2013. Available at: www.unhcr.org/us/media/unhcrs-mental-health-and-psychosocial-support-persons-concern. Accessed April 5, 2024.

Nazer D, Greenbaum J: Human trafficking of children. Pediatr Ann 49(5):e209–e214, 2020 32413148

O'Brien CV, Charura D: Refugees, asylum seekers, and practitioners' perspectives of embodied trauma: a comprehensive scoping review. Psychol Trauma August 1, 2022 35913846 Epub ahead of print

Office of the Director of National Intelligence: Annual Threat Assessment of the U.S. Intelligence Community. April 9, 2021. Available at: www.intelligence.gov/annual-threat-assessment. Accessed July 12, 2024.

Office of the Director of National Intelligence: Annual Threat Assessment of the U.S. Intelligence Community. Washington, DC, Office of the Director of National Intelligence, February 6, 2023. Available at: www.dni.gov/files/ODNI/documents/assessments/ATA-2023-Unclassified-Report.pdf. Accessed July 12, 2024.

Raviola G, Eustache E, Oswald C, et al: Mental health response in Haiti in the aftermath of the 2010 earthquake: a case study for building long-term solutions. Harv Rev Psychiatry 20(1):68–77, 2012 22335184

Raviola G, Naslund JA, Smith SL, et al: Innovative models in mental health delivery systems: task sharing care with non-specialist providers to close the mental health treatment gap. Curr Psychiatry Rep 21(6):44, 2019 31041554

Raviola G, Rose A, Fils-Aimé JR, et al: Development of a comprehensive, sustained community mental health system in post-earthquake Haiti, 2010–2019. Glob Ment Health (Camb) 7:e6, 2020 32180989

Silove D: The ADAPT model: a conceptual framework for mental health and psychosocial programming in post conflict settings. Intervention (Amstelveen) 11(3):237–248, 2013

Singla DR, Kohrt BA, Murray LK, et al: Psychological treatments for the world: lessons from low- and middle-income countries. Annu Rev Clin Psychol 13(1):149–181, 2017 28482687

Tay AK, Miah MAA, Khan S, et al: Theoretical background, first stage development and adaptation of a novel Integrative Adapt Therapy (IAT) for refugees. Epidemiol Psychiatr Sci 29(e47):e47, 2019 31441397

Tol WA, Ager A, Bizouerne C, et al: Improving mental health and psychosocial wellbeing in humanitarian settings: reflections on research funded through R2HC. Confl Health 14(1):71, 2020 33292413

UNICEF: Community-Based Mental Health and Psychosocial Support in Humanitarian Settings: Three-Tiered Support for Children and Families. New York, United Nations Children's Fund, 2018. Available at: www.unicef.org/reports/community-based-mental-health-and-psychosocial-support-guidelines-2019. Accessed April 17, 2023.

United Nations High Commission for Refugees: Global Trends: Forced Displacement in 2021. Geneva, Switzerland, United Nations High Commissioner for Refugees, 2021. Available at: www.unhcr.org/en-us/publications/brochures/62a9d1494/global-trends-report-2021.html. Accessed April 17, 2023.

United Nations High Commission for Refugees: Climate change and disaster displacement. Geneva, Switzerland, United Nations High Commissioner for Refugees, 2023a. Available at: www.unhcr.org/en-us/climate-change-and-disasters.html. Accessed April 17, 2023.

United Nations High Commission for Refugees: Mental health and psychosocial support (MHPSS), in UNHCR Emergency Handbook. Geneva, Switzerland, United Nations High Commissioner for Refugees, 2023b. Available at: https://emergency.unhcr.org/entry/49304/mental-health-and-psychosocial-support. Accessed April 17, 2023.

United Nations High Commission for Refugees: Master Glossary of Terms. Geneva, Switzerland, United Nations High Commissioner for Refugees, 2023c. Available at: www.unhcr.org/glossary. Accessed April 5, 2023.

United Nations Office on Drugs and Crime: Global Report on Trafficking in Persons 2022. New York, United Nations, 2022. Available at: www.unodc.org/documents/data-and-analysis/glotip/2022/GLOTiP_2022_web.pdf. Accessed April 17, 2023.

Weissman MM, Hankerson SH, Scorza P, et al: Interpersonal Counseling (IPC) for depression in primary care. Am J Psychother 68(4)359–383, 2014 26453343

World Health Organization: Psychological First Aid: Guide for Field Workers. Geneva, Switzerland, World Health Organization, 2011. Available at: www.who.int/publications/i/item/9789241548205. Accessed April 17, 2023.

World Health Organization: mhGAP Humanitarian Intervention Guide (mhGAP-HIG): Clinical Management of Mental, Neurological, and Substance Use Conditions in Humanitarian Emergencies. Geneva, Switzerland, World Health Organization, 2015a. Available at: www.who.int/publications/i/item/9789241548922. Accessed April 17, 2023.

World Health Organization: Problem Management Plus (PM+): Individual Psychological Help for Adults Impaired by Distress in Communities Exposed to Adversity. Geneva, Switzerland, World Health Organization, 2015b. Available at: www.who.int/publications/i/item/WHO-MSD-MER-18.5. Accessed July 10, 2024.

World Health Organization: mhGAP Intervention Guide for Mental, Neurological and Substance Use Disorders in Non-Specialized Health Settings—Version 2.0. Geneva, World Health Organization, 2016. Available at: www.who.int/publications/i/item/9789241549790. Accessed April 17, 2023.

World Health Organization: EQUIP—Ensuring Quality in Psychological Support. Geneva, Switzerland, World Health Organization, 2021a. Available at: www.who.int/teams/mental-health-and-substance-use/treatment-care/equip-ensuring-quality-in-psychological-support. Accessed April 17, 2023.

World Health Organization: Self-Help Plus (SH+): A Group-Based Stress Management Course for Adults. Geneva, Switzerland, World Health Organization, 2021b. Available at: www.who.int/publications/i/item/9789240035119. Accessed April 17, 2023.

World Health Organization: Mental health fact sheet. Geneva, Switzerland, World Health Organization, June 17, 2022. Available at: www.who.int/newsroom/fact-sheets/detail/mental-health-strengthening-our-response. Accessed April 17, 2023.

Afterword

Frederick J. Stoddard Jr., M.D.
Craig L. Katz, M.D.
Grant H. Brenner, M.D.

This book provides guidance, as of early 2024, for clinicians serving the mental health and health needs of children, adults, and families and communities impacted by disasters in the world. Originally, our focus was the United States. It is now global. The first edition was translated into (at least) Mandarin, Japanese, and Korean. The contributions, in this book and in their work, of the many authors are, in our view, extraordinary, reflecting their dedication. During preparation of the book, the scope of disasters tragically expanded far beyond anything we expected. Our work originated in services provided to those impacted by fires and floods. It grew after 9/11 and the Boston Marathon bombing to now include the plethora of school and other shootings, massive earthquakes, the coronavirus disease 2019 (COVID-19) pandemic, and war and terrorist events. Refugees and migrating populations represent an increasing population of disaster survivors and victims.

This book was inspired in particular by our awareness of escalating climate change and the enormous challenge it represents to preventing disasters. Hardly a day passes without news of reduced air quality due to carbon emissions, threats to a species, populations affected by drought or fire or unbearable heat, mass migration, or the rapid melting of glaciers in the Arctic and Antarctica. These seemingly Biblical events have effects on both the young and the old, with increased anxiety and depression, much of it realistically anticipatory.

And with wars in Ukraine, the Middle East, and beyond, we are increasingly aware of the devastating impacts of armed conflict, especially for children and their families. This is amplified by the emergence of military weapons, strategies, and tactics enhanced by machine learning and artificial intelligence (AI)–driven technologies, which worsen the impact of conventional warfare. For years we have been grateful to those who serve in military medicine for their leadership in caring for service members, veterans, and their families and what they have taught us about the care they provide to them and to civilians, especially children, affected by war. Furthermore, the role of intergenerational transmission of trauma is highlighted by increased understanding of how war trauma impacts the descendants of those directly involved. With so much going on in the world around us, it can feel as if we are all now practicing with the pace and urgency, if not desperation, of military medicine.

Chapter 10, "Historical, Sociocultural, and Political Considerations," touches on historical and political issues, whose significance in 2024 have become enormous, especially with regard to the importance of responsible citizenship (Shapiro 2020), the future of democracy versus dictatorship, and the example that the leadership of U.S. democracy represents to the world in preventing and mitigating international disasters. Abraham Lincoln's inspiration and courage in sustaining the United States when it was divided by the Civil War may lend inspiration to us now to lead and prevent a political disaster of incalculable scale (Meacham 2022).

An event of an incalculable scale was one of our (F.J.S.) inspirations to begin this work: the decision to use the atomic bomb against Japan, particularly as recounted in Robert J. Lifton's (1986) work on Hiroshima. Recently, there have been escalating impassioned warnings about the existential threat posed by AI and the need to take steps to limit AI in order to safeguard humankind from various threats including, but not limited to, nuclear war (The Economist 2023; Romo 2023). This area merits specific psychological work to aid prevention, similar to that provided by leaders in the Group for the Advancement of Psychiatry (GAP; Committee on Social Issues 1964) and the American Psychiatric Association (APA; American Psychiatric Association 1981) in the 1960s and 1970s. It is time for GAP and the APA to reinstitute committees to update the reports developed in 1964 and 1968, as recommended by the head of the Canadian Security Intelligence Service to one of us (F.J.S.). If we, as a species, are to overcome the challenges facing us, we are called on to evolve beyond our present ways of viewing one another, to develop more effective tools to resolve conflict and share the resources given us, and to embrace complexity (Brenner 2023) in developing novel approaches to finding solutions.

As explained in the Introduction, our personal experiences of loss, grief, and secondary traumatization as caregivers, and our reflections about these experiences, inform what we wrote here. We are particularly grateful for the privilege of providing care for our patients and assistance to disaster-stricken communities and all that they share and have taught us. Our and our families' own experiences receiving psychotherapy and psychiatric care and of living through disasters leaves us particularly grateful to our colleagues who provided care and assistance to us, our families, and our communities. In addition, the psychiatric, neurobiological, organizational, and psychotherapeutic education that we are fortunate to have had has led us down this path to make use of what we learned. In addition, our professional organizations have let us get to know wise colleagues and to receive their guidance and feedback. Among them are GAP, the APA and its district branches, the American Academy of Child and Adolescent Psychiatry and its state councils, and the American College of Psychiatrists.

References

American Psychiatric Association: Psychosocial Aspects of Nuclear Developments (Task Force Rep 20). Washington, DC, American Psychiatric Association, 1981. Available at: www.psychiatry.org/File%20Library/Psychiatrists/Directories/Library-and-Archive/task-force-reports/tfr1981_Nuclear.pdf. Accessed August 29, 2024.

Brenner GH: How embracing complexity could foster enduring peace. Psychology Today, December 4, 2023. Available at: www.psychologytoday.com/us/blog/experimentations/202311/how-embracing-complexity-could-foster-enduring-peace. Accessed February 12, 2024.

Committee on Social Issues: Psychiatric Aspects of the Prevention of Nuclear War (Vol V, Rep No 57). New York, Group for the Advancement of Psychiatry, September 1964

The Economist: Henry Kissinger explains how to avoid World War III. The Economist, May 17, 2023. Available at: www.economist.com/briefing/2023/05/17/henry-kissinger-explains-how-to-avoid-world-war-three. Accessed February 13, 2024.

Meacham J: And There Was Light: Abraham Lincoln and the American Struggle. New York, Random House, 2022

Lifton RJ: Death in Life: Survivors of Hiroshima. New York, Random House, 1986

Romo V: Leading experts warn of a risk of extinction from AI. National Public Radio, May 30, 2023. Available at: www.npr.org/2023/05/30/1178943163/ai-risk-extinction-chatgpt. Accessed February 13, 2024.

Shapiro ER: Finding a Place to Stand. Developing Self-Reflective Institutions, Leaders, and Citizens. Oxfordshire, UK, Phoenix Publishing House, 2020

Index

*Page numbers printed in **boldface** type refer to tables or figures.*